TOXICOLOGIC
BIOMARKERS

TOXICOLOGIC
BIOMARKERS

edited by
Anthony P. DeCaprio
University of Massachusetts Amherst
Amherst, Massachusetts, U.S.A.

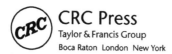

CRC Press
Taylor & Francis Group
Boca Raton London New York

CRC Press is an imprint of the
Taylor & Francis Group, an **informa** business
A TAYLOR & FRANCIS BOOK

First published 2006 by Taylor & Francis

Published 2019 by CRC Press
Taylor & Francis Group
6000 Broken Sound Parkway NW, Suite 300
Boca Raton, FL 33487-2742

© 2006 by Taylor & Francis Group, LLC
CRC Press is an imprint of Taylor & Francis Group, an Informa business

First issued in paperback 2019

No claim to original U.S. Government works

ISBN 13: 978-0-367-45370-1 (pbk)
ISBN 13: 978-0-8247-2351-4 (hbk)

Visit the Taylor & Francis Web site at
http://www.taylorandfrancis.com

and the CRC Press Web site at
http://www.crcpress.com

Library of Congress Cataloging-in-Publication Data

Catalog record is available from the Library of Congress

Contents

Contributors

Daniel Bloomfield Department of Clinical Pharmacology, Merck Research Laboratories, Merck & Co., Inc., Rahway, New Jersey, and Columbia University College of Physicians and Surgeons, New York, New York, U.S.A.

Donna M. Dambach Discovery Toxicology, Pharmaceutical Research Institute, Bristol-Myers Squibb, Princeton, New Jersey, U.S.A.

Anthony P. DeCaprio Environmental Health Sciences Program, School of Public Health and Health Sciences, University of Massachusetts Amherst, Amherst, Massachusetts, U.S.A.

Laura Ferriby ChemRisk, Houston, Texas, U.S.A.

Felix W. Frueh Genomics Team, Office of Clinical Pharmacology and Biopharmaceutics, Center for Drug Evaluation and Research, U.S. Food and Drug Administration, Silver Spring, Maryland, U.S.A.

Jean-Charles Gautier Molecular and Cellular Toxicology, Sanofi-Aventis, Vitry-sur-Seine, France

Federico M. Goodsaid Genomics Team, Office of Clinical Pharmacology and Biopharmaceutics, Center for Drug Evaluation and Research, U.S. Food and Drug Administration, Silver Spring, Maryland, U.S.A.

Joseph L. Hagan Biostatistics Program, School of Public Health, Louisiana State University Health Sciences Center, New Orleans, Louisiana, U.S.A.

Joshua W. Hamilton   Department of Pharmacology and Toxicology and Center for Environmental Health Sciences, Dartmouth Medical School, Hanover, New Hampshire, U.S.A.

Mark Harris   ChemRisk, Houston, Texas, U.S.A.

Stephen W. Looney   Biostatistics Program, School of Public Health, Louisiana State University Health Sciences Center, New Orleans, Louisiana, U.S.A.

Gary E. Marchant   Center for the Study of Law, Science and Technology, Arizona State University College of Law, Tempe, Arizona, U.S.A.

Dennis Paustenbach   ChemRisk, San Francisco, California, U.S.A.

Sofia Pavanello   Occupational Health Section, Department of Environmental Medicine and Public Health, University of Padova, Padova, Italy

Harry Salem   Research and Technology Directorate, U.S. Army Edgewood Chemical Biological Center, Aberdeen Proving Ground, Aberdeen, Maryland, U.S.A.

Annette Santamaria   Environ International Corporation, Houston, Texas, U.S.A.

Edward V. Sargent   Global Safety and the Environment, Merck & Co., Inc., Whitehouse Station, New Jersey, U.S.A.

Ken Sexton   University of Texas School of Public Health, Brownsville, Texas, U.S.A.

William J. Smith   Cell & Molecular Biology Branch, U.S. Army Medical Research Institute of Chemical Defense, Aberdeen Proving Ground, Aberdeen, Maryland, U.S.A.

John A. Wagner   Department of Clinical Pharmacology, Merck Research Laboratories, Merck & Co., Inc., Rahway, New Jersey, and Thomas Jefferson University, Philadelphia, Pennsylvania, U.S.A.

Christopher P. Wild   Molecular Epidemiology Unit, Centre for Epidemiology and Biostatistics, Leeds Institute of Genetics, Health and Therapeutics, University of Leeds, Leeds, U.K.

1

Introduction to Toxicologic Biomarkers

Anthony P. DeCaprio

Environmental Health Sciences Program, School of Public Health and Health Sciences, University of Massachusetts Amherst, Amherst, Massachusetts, U.S.A.

INTRODUCTION AND HISTORICAL PERSPECTIVE

The general concept of measuring a change in some parameter of a biological organism is not new. However, the formalization of the concept in clinical, pharmacological, and toxicological sciences, with the consequent development of unique terminology and conceptual models, is relatively recent. The past two decades have seen a vast expansion of technologies and applications involving these types of measurements, now collectively referred to as "biological markers" or "biomarkers." Indeed, these terms are now so commonly used (some may say overused) in scientific publications (Fig. 1) that their meaning has become diluted. As a result of this generalization, the terms have a myriad of meanings, with some differences subtle and others major, depending on the particular subspecialty where they are employed. The broad coverage of this book reflects the ongoing diversification of the biomarker concept.

One general definition of a biomarker (see below and elsewhere in this book for other definitions) might be "something measured in a biological system as an indicator of exposure, effect, susceptibility, or clinical disease." Predictive and diagnostic disease markers probably represent the oldest type of such measurements. These date back to antiquity, as in the example of "rubor, dolor, calor, and tumor" by Galen in second century Rome. Markers of cardiovascular disease, such as blood pressure measurements, are also

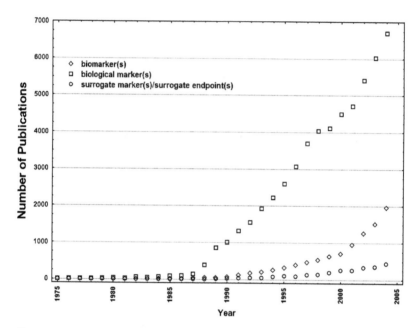

Figure 1 Number of publications identified in Medline containing the terms "biomarker(s)," "biological marker(s)," or "surrogate endpoint(s)/surrogate marker(s)" during the period 1975–2004.

early examples. Such observations were generally descriptive or, at best, semi-quantitative until the advent of modern chemical and physiological measurement techniques beginning in the 1800s. Rudimentary chemical examination of urine from diseased individuals was performed as early as the 1820s, and quantitative chemical analysis of urine, blood, and tissue became widespread with the development of clinical laboratory science in the early 1900s (1). The rapid evolution of analytical chemical methodology, which occurred over the ensuing decades, particularly involving chromatographic separation and colorimetric detection and quantitation, contributed to a subsequent explosion in interest in body fluid-based disease markers.

While clinical disease biomarkers have a long history, systematic efforts to discover and validate markers of adverse exposure to or effects of exogenous chemical agents (i.e., "toxicologic biomarkers") are generally more recent. This concept has its roots primarily in two distinct professional areas; occupational health and forensic toxicology. For example, early efforts to set maximum safe levels of exposure to chemical or physical stressors in the workplace, mostly pioneered by professional organizations and individual private sector manufacturers, led to the development of occupational exposure limits (OELs) and biological exposure indices (BEIs) (2). BEIs, which are direct measurements of xenobiotics or their metabolites in blood or urine, are considered as exposure biomarkers that reflect compliance with OELs. In the forensic arena, descriptive observation of clinical signs of deliberate or accidental poisoning had been performed for centuries. However, major progress in this area was also dependent on advances in clinical laboratory chemistry during the early 20th century.

As indicated earlier, biological measurements that can be classified as toxicologic biomarkers have been performed to some extent for many years. Only recently, however, has there been an expansion of interest in the development and application of markers for prediction or occurrence of specific adverse health endpoints. This interest has been driven primarily by the changing needs of two separate disciplines, environmental epidemiology, and pharmaceutical discovery/development, where parallel evolution and application of the biomarker concept has occurred. In the former discipline, biomarker science has evolved in large part from the recognition that classical "black box" epidemiology may not be able to solve critical questions regarding causation of inherited or environmentally induced disease and that sensitive and validated markers of exposure, effect, and susceptibility are crucial to this process (3–7). In the latter field, interest in biomarkers has accelerated as a direct result of the requirement to more efficiently, rapidly, and economically evaluate and screen new chemical entities and diagnostic tests intended for the therapeutic marketplace (8).

The "biomarker paradigm" as applied to the field of environmental epidemiology (Fig. 2) was initially defined in a 1987 U.S. National Research Council (NRC) report (9). The NRC's construct recognized that a sequence of biological and molecular events occurs following uptake of an exogenous chemical agent (xenobiotic) and development of clinical disease and that measurement of these intermediate events might provide useful and specific biomarkers of exposure or effect. Together, these intermediate stages represent the toxicokinetics and toxicodynamics of a xenobiotic under specified exposure conditions. Previously, epidemiologic methods were too insensitive to identify and characterize all of these events and therefore could not readily be employed for predicting risk associated with environmental (often low-level) exposures.

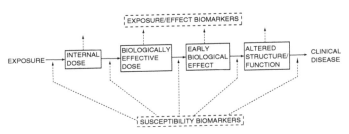

Figure 2 The biomarker paradigm for environmental epidemiology as originally proposed by the U.S. National Research Council. *Source*: From Ref. 9.

NRC further recognized that the kinetics of each step might be governed by additional factors that could mediate individual sensitivity to xenobiotics, and that these factors might represent biomarkers of susceptibility. The NRC report also emphasized that the link between exposure and disease is likely to be a continuum of overlapping events rather than a series of distinct stages. This basic paradigm has subsequently been modified and expanded upon by numerous workers (see Refs. 10–16) and now forms the core of the field of molecular epidemiology as it is currently practiced (17,18).

In the field of pharmaceutical discovery and development, typical costs for a single new drug entity to progress from discovery through approval currently top US$800 million (19). As potential treatments for complex, multifactorial, and degenerative diseases are explored in the coming decades, these costs are expected to rise significantly (20). Biomarkers, including those for toxicity and adverse effect, are now seen both as critical to the success of these ventures and as tools to help control burgeoning costs (21,22). Increasing scientific and regulatory discussion on the potential uses of biomarkers in drug development took place during the 1990s, spurred on to a large extent by the concurrent revolution taking place in genomics and proteomics. A seminal paper published in 2001 by a Biomarkers Definitions Working Group (BDWG) convened by the U.S. National Institutes of Health introduced a conceptual model for appropriate use of biomarkers in this area (Fig. 3) in addition to consensus terminology for the field (23). Major applications of biomarkers were recognized to include those providing information on clinical pharmacology, selection of compounds, clinical trials, guidance in dose selection, and detection of adverse reactions.

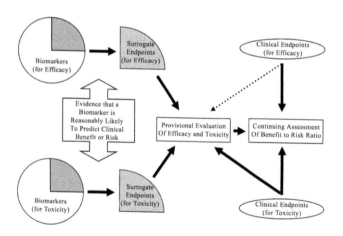

Figure 3 The biomarker paradigm for pharmaceutical development as originally proposed by the Biomarkers Definitions Working Group. *Source*: From Ref. 23, Courtesy of the American Society for Clinical Pharmacology and Therapeutics.

The specific application of toxicity biomarkers (also known as "safety biomarkers") in drug development, such as in lead selection and decisions to terminate compound development at an early stage, has also been addressed in a number of recent publications (24–26). As described by others in this book and elsewhere, toxicologic biomarkers are important in all phases of drug development, including discovery, preclinical assessment, clinical trials, and postmarket surveillance. Markers of organ-specific toxicity (e.g., AST and ALT levels in blood as indicators of hepatotoxicity) have been used for decades in preclinical studies and for clinical monitoring of adverse effects. Major efforts are now being made to supplement these classical markers with newer, more specific and predictive ones, particularly those based on new technologies (discussed later). Toxicity is a significant contributor to both the failure of new therapeutic entities and the withdrawal of approved drugs from the market (25). This fact has led to the recognition by both the pharmaceutical industry and regulatory agencies that toxicologic biomarkers may have much to offer in helping to bring safe drugs to the market (27).

While the concept of biomarkers as applied to these two diverse fields may have evolved independently, recent developments suggest that this may be an instance of convergent evolution. As the techniques of biomarker detection and identification have grown to include highly parallel, high-throughput analytical approaches (such as genomics, proteomics, and metabolomics), in addition to multivariate data processing and informatics, it is clear that these techniques will be key to advances in both environmental epidemiology and pharmaceutical development (28). Perhaps more importantly, some of the goals of these disparate fields are now beginning to overlap, as in the increasing need to assess responses, endpoints, and contributing environmental factors in large human cohort studies (29,30). The apparent merging of the rationale for biomarker use among these disciplines (and the possible benefits associated with this phenomenon) has been addressed in a recent publication (31). Finally, the potential application of biomarkers is now being expanded to other diverse areas, including health risk assessment, toxic tort litigation, and homeland security, in addition to industries such as insurance and health care.

DEFINITIONS AND TERMINOLOGY

It is difficult to determine when and where the terms "biological marker" and "biomarker" originated. Literature search indicates their first appearance in publications from the late 1960s and early 1970s, respectively (Fig. 1). Exponential growth in the use of these terms has occurred since the mid-1980s, when seminal papers on the topic were published. A recent Medline search indicated that almost 8000 papers containing one or both of these terms were published in 2004 alone. Many definitions of biomarkers

(including those for adverse effect) now exist in the literature and in regulatory agency documentation. As mentioned previously, key definitions are
those of the NRC ("... indicators signaling events in biological systems
or samples") (9) and of the BDWG ("... a characteristic that is objectively
measured and evaluated as an indicator of normal biologic processes, pathogenic processes, or pharmacologic responses to a therapeutic intervention")
(23). While each definition reflects the intended use of the data in a particular

Table 1 Selected Literature Definitions and Classifications for Biomarkers

Types of biomarkers	Definition/intended use
Surrogate marker or surrogate endpoint	A biomarker that is intended to substitute for a clinical endpoint. A surrogate endpoint is expected to predict clinical benefit (or harm or lack of benefit or harm) based on epidemiologic, therapeutic, pathophysiologic, or other scientific evidence.
Clinical endpoint	A characteristic or variable that reflects how a patient feels, functions, or survives. Clinical endpoints are distinct measurements or analyses of disease characteristics observed in a study or a clinical trial that reflect the effect of a therapeutic intervention.
Ultimate outcome	A clinical endpoint such as survival, onset of serious morbidity, or symptomatic response that captures the benefits and risks of an intervention
Intermediate endpoint	A clinical endpoint that is not the ultimate outcome but is nonetheless of real clinical benefit
Exposure biomarker	An exogenous substance or its metabolite or the product of an interaction between a xenobiotic agent and some target molecule or cell that is measured in a compartment within an organism
Effect biomarker	Any change that is qualitatively or quantitatively predictive of health impairment or potential impairment resulting from exposure
Susceptibility biomarker	An indicator of an inherent or acquired ability of an organism to respond to the challenge of exposure to a specific xenobiotic substance
Efficacy biomarker or outcome biomarker	Correlates with the desired effect of a treatment, but does not have as much validation as a surrogate endpoint

(*Continued*)

Table 1 Selected Literature Definitions and Classifications for Biomarkers
(*Continued*)

Types of biomarkers	Definition/intended use
Mechanism biomarker	Provides evidence that a drug affects a desired pathway
Pharmacodynamic biomarker	Provides information to determine highest dose in clinical trials, or time-associated measure of a pharmacologic response
Target biomarker	Shows that a drug interacts with a particular molecular target or receptor
Toxicity biomarker or safety biomarker	Indicates potentially adverse effects in in vitro, preclinical, or clinical studies
Bridging biomarker or translational biomarker	Used to measure and compare the same endpoint in preclinical (animal) and clinical studies
Type 0 biomarker	Reflects genotype or phenotype
Type 1 biomarker	Reflects concentration of drug and/or metabolite in blood/tissue
Type 2 biomarker	A marker of molecular target occupancy
Type 3 biomarker	A marker of molecular target activation
Type 4 biomarker	Physiological measurements or laboratory tests
Type 5 biomarker	Measurements of disease processes
Type 6 biomarker	Clinical scales
Type 0 biomarker (Mildvan et al.)	Measures the natural history of a disease and correlates over time with known clinical indicators
Type I biomarker (Mildvan et al.)	Indicates the intervention effect of a therapeutic treatment
Type II biomarker (Mildvan et al.)	Identical to a surrogate endpoint biomarker (see earlier)
Early detection biomarker	Used for screening patients to detect cancer (or other progressive diseases) early
Disease biomarker or diagnostic biomarker	Indicates the presence or likelihood of a particular disease in patients or in animal models
Prognostic biomarker	Used to assess the survival probabilities of patients or to detect an aggressive phenotype and determine how a disease will behave
Predictive biomarker	Used to predict whether a drug or other therapies will be effective, or to monitor the effectiveness of treatment
Genomic biomarker	A reproducible pattern based on gene activity generated by genomic methods
Proteomic biomarker	A reproducible pattern based on protein expression generated by proteomic methods

(*Continued*)

Table 1 Selected Literature Definitions and Classifications for Biomarkers
(*Continued*)

Types of biomarkers	Definition/intended use
Combinatorial biomarker	A combination of one or more individual markers that produces a pattern, usually generated by "-omic" techniques, which confers much more information than the individual measurements alone
Authentic biomarker	Reveals the activity of a pathway that is integrally involved in disease activity or therapeutic action
Kinetic biomarker	An in vivo measurement of flux through the key pathways that drive disease processes and therapeutic response
Known valid biomarker	A biomarker that is measured in an analytical test system with well-established performance characteristics and for which there is widespread agreement in the medical or scientific community about the physiologic, toxicologic, pharmacologic, or clinical significance of the results
Probable valid biomarker	A biomarker that is measured in an analytical test system with well-established performance characteristics and for which there is a scientific framework or body of evidence that appears to elucidate the physiologic, toxicologic, pharmacologic, or clinical significance of the test results
Proximal biomarker	A subset of pharmacodynamic biomarkers that reflects drug action
Distal biomarker	A marker that reflects disease progression
Routine biomarker	A marker that is analyzed in laboratories with well-established methods, such as in diagnostic clinical chemistry
Novel biomarker	Markers that are usually measured in research laboratories and that require specialized reagents or technologies that are not available routinely in a clinical laboratory setting
Screening biomarker	A marker discriminating the healthy state from an early disease state, preferably prior to symptoms
Stratification biomarker	A marker used to predict the likely response to a drug prior to treatment by classifying individuals as responsive or nonresponsive

Source: Refs. 8,9,23,26,27,31–38.

discipline, they are clearly linked by the term "indicator," which, of course, is the primary function of all biomarker measurements.

Numerous classification systems for biomarkers have also been proposed. A number of these are presented in Table 1. Again, important subclasses are those suggested by the NRC (exposure, effect, and susceptibility biomarkers) and the BDWG (clinical endpoints and surrogate endpoints). While some classifications are based on primary intended use of the marker, others reflect mechanism of action, exposure/dose, or pharmacokinetics. It is also clear that many proposed biomarker categories overlap, and that individual markers may fall into more than one category. In particular, markers of adverse effect may include many such classes, including those referred to in Table 1 as effect biomarkers, toxicity or safety biomarkers, bridging or translational biomarkers, mechanism biomarkers, and others. As progress in discovering new markers accelerates in the coming years, further expansion of these categories and classifications can be anticipated.

TOXICOLOGIC BIOMARKERS: PROMISE AND PITFALLS

As will be seen throughout the chapters of this text, we are just beginning to appreciate both the enormous potential and the significant barriers to acceptance of newly discovered biomarkers of adverse effect, regardless of the discipline in which they are designed to be employed. These issues have been covered in a number of editorials and review articles in recent years (27,39–42). Several major relevant points can be summarized here.

One important area where toxicologic biomarkers are poised to make substantial contributions is that of personalized medicine (43,44). This approach takes advantage of the ability of biological markers to be applied on an individual basis. It is widely anticipated that biomarker technology will soon advance to the point where batteries of markers can be assessed in individual people, providing a snapshot of biological status in time. In the case of genomics and proteomics, this has already been done on a limited basis. For prediction or detection of adverse effect, these batteries could provide detailed information on phases I and II metabolic enzyme genotype and phenotype, profiles of existing damage to specific genes, xenobiotic-induced damage to blood and tissue proteins, or any of a multitude of other relevant parameters. Batteries of bridging biomarkers of toxicity (i.e., those that are validated in both preclinical models and clinical studies) would prove particularly valuable for prediction of toxicity. The goal of such studies would be to more accurately define dose thresholds for adverse effect across population groups in addition to identifying characteristics of hyper-responsive individuals.

In conjunction with effect and susceptibility markers, comprehensive environmental exposure profiling could be performed for individual subjects by a combination of biomonitoring, metabolomics, and assessment of DNA and protein modification (covalent adduction) (45–48). This approach reflects the increasing recognition of the importance of environmental exposure factors in contributing to human susceptibility to disease and/or altering individual responses to therapeutic regimens. For example, the modification (induction or suppression) of biotransformation pathways by various classes of xenobiotics is a well-known phenomenon, and individual profiling of exposure to such agents could assist in prediction of adverse drug effects. Comprehensive exposure data would also greatly benefit environmental epidemiology studies, where accurate determination of exposure (particularly retrospective exposure) is often problematic. Recent papers have suggested that human exposure assessment science is poised for a major rebirth and expansion in parallel with the "-omic" technologies (15), and some workers have proposed comprehensive measurement of xenobiotic body burdens as a means to assess the human "exposome" (48). This ambitious goal may now be within reach because of significant advances in analytical technology, particularly mass spectrometry-based methods.

Of course, as with application of any new technology, questions have arisen concerning the ethics of individual subject profiling (discussed later) and approaches to the organization and interpretation of the vast amounts of data generated with these tools. The statistical challenges associated with analysis of biomarker data (discussed in detail in Chapter 2) are widely recognized and have resulted in the creation of entirely new conceptual models for extracting useful information from these data. Many of these models rely upon multivariate analysis techniques that generate patterns from a dataset, usually without a priori establishment of individual testable hypotheses. Some have proposed that a consistent and reproducible pattern derived from a battery of measurements may in and of itself be useful as a biomarker, regardless of the level of understanding of the individual mechanisms that led to the pattern (49,50). This approach may be particularly important for toxicologic biomarkers, since adverse effects often arise from either unknown mechanisms or molecular pathways different from those associated with the beneficial effects of a compound (25). Such so-called "discovery-based" research approaches have generated controversy, although it is generally accepted that some form of initial data reduction is necessary for analysis of these large data sets (51,52). Despite the latter view, there is not yet a clear consensus on what statistical methods are most appropriate for extracting biomarker information from large batteries of measurements.

A major recognized problem in the successful discovery and development of toxicologic biomarkers is that of validation (8,32,41,53–57). Validation of a biomarker requires characterization of parameters such as biological and temporal relevance, sensitivity, specificity, reproducibility, technical feasibility, background rate and variability, and predictive value. The intended use of the marker dictates the relative importance of each factor. For example, sensitivity and specificity are extremely important for exposure biomarker validation in environmental epidemiology. Sensitive markers are necessary to measure the low ambient levels typical of environmental exposures (at least in developed nations). Specificity, which is the probability that the biomarker is indicative of actual exposure to a specific xenobiotic, is also critical to minimizing misclassification in such studies. Validation issues concerning biological relevance, which involves whether and how the marker measures a mechanistic step along the exposure-disease continuum, are critical to developing biomarkers of susceptibility. Other validation factors apply equally to all types of biomarkers proposed for use in epidemiologic studies. Reasonable accessibility is important; invasive sampling procedures are generally unacceptable. Reproducibility of biomarker data temporally within a laboratory and across laboratories is critical and often difficult to demonstrate. Finally, cost and technical feasibility are important considerations in selecting appropriate biomarkers for such applied studies.

Validation is currently considered to be the most significant barrier to exploitation of biomarker information in drug development applications, and this issue has been discussed extensively in recent literature (27,40,58). Pharmaceutical industry use of biomarkers, more so than that for epidemiologic applications (at least at present), depends to a great extent on the "-omic" technologies. Some of the current attention focused on marker validation in the industry has been the result of highly publicized problems associated with proteomic biomarkers proposed for use in ovarian cancer (59). This issue raised concerns regarding reproducibility of marker profiles across studies and platforms, false-positive rates, and biological relevance, which has in turn prompted calls for more extensive validation of new biomarkers. Unfortunately, such validation requires significant industry resources (e.g., larger study sizes and sampling requirements), not the least of which is increased development time. The latter requirement runs counter to the original promise of biomarkers for increasing the efficiency and decreasing lead time in screening potential therapeutic agents. Nevertheless, it is widely recognized that in the long run, batteries of validated biomarkers represent the most promising means of achieving these goals.

As mentioned earlier, the ethical use of biomarkers is a complex issue that involves concerns related to misinterpretation, misapplication, and inappropriate release of such data (60–62). For example, with exposure biomarkers, ethical problems arise when the results of screening studies are implied to reflect health risk rather than exposure. When coupled with our increasing ability to measure lower and lower levels of more and more xenobiotics in human specimens, this problem becomes further amplified. It is often difficult for scientists, regulators and public health professionals, and physicians to interpret the health significance of "body burdens" of xenobiotics. Problems can also arise when claims are made that "excessive" chemical exposure has occurred in a particular group, particularly if the background range of exposure in the general population is not well characterized (63–65). Appropriate use of susceptibility biomarker data presents another serious dilemma. There is significant potential for misuse of biomarker data that predict enhanced individual susceptibility to adverse effects of drugs or environmental contaminants. These ethical issues apply to the use of biomarkers in any discipline and will need to be addressed in coming years as the technology advances.

ORGANIZATION OF THIS BOOK

This book provides a comprehensive discussion of toxicologic biomarkers from the points of view of both basic science and discipline-specific application, with each chapter authored by experts in their particular area. Cross-cutting issues are covered in the present chapter and in those by Looney and Hagan on statistics (Chapter 2), Pavanello on susceptibility (Chapter 6), and Hamilton on toxicogenomics/toxicoproteomics (Chapter 11). The use of toxicological biomarkers specific to epidemiologic applications is discussed in the chapters by Sexton on exposure assessment (Chapter 3) and Wild on environmental epidemiology (Chapter 4). Applications of toxicologic biomarkers in pharmaceutical development are discussed in the chapters by Dambach and Gautier on preclinical assessment (Chapter 7), Bloomfield and Wagner on clinical trials (Chapter 8), and Goodsaid and Frueh on validation and regulatory acceptance (Chapter 9). Finally, more specialized uses of toxicologic biomarkers are addressed in the chapters by Harris and colleagues on risk assessment (Chapter 5), Sargent on occupational health (Chapter 10), Smith and Salem on chemical warfare agents (Chapter 12), and Marchant on toxic tort and litigation aspects of biomarkers (Chapter 13). It is hoped that this organization will allow readers to quickly identify specific topics in their area of interest.

REFERENCES

1. Rosenfeld L. Clinical chemistry since 1800: growth and development. Clin Chem 2002; 48:186–197.
2. Jakubowski M, Trzcinka-Ochocka M. Biological monitoring of exposure: trends and key developments. J Occup Health 2005; 47:22–48.
3. Perera FP. Molecular cancer epidemiology: a new tool in cancer prevention. J Nat Cancer Inst 1987; 78:887–898.
4. Taubes G. Epidemiology faces its limits. Science 1995; 269:164–169.
5. Groopman JD, Kensler TW. The light at the end of the tunnel for chemical-specific biomarker: daylight or headlight? Carcinogenesis 1999; 20:1–11.
6. DeCaprio AP. Biomarkers: coming of age for environmental health and risk assessment. Environ Sci Technol 1997; 31:1837–1848.
7. Perera FP. Molecular epidemiology: on the path to prevention? J Nat Cancer Inst 2000; 92:602–612.

8. Lesko LJ, Atkinson AJ. Use of biomarkers and surrogate endpoints in drug development and regulatory decision making: criteria, validation, strategies. Annu Rev Pharmacol Toxicol 2001; 41:347–366.
9. National Research Council. Biological markers in environmental health research. Environ Health Perspect 1987; 74:3–9.
10. Albertini RJ, Nicklas JA, O'Neill JP. Future research directions for evaluating human genetic and cancer risk from environmental exposures. Environ Health Perspect 1996; 104:503–510.
11. Schulte PA. A conceptual framework for the validation and use of biologic markers. Environ Res 1989; 48:129–144.
12. Hulka BS, Margolin BH. Methodological issues in epidemiologic studies using biologic markers. Am J Epidemiol 1992; 135:200–209.
13. McMichael AJ. "Molecular epidemiology": new pathway or new travelling companion? Am J Epidemiol 1994; 140:1–11.
14. Timbrell J. Overview of biomarkers. In: Robertson DG, Lindon J, Nicholson JK, Holmes E, eds. Metabonomics in Toxicity Assessment. Boca Raton: Taylor and Francis, 2005:27–74.
15. Schwartz DA, Weis B, Wilson SH. The need for exposure health sciences. Environ Health Perspect 2005; 113:A650.
16. Weis BK, Balshawl D, Barr JR, et al. Personalized exposure assessment: promising approaches for human environmental health research. Environ Health Perspect 2005; 113:840–848.
17. Perera FP, Weinstein IB. Molecular epidemiology: recent advances and future directions. Carcinogenesis 2000; 21:517–524.
18. Wild CP, Law GR, Roman E. Molecular epidemiology and cancer: promising areas for future research in the post-genomic era. Mutat Res 2002; 499:3–12.
19. DiMasi JA, Hansen RW, Grabowski HG. The price of innovation: new estimates of drug development costs. J Health Econ 2003; 22:151–185.
20. Naylor S. The biomarker road to redemption. Preclinica 2003; 1:244.
21. Lathia CD. Biomarkers and surrogate endpoints: how and when might they impact drug development? Disease Markers 2002; 18:83–90.
22. Frank R, Hargreaves R. Clinical biomarkers in drug discovery and development. Nature Rev Drug Discov 2003; 2:566–580.
23. Biomarkers Definitions Working Group. Biomarkers and surrogate endpoints: preferred definitions and conceptual framework. Clin Pharm Ther 2001; 69:89–95.
24. Roberts R, Cain K, Coyle B, Freathy C, Leonard J-F, Gautier J-C. Early drug safety evaluation: biomarkers, signatures, and fingerprints. Drug Metab Rev 2003; 35:269–275.
25. Ryan TP, Watson DE, Berridge BR. Toxicology biomarkers in drug development. Pharmaceut Discov 2004:22–28.
26. Koop R. Combinatorial biomarkers: from early toxicology assays to patient population profiling. Drug Discov Today 2005; 10:781–788.
27. Baker M. In biomarkers we trust? Nat Biotechnol 2005; 23:297–304.
28. Ilyin SE, Belkowski SM, Plata-Salamán CR. Biomarker discovery and validation: technologies and integrative approaches. Trends Biotechnol 2004; 22:411–416.

29. Vineis P. A self-fulfilling prophecy: are we underestimating the role of the environment in gene-environment interaction research? Int J Epidemiol 2004; 33:945–946.
30. Potter JD. Toward the last cohort. Cancer Epidemiol Biomarkers Prev 2004; 13:895–897.
31. Gundert-Remy U, Dahl SG, Boobis A, et al. Molecular approaches to the identification of biomarkers of exposure and effect-report of an expert meeting organized by COST Action B15. Toxicol Lett 2005; 156:227–240.
32. Lee JW, Weiner RS, Sailstad JM, et al. Method validation and measurement of biomarkers in nonclinical and clinical samples in drug development: a conference report. Pharmaceut Res 2005; 22:499–511.
33. Mildvan D, Landay A, De Gruttola V, Machado SG, Kagan J. An approach to the validation of markers for use in AIDS clinical trials. Clin Infect Dis 1997; 24:764–774.
34. Manne U, Srivastava RG, Srivastava S. Recent advances in biomakers for cancer diagnosis and treatment. Drug Discov Today 2005; 10:965–976.
35. Turner SM, Hellerstein MK. Emerging applications of kinetic biomarkers in preclinical and clinical drug development. Curr Opin Drug Discov Develop 2005; 8:115–126.
36. International Programme on Chemical Safety. Biomarkers and Risk Assessment: Concepts and Principles; Environmental Health Criteria 155. Geneva: WHO, 1993.
37. Center for Drug Evaluation and Research. Guidance for Industry—Pharmacogenomic Data Submissions (Draft); November. Rockville: U.S. Food and Drug Administration, 2003.
38. Zolg JW, Langen H. How industry is approaching the search for new diagnostic markers and biomarkers. Mol Cell Proteomics 2004; 3:345–354.
39. Naylor S. Biomarkers: current perspectives and future prospects. Expert Rev Mol Diag 2003; 3:525–529.
40. LaBaer J. So, you want to look for biomarkers. J Proteome Res 2005; 4: 1053–1059.
41. Ransohoff DF. Rules of evidence for cancer molecular-marker discovery and validation. Nat Rev Cancer 2004; 4:309–314.
42. Listgarten J, Emili A. Practical proteomic biomarker discovery: taking a step back to leap forward. Drug Discov Today 2005; 10:1697–1702.
43. Hasan RK, Wulfkuhle JD, Liotta LA, Petricoin EF. Molecular technologies for personalized cancer management. J Am Med Assoc 2004; 291:1644–1645.
44. Mukhtar M. Evolution of biomarkers: drug discovery to personalized medicine. Drug Discov Today 2005; 10:1216–1218.
45. Pirkle JL, Osterloh J, Needham LL, Sampson EJ. National exposure measurements for decisions to protect public health from environmental exposures. Int J Hygiene Environ Health 2005; 208:1–5.
46. Sexton K, Needham LL, Pirkle JL. Human biomonitoring of environmental chemicals. Am Sci 2004; 92:38–45.
47. Watson WP, Mutti A. Role of biomarkers in monitoring exposures to chemicals: present position, future prospects. Biomarkers 2004; 9:211–242.

48. Wild CP. Complementing the genome with an "exposome": the outstanding challenge of environmental exposure measurement in molecular epidemiology. Cancer Epidemiol Biomarkers Prev 2005; 14:1847–1850.
49. Diamandis EP. Point—Proteomic patterns in biological fluids: do they represent the future of cancer diagnostics? Clin Chem 2003; 49:1272–1275.
50. Gillette MA, Mani DR, Carr SA. Place of pattern in proteomic biomarker discovery. J Proteome Res 2005; 4:1143–1154.
51. Pritzker KP, Pritzker KPH. Cancer biomarkers: easier said than done. Clin Chem 2002; 48:1147–1150.
52. Luhe A, Suter L, Ruepp S, Singer T, Weiser T, Albertini S. Toxicogenomics in the pharmaceutical industry: hollow promises or real benefit? Mutat Res 2005; 575:102–115.
53. Schulte PA, Talaska G. Validity criteria for the use of biological markers of exposure to chemical agents in environmental epidemiology. Toxicology 1995; 101:73–88.
54. Wahrendorf J. Design of studies for validation of biomarkers of exposure and their effective use in environmental epidemiology. Toxicology 1995; 101:89–92.
55. DeCaprio AP. Biomarkers of exposure and susceptibility. In: Ballantyne B, Marrs TC, Syversen T, eds. General and Applied Toxicology, 2nd ed. London: Macmillan Reference Ltd., 2000:1875–1898.
56. Bonassi S, Neri M, Puntoni R. Validation of biomarkers as early predictors of disease. Mutat Res 2001; 480–481:349–358.
57. Colburn WA, Lee JW. Biomarkers, validation and pharmacokinetic-pharmacodynamic modelling. Clin Pharmacokin 2003; 42:997–1022.
58. Armstrong WB, Taylor TH, Meyskens FL. Point: Surrogate end point biomarkers are likely to be limited in their usefulness in the development of cancer chemoprevention agents against sporadic cancers. Cancer Epidemiol Biomarkers Prev 2003; 12:589–592.
59. Robbins RJ, Villanueva J, Tempst P. Distilling cancer biomarkers from the serum peptidome: high technology reading of tea leaves or an insight to clinical systems biology? J Clin Oncol 2005; 23:4835–4837.
60. Schulte PA. Biomarkers in epidemiology: scientific issues and ethical implications. Environ Health Perspect 1992; 98:143–147.
61. Schulte PA, Lomax GP, Ward EM, Colligan MJ. Ethical issues in the use of genetic markers in occupational epidemiologic research. J Occup Environ Med 1999; 41:639–646.
62. Sharp RR. Ethical issues in environmental health research. Environ Health Perspect 2003; 111:1786–1788.
63. Belzer RB. Exposure assessment at a crossroads: the risk of success. J Exposure Anal Environ Epidemiol 2002; 12:96–103.
64. Stokstad E. Biomonitoring: pollution gets personal. Science 2004; 304:1892–1894.
65. Paustenbach DJ, Galbraith D. Biomonitoring: measuring levels of chemicals in people - and what the results mean. New York: American Council on Science and Health, 2005.

2

Challenges in the Statistical Analysis of Biomarker Data

Stephen W. Looney and Joseph L. Hagan

Biostatistics Program, School of Public Health, Louisiana State University Health Sciences Center, New Orleans, Louisiana, U.S.A.

INTRODUCTION

Overview

In this chapter, we provide a description of some challenges that may be encountered in the analysis of biomarker data, and offer advice on how best to deal with these challenges. Our treatment is not intended to be comprehensive; rather, it is hoped that we have successfully identified some of the more commonly occurring issues in the statistical analysis of biomarker data and that we have addressed them in a way that will be helpful to those who perform statistical analyses of biomarker data on a regular basis. This chapter is not intended to be a primer on how to perform the statistical analysis of biomarker data. Basic statistical methods, when properly applied, will usually suffice for this purpose. For a good treatment of basic statistical methods and their proper application to environmental exposure data (for which biomarkers are frequently used), see Griffith et al. (1).

To the greatest extent possible, we have based our recommendations in this chapter on the published advice of recognized authorities in the field of statistics. Our emphasis is on statistical methods and procedures that can be implemented using widely available statistical software, and we have indicated how commonly used statistical packages can be used to carry out the recommended analyses. However, since statistics is a dynamic field, many of the recommendations contained in this chapter may soon prove to be obsolete because of new developments in the discipline and/or new advancements in statistical software.

In many instances, we have illustrated what we consider to be inadequate treatment of biomarker data with examples taken from the scientific literature. It is not our intention to be critical of these investigators, but rather to demonstrate that many of the challenges that we have discussed in this chapter are encountered on a regular basis by those who analyze biomarker data. It is often the case that the statistical analyses that are performed are the best that are available at that time due to time, personnel, or resource constraints and that a better job could have been done under different circumstances. It is hoped, however, that readers of this chapter will be better equipped to analyze biomarker data in their future endeavors.

Validation of Biomarkers

The proper statistical analysis of biomarker data cannot proceed unless it has been established that the biomarker has been validated, i.e., that it is known to be both valid and reliable. Reliability refers to "the degree to which the results obtained by a measurement procedure can be replicated" (2). The reliability of a measurement process is most often described in terms of intrarater and interrater reliability. Intrarater reliability refers to the agreement between two different determinations made by the same individual, and interrater reliability refers to the agreement between the determinations made by two different individuals. A reliable biomarker must exhibit adequate levels of both types of reliability. The reliability of a biomarker must be established before validity can be examined; if the biomarker cannot be assumed to provide an equivalent result upon repeated determinations on the same biological material, it will not be useful for practical application.

The validity of a biomarker is defined to be the extent to which it measures what it is intended to measure. For example, Qiao et al. (3) proposed that the expression of a tumor-associated antigen by exfoliated sputum epithelial cells could be used as a biomarker in the detection of preclinical, localized lung cancer. For their biomarker to be valid, there must be close agreement between the classification of a patient (cancer/no cancer) using the biomarker and the diagnosis of lung cancer using the gold standard (in this case, consensus diagnosis using "best information"). As another example, body fluid levels of cotinine have been proposed for use as biomarkers of environmental tobacco smoke exposure (4). For cotinine level to be a valid biomarker of tobacco exposure, it must be the case that high levels of cotinine consistently correspond to high levels of tobacco exposure and low levels of cotinine consistently correspond to low levels of exposure.

The appropriate statistical methods for assessing the reliability and validity of a biomarker are discussed in detail in Looney (5) and elsewhere in this book and therefore will not be examined in detail in this chapter.

Designing Biomarker Studies

Issues that arise in designing studies that involve biomarkers are the same as those that must be dealt with in any type of research that involves the quantitative examination of data. One must first formulate a research question involving one or more measurable entities (e.g., second-hand smoke and lung cancer). Then, one must decide how best to detect or measure these entities (cotinine levels in urine, lung biopsy, etc.). For the purposes of this chapter, at least one of the measures will involve a biomarker. Once the processes to be used in measuring the entities under consideration have been specified and described very carefully in the study protocol, attention must be given to how the study will be conducted. This involves (i) selection of a study design (cross-sectional, case–control, cohort, randomized trial, etc.); (ii) identification of a target population, accessible population, intended sample, and actual sample; (iii) a careful description of how the study data will be collected from the actual sample; (iv) a description of the statistical analyses to be used once the data have been collected; and (v) determination of the sample size required for the intended study. (see Hulley and Cummings (6) for an excellent description of the design of clinical research studies.) Each of the above steps (i)–(v) should be carried out prior to collecting any data.

Once steps (i)–(v) above have been carried out and it has been determined that sufficient resources are available to conduct the study, the study may begin. Eventually, the study will be completed and the study data will be prepared for analysis. (This almost always requires some data "cleaning" to remove misentered or otherwise faulty data points.) Our focus in this chapter will be on what is to be done once the data are ready to be analyzed. Of course, it is extremely important that the sample size that was used in the study was appropriately determined: an n that is too small can result in insufficient statistical power and imprecise estimation; an n that is too large leads to waste of resources and statistically significant results that have no practical meaning. This chapter will be primarily devoted to appropriate methods of analysis of biomarker data; however, we will touch on issues of sample size determination as needed since even the most carefully selected statistical procedures will not perform properly if the sample size is too small.

Designing Analyses of Biomarker Study Data

The design of the data analysis for a study is an important part of the overall study design. Knowledge of what statistical tests will be performed ultimately is required before one can carry out the correct sample size calculation (7).

An approach that we have found useful is to write the statistical analysis plan before any data are collected. This plan can then be used as a preliminary draft of the Statistical Analysis section of any manuscripts that result from the study. Going through the formal exercise of stating exactly what statistical analyses will be performed is helpful in identifying key data elements that have not been previously identified. For example, carefully describing the analyses to be used in accounting for the effects of confounding variables may remind the investigator to include an appropriate measure of exposure to cigarette smoke in the data to be collected. Developing the statistical analysis plan prior to collecting the study data is just as important to the validity of the study as developing a detailed data collection protocol prior to beginning the study. It is useful to follow the model of developing a fundable proposal for extramural support, in which it is just as important to clearly describe how the study data will be analyzed as it is to clearly describe how the study data will be collected.

Of course, once the study data have been collected, it may be necessary to make modifications to the data analysis protocol, just as it is often necessary to make adjustments to the study protocol in the middle of the study. One should keep such modifications to a bare minimum; on the other hand, an appropriate analysis can be developed for almost any set of data, even if the original study protocol has been extensively modified. Data analysts should be flexible enough that they can adapt their planned analyses to fit whatever alterations were made to the study design or data collection procedures (8).

Sample Size Issues

A justification for the sample size that was used should be a required part of the Methods section of any manuscript based on a study in which biomarker data were collected. Published studies that have used biomarker data have generally been deficient in this regard. Notable exceptions include Lagorio et al. (9), who provide curves showing the sample size required to obtain precise estimates of population mean concentrations of urinary benzene and urinary t, t-muconic acid, and Stengel et al. (10), who provide tables examining the effect of the number of repeated measurements on both sample size and power when using any one of three different biomarkers of early detection of renal injury. A good source for practical advice on carrying out sample size calculations and statistical power analyses is Goldsmith (7); this author also provides an extensive list of references in these areas.

Presenting Statistical Results

Once the study has been performed, the data have been "cleaned," and the appropriate statistical analysis has been performed, it then becomes necessary to prepare the results for presentation. Generally speaking, the following information should be presented for the results of *any* statistical analysis: summary measure(s), test statistic [if different from the summary measure(s)], degrees of freedom (if appropriate), *p*-value, and confidence interval (CI) (11). In many published articles in the biomarker literature, the emphasis is on *p*-values; while *p*-values are certainly important for determining statistical significance, they contribute nothing in terms of describing the precision of the statistical result. CIs serve this purpose and also provide a range of reasonable values for the population parameter (mean, variance, correlation, etc.).

To illustrate, consider the study by Pérez-Stable et al. (12), in which the authors examined the association of number of cigarettes smoked per day and serum cotinine levels with several biochemical, physical examination, and depression assessments. They used the Pearson correlation coefficient (r) to measure these associations. In their Table 3, they present the value of r and indicate statistical significance by using an asterisk (*) if the *p*-value is less than 0.01 and a cross (†) if $p \leq 0.05$. However, using these symbols tells us nothing about the strength of evidence against the null hypothesis that the population correlation is zero; a *p*-value of 0.049 is treated the same as 0.011. In addition, there is no indication of the precision of these correlation estimates, and hence no information is available on the range of possible values for the population correlation that a CI would provide. In a related study, Henderson et al. (13) found a correlation of 0.68 ($p = 0.005$) between residential air nicotine level and urinary cotinine/ creatinine ratio in their sample of 15 children who lived in homes with smokers. A 95% CI for the population correlation in this case is (0.26–0.88), i.e., it is likely that the population correlation is somewhere between 0.26 and 0.88. Such a wide CI tells us that the estimate of the population correlation (0.68) is not very precise. The analysis of correlation coefficients is discussed in more detail in section "Challenges in Using Correlation Coefficients to Analyze Biomarker Data" in this chapter.

THE IMPORTANCE OF DISTRIBUTIONAL ASSUMPTIONS

The Effects of Nonnormality

It is well known that violating the distributional assumption(s) underlying a statistical procedure can have serious adverse effects on the performance of the procedure (14). Therefore, it is beneficial to attempt to verify such assumptions prior to beginning data analysis. The assumption that the data are normally distributed is the most common distributional assumption and underlies many commonly used statistical methods, including the *t*-test and analysis of variance (ANOVA), simple linear and multiple regression, and the Pearson correlation coefficient. However, checking distributional assumptions is often overlooked in many analyses of biomarker data and the underlying distributional assumptions are typically ignored. Some authors may state something to the effect that "due to the skewed nature of the data, nonparametric statistical methods were used," but usually no formal test of the distributional assumption was ever reported. For example, in their evaluation of hemoglobin adducts as biomarkers of exposure to tobacco smoke, Atawodi et al. (15) state that "because the distribution of HPB-Hb adduct levels was not normal, we used the nonparametric Kruskal-Wallis test..." (p. 819); however, they offer no justification for why they concluded that the adduct levels were not normally distributed.

Verifying the Assumption of Normality

Several graphical methods for verifying the assumption of normality have been proposed (16). One commonly used method is the probability plot (17), of which the quantile–quantile (Q–Q) plot is a special case. Another graphical method that is not as widely used as the probability plot is the normal density plot (18,19a,b), which is easier to interpret than a probability plot because it is based on a direct comparison of a certain plot of the sample data versus the familiar bell-shaped curve of the normal distribution.

Because the interpretation of any plot or graph is inherently subjective, it is not sufficient to base the assessment of a distributional assumption on a graphical device. Bernstein et al. (20) evaluated the use of a bile acid-induced apoptosis assay as a measure of colon cancer risk. They determined that their apoptotic index (AI) "had a Gaussian distribution, as assessed by a box plot, quantile–quantile plot, and histogram" (p. 2354). However, each of these methods is a graphical technique, and different data analysts could interpret the plots differently. One should always supplement the graphical examination of a distributional assumption with a formal statistical test, which may itself be based on the results of the graphical device that was used. For example, correlation coefficient tests based on probability plots have been shown to have good power for detecting departures from normality against a wide variety of nonnormal distributions (21). Formal tests of the distributional assumption can also be based on a normal density plot (18,19a,b).

A formal test of the assumption of normality that we recommend for general use is the Shapiro–Wilk (S-W) test (22). Several studies have demonstrated that the S-W test has good statistical power against a wide variety of nonnormal distributions; while it is not based directly on a graphical method for assessing normality, it is a valuable adjunct to such methods. The S-W test can be performed using the UNIVARIATE procedure within the Statistical Analysis System (SAS) (23) and other commercially available statistical software packages. It has been used in several studies involving biomarker data (9,24,25). Caution must be taken, however, in interpreting the p-value for the S-W test; low p-values indicate a departure from the normality assumption, whereas higher values indicate that there is insufficient evidence to reject the normality assumption. In their evaluation of a urinary biomarker for environmental exposure to benzo[*a*]pyrene (BaP), Buckley et al. (24) tested the assumption of normality for their data on potential BaP inhalation dose using the S-W test. The *p*-value was 0.07, leading them to conclude that their data were *not* normally distributed when, in fact, any *p*-value greater than 0.05 would indicate that the normality assumption is reasonable.

Remedial Measures for Violation of a Distributional Assumption

If it has been determined that a violation of the distributional assumption has occurred, and that this departure is important enough to adversely affect the results of the proposed statistical analyses, there are three recommended approaches: (i) attempt to find a data transformation method that will result in a new random variable that does appear to follow the assumed underlying distribution (usually the normal), (ii) attempt to find a statistical procedure that is more robust; that is, one that is not as seriously affected by the violation of the underlying distributional assumption as the procedure originally selected, or (iii) use a statistical test that is not dependent *at all* on the assumption of an underlying statistical distribution (such tests are generally referred to as being nonparametric). Each of these approaches will be discussed below.

Choosing a Data Transformation

A transformation based on the logarithm (usually the "natural" logarithm $\log_e$) is commonly used in the analysis of biomarker data (15,25,26). However, there is usually no justification given for such a transformation other than that it is commonly used in analyzing the type of data collected in the study. At the very least, the log-transformed data should be tested for normality as described in subsection "Verifying the Assumption of Normality" (this is equivalent to testing the assumption that the original data were log-normally distributed). If one concludes that the log-transformed data are not normally distributed, then there are many other possible transformations available. Several families of possible transformations have been proposed, including the Box–Cox family (27), the Tukey "ladder of powers" (28), the Johnson S_u family (29), and the Pearson family (30). The Box–Cox approach is particularly attractive, in that there is a formal statistical test for determining if the chosen transformation is "statistically significant"; however, selecting the appropriate transformation can be computationally difficult (31). The Tukey ladder of powers is also attractive in that it requires that one consider only a small number of possible transformations. Whatever method is used to select a transformation, the transformed data should be tested for normality before proceeding to the next stage of the analysis [e.g., MacRae et al. (25)].

Using a More Robust Procedure

Some statistical procedures are more robust than others. Generally, tests for comparing means (*t*-test, ANOVA) are reasonably robust to violations of the assumption of normality, whereas tests for comparing variances (the *F*-test, Bartlett's test) are much less robust (32). Robust alternatives have been proposed for many estimation and hypothesis testing situations (33), but very few of them are available in commonly used statistical packages.

Nonparametric Alternatives

The field of nonparametric statistical analysis is rich with many alternative procedures that are not dependent on distributional assumptions, yet are comparable to methods that are based on distributional assumptions, even when the distributional assumption is satisfied. Table 1 contains a listing of statistical methods that are based on the assumption of normality, along with some generally accepted nonparametric alternatives. All of these nonparametric tests can be performed using StatXact software (34) or StatXact procs within SAS (23). Nonparametric alternatives for comparing mean biomarker levels in two or more groups are discussed in subsection "Importance of Distributional Assumptions in the Comparison of Means," and a nonparametric alternative to the Pearson correlation coefficient is discussed in section "Challenges in Using Correlation Coefficients to Analyze Biomarker Data" in this chapter.

EXAMINING THE ASSOCIATION BETWEEN PREDICTOR AND OUTCOME

Issues that arise in determining the appropriate statistical method(s) to use in analyzing biomarker data are the same as those that must be dealt with in any type of research that involves the quantitative examination of data. For each research question or hypothesis, one must first identify the measurable entities that are to be included in the study and then clearly describe how the entities are to be measured. In this chapter, we will use the generic terms

Table 1 Nonparametric Alternatives for Some Commonly Used Tests That Are Based on the Assumption of Normality

Normal-theory test	Nonparametric alternatives
Paired *t*-test	Wilcoxon signed-ranks test
2-Sample *t*-test	Mann–Whitney–Wilcoxon test
ANOVA	Kruskal–Wallis test
Pearson correlation	Spearman correlation

Abbreviation: ANOVA, analysis of variance.

predictor and *outcome* to refer to the two entities to be examined. Predictor will typically be used to refer to the entity that occurs first chronologically. (In this context, the predictor is equivalent to the independent variable and the outcome is equivalent to the dependent variable.) In analyzing biomarker data, of course, either the predictor or the outcome (or both) will be the observed value of a biomarker, perhaps a biomarker of exposure to a potentially harmful agent.

A given biomarker may serve as the outcome in one phase of a study and the predictor in another phase. For example, Cook et al. (35) examined the association between passive smoking and spirometric indices in children. In the validation phase, they examined the association between the true level of passive smoking, as measured by the number of smokers to whom the child was exposed (the predictor), and the biomarker, which was salivary cotinine (the outcome). In the experimental phase, they examined the association between the biomarker (the predictor) and spirometric indices as measures of lung function (the outcome).

To design (and eventually carry out) a proper statistical analysis of the data collected from such a study, one must complete the following steps (in this order): (i) determine the appropriate numerical measure(s) to be used to describe the association between the predictor and the outcome, (ii) determine the appropriate statistical method to apply when analyzing the data that will ultimately be obtained from the study, and (iii) determine the appropriate sample size to be used in the study. Data collection should not begin until each of these steps has been completed. We describe each of these steps separately in the following three sections.

Choosing the Appropriate Measure of Association Between Predictor and Outcome

Table 2 provides guidance for selecting the appropriate statistical method to use to measure the association between exposure and outcome. It is often the case in biomarker studies that both the predictor and the outcome are dichotomous. The predictor might be exposure to a hazardous substance, classified as "high" or "low" according to the value of a particular biomarker, and the outcome might be the presence or absence of a disease or condition. For example, Tunstall-Pedoe et al. (36) examined the association between passive smoking, as measured by level of serum cotinine, and the presence or absence of several adverse health outcomes [chronic cough, coronary heart disease (CHD), etc.]. Serum cotinine level was classified into four ordinal categories: "nondetectable," and 0.01 to 1.05, 1.06 to 3.97, or 3.98 to 17.49 ng/mL. As indicated in Table 2, the authors correctly calculated odds ratios for the comparison of each serum cotinine category versus non-detectable in terms of the prevalence of each adverse health outcome in that serum cotinine category.

Table 2 Determining Which Measure of Association to Use

Predictor variable	Outcome variable		
	Dichotomous	Ordinal	Continuous
Dichotomous	OR[a]	Spearman's r_s	Point biserial correlation or Spearman's r_s[b]
Ordinal	Spearman's r_s	Spearman's r_s	Spearman's r_s
Continuous	Point biserial correlation or Spearman's r_s[b]	Spearman's r_s	Pearson's r or Spearman's r_s[b]

[a]The risk ratio should be used for cohort and intervention studies.
[b]Use the measure listed first if the continuous variable(s) is (are) normally distributed. Use the test listed second if the continuous variable(s) is (are) not normally distributed.
Abbreviation: OR, Odds ratio.

Table 3 Determining Which Method of Statistical Analysis to Use

Predictor variable	Outcome variable			
	Dichotomous	Nominal	Ordinal	Continuous
Dichotomous	Logistic regression or Fisher's exact test[a]	Fisher–Freeman–Halton test	Mann–Whitney–Wilcoxon test	t-test or Mann–Whitney–Wilcoxon test[b]
Nominal	Fisher–Freeman–Halton test	Fisher–Freeman–Halton test	Kruskal–Wallis test	ANOVA or Kruskal–Wallis test[b]
Ordinal	Cochran–Armitage test for trend	Fisher–Freeman–Halton test	Linear-by-linear association test	Linear-by-linear association test
Continuous	Logistic regression	Polytomous logistic regression	Spearman's r_s	Pearson's r or Spearman's r_s[b]

[a]Use logistic regression if the odds ratio is being used as the measure of association. Use Fisher's exact test for testing the equality of binomial proportions.
[b]Use the measure listed first if the continuous variable(s) is (are) normally distributed. Use the test listed second if the continuous variable(s) is (are) not normally distributed.
Abbreviation: ANOVA, analysis of variance.

Choosing the Appropriate Statistical Analysis

Once the appropriate measure of association has been chosen, statistical methods must then be used to determine if the result is statistically significant. Table 3 can be consulted to help determine the appropriate statistical method to use when examining the association between a predictor and an outcome. For example, in the study by Tunstall-Pedoe et al. (36) described in the previous section, the authors correctly used the results from logistic regression to calculate CIs and *p*-values for the odds ratios in their study (Table 3). An advantage of using logistic regression in the analysis of odds ratios is that the effects of confounding variables can also be taken into account (37). For example, Tunstall-Pedoe et al. adjusted their odds ratios for the effect of age, housing tenure, cholesterol, and diastolic blood pressure (36).

Sample Size Concerns

As discussed in subsections "Designing Biomarker Studies" and "Sample Size Issues," once the statistical analysis for a study has been designed, one should then determine the appropriate sample size to be used. Both of these steps should be performed prior to beginning data collection. Sample size determination is specific to the statistical method to be used; for example, methods such as those described in Fleiss (38), which have been implemented in the Epi Info^{TM} software (39), could have been used to determine the appropriate sample size to use in the study by Tunstall-Pedoe et al. (36) described earlier (sample size determination was not discussed in that report). StatXact also has extensive capabilities for determining the appropriate sample size to use when applying various methods for analyzing categorical data. From a more general perspective, Goldsmith (7) provides practical advice on which statistical packages to use for sample size calculations for many of the statistical procedures described in this chapter.

CHALLENGES IN THE ANALYSIS OF CROSS-CLASSIFIED CATEGORICAL DATA

Both the Predictor and the Outcome are Dichotomous

We have already discussed the proper handling of odds ratios, in which the predictor typically precedes the outcome chronologically, in subsections "Choosing the Appropriate Measure of Association Between Predictor and Outcome" and "Choosing the Appropriate Statistical Analysis." Another situation that occurs frequently in studies involving biomarkers is that there is no clear temporal relationship between predictor and outcome (e.g., in cross-sectional studies). In this case, it may be of interest to compare two groups in terms of binomial proportions (or percentages). The data for such a comparison can be represented as cross-classified data with the rows corresponding to groups and the columns corresponding to the "success" and "failure" categories. For example, Pérez-Stable et al. (12) compared smokers and nonsmokers in terms of the percentage diagnosed with depression. As is commonly done with data of this type, they performed the comparison using the χ^2 (chi-squared) test. However, this test is known to have very poor statistical properties, especially if the number of subjects in either group is small (40), and is therefore not recommended for general use. A preferred method is Fisher's exact test (34), as implemented in StatXact or StatXact procs in SAS.

Choice of a Statistical Method When the Predictor Is Ordinal and the Outcome Is Dichotomous

As described previously, one study (36) examined the association between level of serum cotinine and the presence or absence of several adverse health outcomes. The authors calculated odds ratios for the comparison of each serum cotinine category versus nondetectable in terms of the prevalence of each health outcome. However, an additional analysis that is recommended for data of this type is to perform a test for trend across the serum cotinine categories in terms of the prevalence of the outcomes (Table 3). Such an analysis would be especially helpful in establishing dose–response relationships between passive smoking and the adverse outcomes. The authors speak in terms of a "gradient" across exposure categories, but report no statistical test to determine if their data support the existence of such a gradient.

Recommended procedures for testing for trend include the permutation test [(41), Chapter 8], in which scores can be assigned to the ordinal levels of the predictor variable, and the Cochran–Armitage test (42,43), which should be used if no such scores are available. In the study referred to above (36), scores corresponding to the midpoint were assigned to each serum cotinine category (0.00, 0.53, 2.52, and 10.74 ng/mL) and then the permutation test was performed. The results indicated a highly significant increasing trend in the prevalence of "diagnosed coronary heart disease" as serum cotinine level increases ($p < 0.001$), a finding that was not reported by the authors. Both the permutation test and the Cochran–Armitage test are available in StatXact, which also has the capability of determining the appropriate sample size to use when performing these tests.

Choice of a Statistical Method When Both the Predictor and the Outcome are Ordinal

Cook et al. (35) examined the association between the number of smokers to whom children had been exposed and their salivary cotinine measured in ng/mL. "Number of smokers" was categorized as 0, 1, 2, and ≥ 3, and salivary cotinine was categorized as nondetectable, 0.1 to 0.2, 0.3 to 0.6, 0.7 to 1.7, 1.8 to 4.0, 4.1 to 14.7, and >14.7. The authors stated that "salivary cotinine concentration was strongly related to the number of smokers to whom the child was usually exposed". However, they provide no numerical summary or statistical test to justify this assertion. According to our Table 3, an appropriate method for testing for significant association between these two variables would be the linear-by-linear association test (44). In addition, Spearman's correlation could be used to produce a single numerical summary of this association (Table 2), and a statistical test then performed to determine if the population value of Spearman's correlation is different from zero. For the data presented in Table 1 of Cook et al. (35), the linear-by-linear association test indicated a strongly significant association between number of smokers and salivary cotinine ($p<0.001$). Similar results were obtained for Spearman's correlation: $r_s = 0.72$, 95% CI $0.70 - 0.74$, $p<0.001$. Software such as StatXact is capable of performing each of these analyses.

CHALLENGES IN COMPARING MEAN LEVELS OF BIOMARKERS ACROSS GROUPS

According to Table 3, if the predictor variable is dichotomous and the outcome is continuous, the appropriate statistical method to use is the *t*-test. If the predictor variable is nominal and the outcome is continuous, the appropriate method is ANOVA. The proper application of both the *t*-test and ANOVA as they are usually formulated is based on two assumptions: (i) that the data in all groups being compared are normally distributed, and (ii) that the population variances in all groups being compared are equal (45). In this section, we discuss the importance of these assumptions and provide recommendations for alternative procedures to use when these assumptions appear to be violated.

Importance of Distributional Assumptions in the Comparison of Means

The performance of both the *t*-test and ANOVA is generally robust against violations of the normality assumption; however, the presence of certain types of departures from normality can seriously affect their performance (46). If the methods for testing the assumption of normality described in subsection "Verifying the Assumption of Normality" indicate a significant departure from normality in any of the groups being compared, one should consider the nonparametric alternatives indicated in Table 1 (47).

For example, the Mann–Whitney–Wilcoxon (M-W-W) test has been used in biomarker studies when comparing two groups in terms of a continuous variable that appears to be nonnormally distributed (3,48). The equivalent procedure for comparing more than two groups is the Kruskall–Wallis

(K-W) test, which has also been used with biomarker data (15,49). However, an assumption underlying both the M-W-W and K-W tests that is often over-looked is that the populations being compared have identical shapes; that is, each population is a "shifted" version of each of the others. This assumption should be tested prior to applying either the M-W-W or K-W tests; a preferred method for doing this is the Kolmogorv–Smirnov test (41). One interesting, but sometimes overlooked (15), feature of any nonparametric test based on ranks (of which the M-W-W and K-W tests are examples) is that applying a monotonic transformation (such as the logarithm) to the data does not affect the results of the analysis.

All of the nonparametric methods mentioned in this section for com-paring groups in terms of location are available in StatXact and StatXact procs in SAS. It is recommended that StatXact be used to perform these tests since it produces exact p-values and CIs whenever possible; many com-monly used statistical packages are only able to produce approximate p-values and CIs when applying nonparametric methods. This may explain discrepancies found by some workers, such as those reported by Atawodi et al. (15) when they compared the results of the K-W test for the original and log-transformed data.

Importance of Heterogeneity in the Comparison of Means

Two-Group Comparisons

The performance of the "usual" t-test (sometimes called the "equal variance t-test") depends very strongly on the underlying assumption of equal popu-lation variances (sometimes called homogeneity) between the groups (50). One approach would be to attempt to use the F-test for testing equality of population variances to verify the homogeneity assumption before apply-ing the equal variance t-test (51). If the hypothesis of equal variances is not rejected, then one would apply the usual t-test. If the hypothesis of equal variances is rejected, then one would use an alternative approach that does not depend on the homogeneity assumption. One such alternative is the "unequal variance t-test" [sometimes referred to as the "Welch test" or "Satterthwaite approximation" (51)], which is generally available in any statistical package that can perform the equal variance t-test. However, Moser and Stevens (51) demonstrated that the preliminary test of equality of variances contributes nothing of value and that, in fact, the unequal variance t-test can be used any time the means of two groups are being compared, since the test performs almost as well as the equal variance t-test when the population variances in the two groups are equal and outperforms the equal variance t-test when the variances are unequal. Hence, we follow their advice and recommend that the unequal variance t-test be used routinely whenever the means of two groups are being compared and the data appear to be normally distributed. If the data are not normally distributed, a nonparametric alternative to the *t*-test such as the M-W-W test (section "Importance of Distributional Assumptions in the Comparison of Means") can be used instead.

Salmi et al. (52) evaluated the potential usefulness of soluble vascular adhesion protein-1 (sVAP-1) as a biomarker to monitor and predict the extent of ongoing artherosclerotic processes. These investigators compared two groups; diabetic study participants on insulin treatment only ($n = 7$) versus diabetic study participants on other treatments ($n = 41$). They used the usual (equal-variance) *t*-test to compare the mean sVAP-1 levels of the two groups: mean $\pm$ S.D. 148 ± 114 versus 113 ± 6; $t = 2.06$, df $= 46$, one-tailed $p = 0.023$, a statistically significant result. However, they overlooked the fact that the variances in the two groups they were comparing were quite different (12,996 versus 36, $F = 361$, df $= (6,40)$, $p < 0.001$). If the unequal variance *t*-test as recommended by Moser and Stevens (51) had been used, a nonsignificant result ($t = 0.81$, df $= 6$, one-tailed $p = 0.224$) would have been obtained. Given the extremely strong evidence that the two population variances are unequal, the latter result provides a more valid comparison of the two study groups.

Multiple Comparisons

It is often of interest to compare three or more groups in terms of the mean level of a certain biomarker. For example, Bernstein et al. (20) compared the mean levels of their AI across three groups: (i) "normal" subjects, that is, those with no previous history of polyps or cancer; (ii) patients with a history of colorectal cancer; and (iii) patients with colorectal adenomas. They used the Tukey method to perform all possible pairwise comparisons among the three groups. The Tukey method is the technique of choice if the population variances of the three groups are equal (53); however, if they are not equal, the methods known as Dunnett's C and Dunnett's T3 are preferable (54). These two methods are very similar to the unequal variance *t*-test recommended in the previous section. The Tukey, Dunnett's C, and Dunnett's T3 procedures are all available in the Statistical Package for the Social Sciences (SPSS) (55).

CHALLENGES IN USING CORRELATION COEFFICIENTS TO ANALYZE BIOMARKER DATA

It is often of interest in studies involving biomarker data to examine the association between two continuous variables, at least one of which is the value of a particular biomarker. For example, Salmi et al. (52) correlated observed levels of sVAP-1 with risk factors for coronary heart disease, measures of liver dysfunction, diabetic parameter levels, etc. As indicated in Table 2, the appropriate measure of association to use if the data for both variables are normally distributed is the Pearson correlation coefficient. As indicated in Table 1, if the data for either variable appear to be nonnormally distributed, then Spearman's correlation is the recommended method. In the study by Buss et al. (56), the authors correctly used Spearman's correlation in their evaluation of 3-chlorotyrosine in tracheal aspirates from preterm infants as a biomarker for protein damage by myeloperoxidase; they stated that they used Spearman's r_s "because the data were not normally distributed" (p. 5).

In the following section, we address three challenges frequently encountered when correlation coefficients are used in the analysis of biomarker data: (i) proper methods of analysis and interpretation of the results, (ii) sample size determination, and (iii) comparison of related correlation coefficients.

Proper Methods of Analysis and Interpretation of the Results

In their study, Salmi et al. (52) determined the "significance" of their correlation coefficients by testing the null hypothesis that the population correlation coefficient is equal to zero. However, there are several problems with this approach, the primary one being that correlations of no practical significance may be declared to be "significant" simply because the p-value is less than 0.05 (57). We have found the classification scheme presented by Morton et al. (58) to be useful in interpreting the magnitude of correlation coefficients in terms of their practical significance. They classify correlations between 0.0 and 0.2 as "negligible," between 0.2 and 0.5 as "weak," between 0.5 and 0.8 as "moderate," and between 0.8 and 1.0 as "strong." In their sample of 411 Finnish men, Salmi et al. (52) found a significant correlation of 0.108 between sVAP-1 and carbohydrate-deficient transferrin, a measure of liver dysfunction. While this correlation is statistically significant ($p = 0.029$), it would be considered negligible according to the Morton et al. criteria mentioned earlier, raising doubt about the practical, biological significance of the result.

In addition to testing the hypothesis that the population correlation is zero, one should also construct a CI for the population correlation in order to get a sense of the precision of the correlation estimate, as well as a reasonable range of possible values for the population correlation. In the example taken from Salmi et al. (52) mentioned earlier, the 95% CI is (0.01–0.20). Thus, the entire CI falls within the negligible range according to the Morton et al. criteria, casting further doubt on the practical significance of the result.

As discussed in Looney (57), another problem with declaring a correlation to be significant simply because $p < 0.05$ is that smaller correlations may be declared to be significant even when n is fairly small, resulting in CIs that are too wide to be of any practical usefulness. In the study by Salmi et al. (52) mentioned earlier, the value of r for the correlation between sVAP-1 and ketone bodies in a sample of 38 observations taken from diabetic children and adolescents was 0.34 ($p = 0.037$), a statistically significant result. However, a 95% CI for the population correlation is (0.02–0.60), which indicates that the population correlation could be anywhere between negligible and moderate according to the Morton et al. criteria. A CI of such large width provides little useful information about the magnitude of the population correlation.

Sample Size Issues in the Analysis of Correlation Coefficients

One way to avoid the difficulties described in the previous section is to follow the recommendations presented in subsections "Designing Biomarker Studies" and "Sample Size Issues" and perform a sample size calculation prior to beginning the study. Looney (57) describes several approaches that typically yield sample sizes that provide more useful information about the value of the population correlation coefficient and the practical significance of the results than if one simply bases the sample size calculation on achieving adequate power for the test that the population correlation is zero. These include basing the sample size calculation on (i) the desired width of the CI for the population correlation, or (ii) tests of null hypotheses other than that the population correlation is zero. For example, one might test the null hypothesis that the population correlation is less than or equal to 0.20; rejecting this null hypothesis would indicate that the population correlation is nonnegligible.

Comparison of Several Correlation Coefficients

In some studies involving biomarker data, it has been of interest to compare "related" correlation coefficients, that is, the correlation of variable X with Y versus the correlation of variable X with Z. For example, Salmi et al. (52) reported significant correlations of sVAP-1 with both glucose ($r = 0.57, p < 0.001$) and ketone bodies ($r = 0.34, p = 0.037$) in their sample of 38 observations taken from diabetic children and adolescents. They concluded that there was a "less marked" correlation of sVAP-1 with ketone bodies than with glucose. However, they did not report the results of any statistical tests to determine if, in fact, the corresponding population correlation coefficients were different from each other. Had they performed such a test, as described in Steiger (59), they would have found no significant difference between the two correlations ($p = 0.093$). (SAS code for performing comparisons of related correlation coefficients is available from the first author of this chapter.) In general, it is preferable to perform a formal statistical test when comparing parameters (means, variances, correlation coefficients, etc.), than to simply use a qualitative comparison based on subjective judgment.

CHALLENGES IN THE STATISTICAL COMPARISON OF BIOMARKERS

It is often of interest to compare two or more biomarkers. One may wish to determine which of several newly proposed biomarkers are the most accurate, or to compare one or more newly proposed biomarkers to an existing biomarker. General methods for validating biomarkers are discussed in detail in Looney (5) and elsewhere in this book, so they will not be treated in depth here. However, there are two types of analyses involving biomarker comparisons that we feel are worthy of a separate treatment in this chapter. These are discussed in the following two sections.

Comparing the Accuracies of Several Biomarkers

Qiao et al. (3) used the "paired χ^2 test" to compare the accuracies of three different screening tests for lung cancer based on biomarkers. When analyzing paired data of this type, the appropriate method for comparing two biomarkers in terms of accuracy is McNemar's test (47). There is no statistical method that is commonly known as the paired χ^2 test. Although a χ^2 approximation is available for McNemar's test, it is preferable to use the exact version of the test (60,61). When comparing the accuracies of three or more biomarkers, the preferred method to use is the Cochran Q test (62).

Measuring Agreement Among Biomarkers

Dichotomous Biomarkers

Tockman et al. (63) examined the use of murine monoclonal antibodies to a glycolipid antigen of human lung cancer as a biomarker in the detection of early lung cancer. As part of their assessment of the interrater reliability of scoring stained specimens, they compared the results obtained on 123 slides read by both a pathologist and a cytotechnologist. The authors stated that they used McNemar's test to test for "significant agreement ($p = 1.000$)" between the readers. However, what was actually tested for was a significant difference in classification accuracy between the two readers. While such a test is often informative, one should also measure the degree of agreement between the readers (64). The generally accepted method for assessing agreement between two dichotomous biomarkers, neither of which can be assumed to be the gold standard, is Cohen's kappa (5). When measuring agreement between three or more dichotomous biomarkers, we recommend the methods described in Shoukri (65).

Continuous Biomarkers

Bartczak et al. (66) compared a high-pressure liquid chromatography-based assay with a gas chromatography-based assay for urinary muconic acid, both of which have been used as biomarkers of exposure to benzene. They used Pearson's correlation coefficient r and the slope of the fitted regression line in their assessment of the agreement between the two methods (p. 255). However, at least as far back as 1973, it was recognized that r is not appropriate for assessing agreement in what are typically called "method comparison studies," i.e., studies in which neither method of measurement can be considered to be the gold standard (67). In fact, Westgard and Hunt go so far as to state that "the correlation coefficient ... is of no practical use in the statistical analysis of comparison data" (67). The use of linear regression coefficients is also inappropriate for assessing agreement between continuous biomarkers, as discussed by several authors (68).

CONCLUDING REMARKS

In this chapter, we have focused our discussion on some challenges that we have encountered in our analyses of biomarker data, and on some statistical techniques that we have found useful in meeting those challenges. We have not attempted to provide a comprehensive treatment of statistical methods that could be used in analyzing biomarker data; certainly, this entire volume could have been devoted to this task. It is hoped that the recommendations provided here will prove to be useful to statisticians and other analysts who are faced with the often challenging task of working with biomarker data.

REFERENCES

1. Griffith J, Aldrich TE, Duncan RC. Epidemiologic research methods. In: Aldrich T, Griffith J, Cooke C, eds. Environmental Epidemiology and Risk Assessment. New York: Van Nostrand Reinhold, 1993:27–60.
2. Last JM. A Dictionary of Epidemiology. 3rd ed. New York: Oxford University Press, 1995.
3. Qiao Y, Tockman MS, Li L, et al. A case-cohort study of an early biomarker of lung cancer in a screening cohort of Yunnan tin miners in China. Cancer Epidemiol Biomarker Prev 1997; 6:893–900.
4. Benowitz L. Biomarkers of environmental tobacco smoke exposure. Environ Health Perspect 1999; 107(Suppl 2):349–355.
5. Looney SW. Statistical methods for assessing biomarkers. In: Looney SW, ed. Methods in Molecular Biology, Biostatistical Methods. Totowa, NJ: Humana Press 2001: Vol. 184:81–109.
6. Hulley SB, Cummings SR. Designing Clinical Research Baltimore. : Williams & Wilkins 1988.
7. Goldsmith LJ. Power and sample size considerations in molecular biology. In: Looney SW, ed. Methods in Molecular Biology, Biostatistical Methods. Totowa, NJ: Humana Press 2001:184:111–130.
8. Boen JR, Zahn DA. The Human Side of Statistical Consulting. Belmont, CA: Lifetime Learning Publications, 1982.
9. Lagorio S, Crebelli R, Ricciarello R, et al. Methodological issues in biomonitoring of low level exposure to benzene. Occup Med 1998; 8:497–504.
10. Stengel B, Watier L, Chouquet C, Cénée S, Philippon C, Hémon D. Influence of renal biomarker variability on the design and interpretation of occupational or environmental studies. Toxicol Lett 1999; 106:69–77.
11. Lang TA, Secic M. How to Report Statistics in Medicine. Philadelphia: American College of Physicians, 1997.

12. Pérez-Stable EJ, Benowitz NL, Marín G. Is serum cotinine a better measure of cigarette smoking than self-report. Prev Med 1995; 24:171–179.
13. Henderson FW, Reid HF, Morris R, et al. Home air nicotine levels and urinary cotinine excretion in preschool children. Am Rev Respir Dis 1989; 140: 197–201.
14. Wilcox RR. New Statistical Procedures for the Social Sciences. Hillsdale, NJ: Lawrence Erlbaum Associates, 1987.
15. Atawodi SE, Lea S, Nyberg F, et al. 4-Hydroxyl-1-(3-pyridyl)-1-butanone-hemoglobin adducts as biomarkers of exposure to tobacco smoke: Validation of a method to be used in multicenter studies. Cancer Epidemiol Biomark Prev 1998; 7:817–821.
16. D'Agostino RB. Graphical analysis. In: D'Agostino RB, Stephens MA, eds. Goodness-of-Fit Techniques. New York: Marcel Dekker, 1986:7–62.
17. Gerson M. The techniques and uses of probability plots. The Statistician 1975; 24:235–257.
18. Jones MC, Daly F. Density probability plots. Commun Stat—Simul C 1995; 24:911–927.
19a. Hazelton ML. A graphical tool for assessing normality. Am Stat 2003; 57:285–288.
19b. Letter to the editor and reply Am Stat 2004; 58:176–177.
20. Bernstein C, Bernstein H, Garewal H, et al. A bile acid-induced apoptosis assay for colon cancer risk and associated quality control studies. Cancer Res 1999; 59: 2353–2357.
21. Looney SW, Gulledge TR. Use of the correlation coefficient with normal probability plots. Am Stat 1985; 39:75–79.
22. Shapiro SS, Wilk MB. An analysis of variance test for normality (complete samples). Biometrika 1965; 52:591–611.
23. Statistical Analysis System (SAS), Version 9.0. Cary, NC: SAS Institute Inc, 2002. http://www.sas.com/.
24. Buckley TJ, Waldman JM, Dhara R, Greenberg A, Ouyang Z, Lioy PJ. An assessment of a urinary biomarker for total human environmental exposure to benzo[a]pyrene. Int Arch Occup Environ Health 1995; 67:257–266.
25. MacRae AR, Gardner HA, Allen LC, Tokmakejian S, Lepage N. Outcome validation of the Beckman Coulter access analyzer in a second-trimester Down Syndrome serum screening application. Clin Chem 2003; 49:69–76.
26. Strachan DP, Jarvis MJ, Feyerabend C. The relationship of salivary cotinine to respiratory symptoms, spirometry, and exercise-induced bronchospasm in seven-year-old children. Am Rev Respir Dis 1990; 142:147–151.
27. Box GEP, Cox DR. An analysis of transformations. J Roy Stat Soc B 1964; 26:211–252.
28. Tukey JW. Exploratory Data Analysis. Reading, MA: Addison-Wesley, 1977.
29. Johnson NL. Systems of frequency curves generated by methods of translation. Biometrika 1949; 36:149–176.
30. Stuart A, Ord JK. Kendall's Advanced Theory of Statistics. New York: Oxford University Press, 1987.
31. Atkinson AC. Testing transformations to normality. J Roy Stat Soc B 1973; 35:473–479.

32. Milliken GA, Johnson DE. Analysis of Messy Data Vol. 1. Designed Experiments. New York: Van Nostrand Reinhold 1984.
33. Huber PJ. Robust Statistical Procedures. 2nd ed. Philadelphia: Society for Industrial and Applied Mathematics, 1996.
34. Mehta C, Patel N. StatXact 6. Cambridge, MA: CYTEL Software Corporation, 2003. www.cytel.com.
35. Cook DG, Whincup PH, Papacosta O, Strachan DP, Jarvis MJ, Bryant A. Relation of passive smoking as assessed by salivary cotinine concentration and questionnaire to spirometric indices in children. Thorax 1993; 48:14–20.
36. Tunstall-Pedoe H, Brown CA, Woodward M, Tavendale R. Passive smoking by self-report and serum cotinine and the prevalence of respiratory and coronary heart disease in the Scottish heart health study. J Epidemiol Commun H 1995; 49:139–143.
37. Kleinbaum DG, Kupper LL, Morgenstern H. Epidemiologic Research. New York: Van Nostrand Reinhold, 1982.
38. Fleiss JL. Statistical Methods for Rates and Proportions. 2nd ed. New York: John Wiley, 1981.
39. Epi Info, Version 3.2.2. Atlanta: Centers for Disease Control and Prevention, 2004. http://www.cdc.gov/epiinfo/
40. Mehrotra DV, Chan ISF, Berger RL. A cautionary note on exact unconditional inference for a difference between two independent binomial proportions. Biometrics 2003; 59:441–450.
41. Gibbons JD. Nonparametric Statistical Inference. 2nd ed. New York:Marcel Dekker, 1985
42. Cochran WG. Some methods for strengthening the common χ^2 tests. Biometrics 1954; 10:417–454.
43. Armitage P. Test for linear trend in proportions and frequencies. Biometrics 1955; 11:375–386.
44. Agresti A, Mehta CR, Patel NR. Exact inference for contingency tables with ordered categories. JASA 1990; 85:453–458.
45. Sheskin DJ. In: Handbook of Parametric and Nonparametric Statistical Procedures. Boca Raton, FL: CRC Press, 1997.
46. Algina J, Oshima TC, Lin W. Type I error rates for Welch's test and James's second-order test under nonnormality and inequality of variance when there are two groups. J Educ Behav Stat 1994; 19:275–291.
47. Conover WJ. Practical Nonparametric Statistics. 3rd ed. New York: John Wiley, 1999.
48. Granella M, Priante E, Nardini B, Bono R, Clonfero E. Excretion of mutagens, nicotine and its metabolites in urine of cigarette smokers. Mutagenesis 1996; 11:207–211.
49. Amorim LCA, Alvarez-Leite EM. Determination of *o*-cresol by gas chromatography and comparison with hippuric acid levels in urine samples of individuals exposed to toluene. J Toxicol Environ Health 1997; 50:401–407.
50. Moser BK, Stevens GR, Watts CL. The two-sample t test versus Satterthwaite's approximate F test. Commun Stat A—Theor 1989; 18:3963–3975.
51. Moser BK, Stevens GR. Homogeneity of variance in the two-sample means test. Am Stat 1992; 46:19–21.

52. Salmi M, Stolen C, Jousilahti P, et al. Insulin-regulated increase of soluble vascular adhesion protein-1 in diabetes. Am J Pathol 2002; 161:2255–2262.
53. Dunnett CW. Pairwise multiple comparisons in the homogeneous variance, unequal sample size case. JAMA 1980; 75:789–795.
54. Dunnett CW. Pairwise multiple comparisons in the unequal variance case. JAMA 1980; 75:796–800.
55. SPSS for Windows, Version 11.0.1. Chicago: SPSS Inc., 2001. http://www.spss.com/
56. Buss IH, Senthilmohan R, Darlow BA, Mogridge N, Kettle AJ, Winterbourn CC. 3-chlorotyrosine as a marker of protein damage by myeloperoxidase in tracheal aspirates from preterm infants: association with adverse respiratory outcome. Pediat Res 2003; 53:455–462.
57. Looney, SW. Sample size determination for correlation coefficient inference: Practical problems and practical solutions. In: Proceedings of the Statistical Computing Section, American Statistical Association. Alexandria, VA: American Statistical Association, 1996:240–245.
58. Morton RF, Hebel JR, McCarter RJ. A Study Guide to Epidemiology and Biostatistics. 4th ed. Gaithersburg, MD: Aspen Publishers, 1996.
59. Steiger JH. Tests for comparing elements of a correlation matrix. Psychol Bull 1980; 87:245–251.
60. Siegel S, Castellan NJ. Nonparametric Statistics for the Behavioral Sciences. New York: McGraw-Hill, 1988.
61. Suissa S, Shuster J. The 2x2 matched-pairs trial: Exact unconditional design and analysis. Biometrics 1991; 47:361–372.
62. Lehmann EL. Nonparametrics: Statistical Methods Based on Ranks. San Francisco: Holden-Day 1975:267–270.
63. Tockman MS, Gupta PK, Myers JD, et al. Sensitive and specific monoclonal antibody recognition of human lung cancer antigen on preserved sputum cells: A new approach to early lung cancer detection. J Clin Oncol 1988; 6:1685–1693.
64. Kraemer HC. Extension of the kappa coefficient. Biometrics 1980; 36:207–216.
65. Shoukri MM. In: Measures of Interobserver Agreement. Boca Raton, FL: Chapman & Hall/CRC, 2004.
66. Bartczak A, Kline SA, Yu R, Weisel CP, Goldstein BD, Witz G. Evaluation of assays for the identification and quantitation of muconic acid, a benzene metabolite in human urine. J Toxicol Environ Health 1994; 42:245–258.
67. Westgard JO, Hunt MR. Use and interpretation of common statistical tests in method-comparison studies. Clin Chem 1973; 19:49–57.
68. Cornbleet PJ, Gochman N. Incorrect least-squares regression coefficients in method comparison analysis. Clin Chem 1979; 25:432–438.

3

Biomarkers of Toxicant Exposure

Ken Sexton

University of Texas School of Public Health, Brownsville, Texas, U.S.A.

INTRODUCTION

Every day we are exposed to low levels of thousands of toxic chemicals in the air we breathe, the food we consume, the water and beverages we drink, the products we use, and the surfaces we touch. Each individual's personalized risk of developing an environmentally-related disease results from each person's unique combination of exposure level, genetic susceptibility, age, sex, nutritional status, and lifestyle. Although in most cases the complicated interactions that ultimately give rise to environmentally induced health effects are not well elucidated, it is clear that exposure is a key factor in determining risk. A fundamental goal of environmental health policies is to prevent or at least reduce exposures that contribute to death, disease, disability, dysfunction, or discomfort (1–4).

Exposure to an environmental chemical is commonly defined as contact of that chemical with the outer surface of the human body, such as the skin, mouth, or nostrils, for a defined period of time (2–7). For risk assessment purposes, the most important attributes of exposure are magnitude (i.e., what is the concentration?), duration (i.e., how long does contact last?), frequency (i.e., how often do exposures occur?), and timing (i.e., at what age do exposures occur?). Assessing people's actual exposure is often a complex endeavor that requires obtaining and analyzing a diversity of real-world information, including data on specific environmental chemicals (e.g., pesticides), sources (e.g., agricultural applications), transport or carrier media (e.g., water), and pathways (e.g., drinking contaminated well water). Data on people's activity patterns, eating and drinking habits, and lifestyle-related behaviors must be combined with data on concentrations of chemicals in environmental media (e.g., air, water, beverages, food, dust, oil) to obtain a realistic estimate of actual exposure. The nature, quantity, and quality of required information will depend on the intended use or uses of the assessment (5–8).

Exposure assessment for most environmental chemicals is typically limited by a scarcity of relevant data on the populations and chemicals of interest, and by a lack of understanding about important exposure-related mechanisms, such as transport and transformation processes in the atmosphere. Although direct measurement, as for example placing a monitor in the breathing zone to record airborne concentrations, is the only way to establish exposure levels unequivocally, it is usually technically infeasible or prohibitively expensive. Also, while these monitors establish exposure they tell us nothing about the individual's uptake of these chemical concentrations into the body (1–8).

Historically, the vast majority of exposure assessments have relied on indirect methods, like questionnaires, diaries, interviews, centralized environmental monitoring in community air or drinking water, and limited environmental measurements in combination with data on human activity patterns (5,7). Although these indirect approaches have the advantage of being practical and relatively inexpensive, they tend to introduce substantial uncertainty into resulting exposure estimates. This increases the potential for misclassification errors, such as classifying a person as "not exposed" when in fact that person is "exposed," or vice versa (1–7). Today, advances in biomedical sciences and analytical chemistry make it possible to estimate exposure using a different method altogether, one that provides information on both exposure and dose: namely, measurement of biologic markers in human tissues and fluids (1,5,7,9–16).

BASICS OF EXPOSURE ESTIMATION

There are several critical events that are an inherent part of understanding how, why, when, to what extent, and for whom exposures occur: release of an agent into the environment; its ensuing transport, transformation, and fate in various environmental media; contact with people; entry into the body; and the resulting internal dose. The environmental health paradigm, a simplified representation of key steps between emissions of toxic chemicals into the environment and adverse outcomes in people, is depicted in Figure 1 (7). The figure also shows the domain of exposure assessment, which includes important events, processes, and mechanisms that provide context for understanding and estimating people's actual exposure (2,7). Definitions for significant events in the environmental health paradigm are summarized below.

The point or area of origin for an environmental agent is known as a "source." Agents are released into the environment from a wide variety of

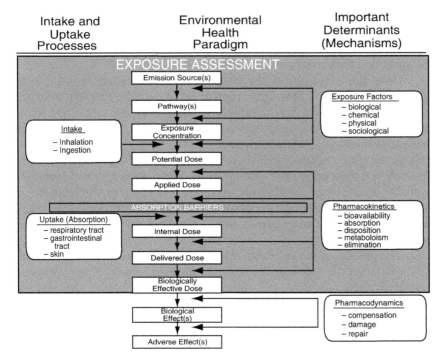

Figure 1 Important events in the environmental health paradigm, with the domain of exposure assessment designated by the shaded area. *Source*: From Ref. 7.

sources, which are often placed in dichotomous categories: point (e.g., incinerator) versus area sources (e.g., urban runoff), stationary (e.g., refinery) versus mobile sources (e.g., automobile), or anthropogenic (e.g., landfill) versus non-anthropogenic sources (e.g., natural vegetation) (2,7).

An exposure pathway is the physical course taken by an agent as it moves from a source to a point of contact with a person (e.g., mercury attached to airborne particles deposited in a reservoir used as a drinking water supply by a city). Exposure concentration is the concentration of an agent in a carrier medium at the point of contact with the outer boundary of the human body. Most exposure assessments go beyond exposure concentration and estimate how much of an agent is expected to enter the body (i.e., dose) (2,7).

The transfer of an environmental agent from the exterior to the interior of the body can occur by either or both of two basic processes: intake and uptake. Intake is associated with ingestion and inhalation, wherein the agent enters the body through the nose (e.g., bulk transport by air) or the mouth (e.g., bulk transport by water or food). The rates of bulk transport into the body are assumed to be the same for both the agent and the carrier medium (2,7). Uptake occurs when an agent (usually as part of a carrier medium) enters the body by crossing an absorption barrier, such as the skin (e.g., dermal contact), respiratory tract, or gastrointestinal tract. The rates of bulk transport across the absorption barriers are generally not the same for the agent and the carrier medium (2,7).

Once the agent enters the body by either intake or uptake, it is described as a "dose." Several different types of dose are relevant to exposure estimation. Potential (or administered) dose is the amount of the agent that is actually ingested, inhaled, or applied to the skin. Applied dose is the amount of the agent directly in contact with the body's absorption barriers, such as the skin, respiratory tract, and gastrointestinal tract, and therefore available for absorption. The amount of the agent absorbed, and therefore available to undergo metabolism, transport, storage, or elimination, is referred to as the "internal" or "absorbed" dose. The portion of the internal (absorbed) dose that reaches a tissue of interest is called the "delivered dose" (2,7).

The portion of the delivered dose that reaches the site or sites of toxic action is called the "biologically effective dose." The link, if any, between biologically effective dose and subsequent disease or illness depends on the relationship between dose and response (e.g., shape of the dose–response curve), underlying pharmacodynamic mechanisms (e.g., compensation, damage, repair), and important susceptibility factors (e.g., health status, nutrition, stress, genetic predisposition) (2,7).

BIOLOGIC MARKERS (BIOMARKERS) OF HUMAN EXPOSURE

Many of the dose-related and health-related events in the environmental health paradigm occur at inaccessible sites in the body (e.g., liver, developing organs). Biologic markers (biomarkers) are indicators of these significant but inaccessible events that can be measured in accessible human tissues (e.g., blood, urine, saliva). Categories of biomarkers include the following (7,15):

- Unchanged exogenous agents: solvents, asbestos fibers, PCBs, ethanol, nicotine, and heavy metals;
- Metabolized exogenous agents (precursors in parentheses): phenol (benzene), DDE (DDT), cotinine (nicotine);
- Endogenously produced molecules (exposure in parentheses): acetyl cholinesterase (organic phosphate pesticides), porphyrin ratios (lead and other metals);
- Molecular changes (exposure in parentheses): DNA adducts (chemical carcinogens), alkylated amino acids (electrophilic chemicals);
- Cellular/tissue changes (in response to various toxins): cell histology, lymphocyte ratios, sperm mobility, sperm counts, macrophage activity, and red blood cell counts.

According to the National Research Council (11–13), a biologic marker of exposure is an exogenous substance or its metabolite(s) or the product of an interaction between a xenobiotic agent and some target molecule or cell that is measured in a compartment within an organism. Exposure biomarkers can be obtained from many human tissues and excreta by either invasive or noninvasive methods (1,7,9). The term "noninvasive" indicates that sample collection does not require penetration of the body envelope, although a complete definition of invasive/noninvasive must also include consideration of social, cultural, and psychological factors. Collection of saliva, expired air, semen, urine, sputum, hair, feces, breast milk, or fingernails is typically considered noninvasive. Invasive methods, on the other hand, require incursion into the body and may involve collection of blood, lung tissue, bone marrow, amniotic fluid, liver tissue, bone, follicular fluid, adipose tissue, or blood vessels (1,7,9).

Biologic markers historically have played a relatively small role in most exposure assessments because of the nature of the risks being assessed (e.g., using "average" life-time exposure to estimate life-time cancer risk); the types of questions being asked (e.g., what incremental risks are associated with a single source/pathway/route?); the lack of appropriate human tissue data (e.g., no data for the population/situation of interest); and incomplete understanding of pharmacokinetics (e.g., problems relating biomarker measurements to exposure-related events) (7,9). This is changing, however, as more sensitive and specific biomarkers become available for a growing list of environmental chemicals, including dioxins, furans, heavy metals, pesticides, polychlorinated biphenyls (PCBs), phthalates, and phytoestrogens (9). Moreover, pharmacokinetic understanding is improving (10–13); there are better data on concentrations of various biomarkers in human populations (17–22), and technical advances make it possible to measure lower concentrations of more chemicals at less cost (1,7,9).

Interpreting Biomarkers for Exposure Assessment

An overview of the major pathways by which people come into contact with environmental chemicals is provided in Figure 2 (6). Although it does not include nontraditional pathways, such as infant exposures to contaminated breast milk and dermal contact with consumer products, Figure 2 demonstrates the diversity of traditional pathways that need to be considered when assessing human exposure. It also illustrates the fact that a biologic marker of exposure is an aggregate measure of dose, which integrates across all pathways and routes of exposure. Biomarkers are valuable tools for exposure assessment because they provide unequivocal evidence that exposure and uptake have occurred, and they are quantitative measures of the amount of chemical, its metabolites, or its reaction products (e.g., protein adducts) present in the body (1,2,7,9–14).

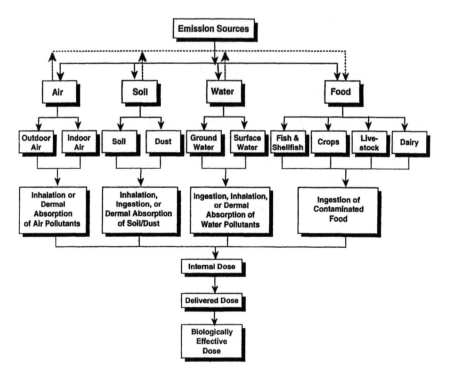

Figure 2 Major human exposure pathways and the integrative function of exposure biomarkers. *Source*: From Ref. 6.

The utility of biomarkers for exposure assessment depends on whether we understand the relevance of measured levels in relation to other important events in the environmental health paradigm (e.g., exposure concentration) (2,6,7,9). Our ability to interpret the significance of exposure biomarkers depends on answers to several important questions (7,23,24).

How is the biomarker related to different aspects of exposure?

- How are exposure magnitude, duration, and frequency related to the biomarker?
- How soon after exposure will the biomarker appear?
- How soon after exposure will the biomarker reach its maximum value?
- How soon after exposure will the biomarker reach its steady-state value?
- How long will the biomarker persist after exposure ends?
- What is the sensitivity and specificity of the biomarker?
- What is the intraindividual, interindividual, and between-group variability?

How is the biomarker related to the different aspects of dose?

- Is the marker a measure of internal, delivered, or biologically effective dose?
- How is the marker related to other dose events?

Is the biomarker specific?

- For a particular agent (e.g., lead)?
- For a particular source (e.g., coal-fired power plant)?
- For a particular source category (e.g., combustion sources)?
- For a particular exposure setting (e.g., occupational)?

Overall, the advantages of biomarkers for human exposure assessment are fivefold (2,7,14): (i) biomarkers may reflect exposures accumulated over time, (ii) biomarkers account for all routes of exposure (inhalation, ingestion, dermal absorption), including some, such as hand-to-mouth ingestion by young children, that are difficult to assess with environmental measurements, (iii) biomarkers of exposure have undergone the modifying effects of physiology and biologic availability, (iv) some environmental chemicals are more concentrated in biological samples and are therefore more readily detectable, and (v) biological samples provide an opportunity within a specific individual to correlate biomarkers of exposure with biomarkers of effect or susceptibility that might be predictive of illness or injury (14).

Choosing the Right Exposure Biomarker

Biomarker analysis for exposure assessment purposes generally involves measurement of the concentration of the toxicant, its primary metabolite(s), or its reaction products in a biological specimen, such as blood or urine. The choice of a specimen for measuring the internal dose is based primarily on the chemical and physical properties of the toxicant and, in some cases, on the time interval since the last exposure (1,9,25,26). Highly lipophilic compounds, such as dioxins, PCBs, and organochlorine pesticides, tend to have long biological half-lives and to sequester in the lipid portions of the body, such as adipose tissue. They are often referred to as "persistent" compounds. Lipophilic toxicants equilibrate between the lipids in adipose tissue and the lipids in blood because of blood flow through the adipose tissue. The 1:1 partitioning of 2,3,7,8-tetrachlorodibenzo-p-dioxin in humans between the lipids in adipose tissue and the lipids in serum is a good example of this equilibration (27). Typically, concentrations of lipophilic chemicals are reported in terms of their amount in the entire matrix (whole weight) or in the lipid portion (lipid-adjusted) (9).

Lipophobic (i.e., hydrophilic) compounds, which are referred to as non-persistent, have relatively short biological half-lives and tend to metabolize rapidly. Their metabolites are usually even more lipophobic and are excreted in the urine. Consequently, assessment of exposure to nonpersistent chemicals is generally conducted using urinary biomarkers, and concentrations are reported as the amount in urine or on an adjusted basis using creatinine, specific gravity, or osmolality. Pentachlorophenol is an example of a chemical that has both a lipophilic moiety and a lipophobic moiety, and exposure can be assessed in blood or urine (28). Similarly, exposure assessments for volatile organic compounds (VOCs) have used biomarkers in blood, urine, and exhaled breath (29,30).

The time interval since the last exposure can also affect the choice of an appropriate matrix (i.e., blood vs. urine) for assessing exposure to environmental chemicals. This is illustrated schematically in Figure 3 for a hypothetical persistent toxicant and in Figure 4 for a hypothetical nonpersistent toxicant. The nonpersistent chemical (or its metabolite) is only present in appreciable quantities in blood for a relatively short time (less than a day), while the persistent chemical (or its metabolite) is in the blood at substantial levels for a much longer time (more than 100 days). The persistent chemical does not form urinary metabolites to a significant degree, while the nonpersistent chemical does. It is important to keep in mind that even nonpersistent chemicals can be measured in blood if (i) the sample is collected soon after exposure or (ii) the method has sufficient sensitivity to measure the small portion of the nonpersistent toxicant that is in the

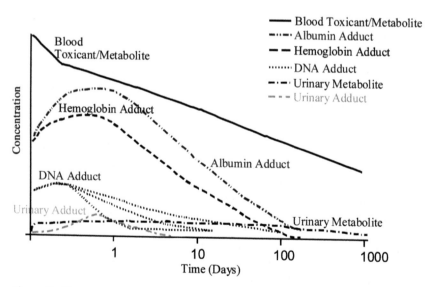

Figure 3 Postexposure fate of a hypothetical persistent toxicant in blood and urine. *Source*: From Ref. 9.

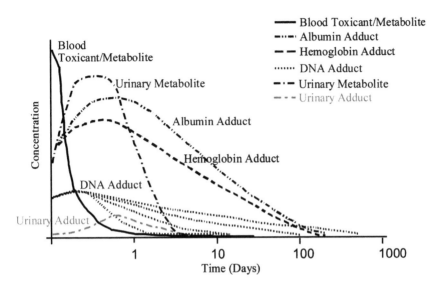

Figure 4 Postexposure fate of a hypothetical nonpersistent toxicant in blood and urine. *Source*: From Ref. 9.

blood for several days after the exposure. An example of this is the analysis of VOCs in blood at the parts-per-trillion levels by purge-and-trap/mass spectrometry (29).

Biomarkers of exposure also include the products of attack of a reactive parent compound or metabolite with biological macromolecules such as DNA and protein. These products are typically called "adducts." Various adducts can form between blood components and both persistent and nonpersistent chemicals, as shown in Figures 3 and 4 (9). Only those chemicals or their metabolites that have an electrophilic center, which reacts with the nucleophilic center of nucleic acids (such as DNA) and proteins (such as hemoglobin and albumin), are capable of forming adducts. Protein adducts generally have greater sensitivity over a longer postexposure time than DNA adducts, and are therefore preferred for exposure assessment (31). The increased amounts of the proteins relative to DNA are responsible for this better sensitivity. For example, in 10 mL of blood, there are gram amounts of hemoglobin and albumin, but only about 1 mg of leukocyte DNA. DNA adducts usually have shorter half-lives than protein adducts because of rapid DNA-repair mechanisms and subsequent excretion. The half-life for certain DNA adducts can, however, be substantial (e.g., four months for polyaromatic hydrocarbon–DNA adducts) (32).

Figures 3 and 4 show the potential formation of hemoglobin adducts and their demise with the death of the red blood cell, which has a lifespan of approximately 120 days (9). Adducts can also form with albumin, the most abundant serum protein. Albumin adducts decay with the decay of albumin, which has an average half-life of 14 to 20 days. Although the analytical sensitivities for both types of adducts vary by chemical, hemoglobin is generally preferred over albumin as an exposure biomarker (31).

Because of the equilibrium of a persistent compound between the lipids in adipose tissue and blood, as adducts are formed in the blood more of the compound becomes available from the adipose tissue, which in turn allows more adduct to form in the blood. This means that as analytical methods become more sensitive, it will be possible to monitor persistent compounds over a longer postexposure time period. Although nucleic acid adducts have been monitored in urine to assess exposure to several carcinogens, urinary adducts have not been used extensively as exposure biomarkers (33,34).

Chemical Analysis of Exposure Biomarkers

The inventory of exposure biomarkers continues to expand as analytical techniques keep improving. Examples of chemical analyses of biological matrices carried out by the National Center for Environmental Health, Centers for Disease Control and Prevention, including the amount of sample needed and the limit of detection of the analytical method, are provided in Tables 1 to 5 (9).

Twenty-eight organophosphate pesticides approved by the U.S. Environmental Protection Agency (EPA) for agricultural use, along with their corresponding phosphorus-containing urinary metabolites, are listed in Table 1 (9). Although these metabolites are not specific for a particular organophosphate pesticide, their quantification provides important information about cumulative exposure/dose for this group of pesticides (9).

Nonpersistent pesticides that can be measured in urine are summarized in Table 2 (9). The list includes representatives of the organophosphate, carbamate, amide, carboxylic acid, phenol, pyrethroid, aromatic, and triazine classes. The metabolite is the analyte most often measured in urine, and the analytical technique is either gas chromatography/mass spectrometry/mass spectrometry (GC/MS/MS) or liquid chromatography/mass spectrometry/mass spectrometry (LC/MS/MS). With the exception of deltamethrin and permethrin, all of the analytes measured by LC/MS/MS can be quantified in a single 5 mL sample of urine (36). Other nonpersistent organic toxicants measured in the current NHANES are listed in Table 3 (9), including two groups of potential endocrine modulators: the synthetic phthalates, which are widely used as plasticizers in plastics, particularly polyvinyl chloride (40); and the naturally occurring phytoestrogens (41).

Persistent chemicals that can be measured in serum are shown in Table 4, including chemicals like polychlorinated dibenzo-*p*-dioxins,

Table 1 Organophosphate Pesticides and Their Phosphorus-Containing Metabolites (LOD in ng/mL for 4 mL Urine Sample)

Pesticide	DMP (0.51)	DMPT (0.18)	DMDTP (0.08)	DEP (0.2)	DEPT (0.09)	DEDTP (0.05)
Azinphos methyl	X	X	X			
Chlorethoxyphos				X	X	
Chlorpyrifos				X	X	
Chlorpyrifos methyl	X	X				
Coumaphos				X	X	
Dichlorvos (DDVP)	X					
Diazinon				X	X	
Dicrotophos	X					
Dimethoate	X	X	X			
Disulfoton				X	X	X
Ethion				X	X	X
Fenitrothion	X	X				
Fenthion	X	X				
Isazaphos-methyl	X	X				
Malathion	X	X	X			
Methidathion	X	X	X			
Methyl parathion	X	X				
Naled	X					
Oxydemeton-methyl	X	X				
Parathion				X	X	
Phorate				X	X	X
Phosmet	X	X	X			
Pirimiphos-methyl	X	X				
Sulfotepp				X	X	
Temephos	X	X				
Terbufos				X	X	X
Tetrachlorvinphos	X					
Trichlorfon	X					

Abbreviations: LOD, Limit of detection; DMP, dimethylphosphate; DMPT, dimethylthiophosphate; DMDTP, dimethyldithiophosphate; DEP, diethylphosphate; DEPT, diethylthiophosphate; DEDTP, diethyldithiophosphate.
Source: From Refs. 9, 35.

polychlorinated dibenzofurans, PCBs, and organochlorine pesticides that have long half-lives in the body (9). Needham et al. (19) have reported reference range concentrations for many of these chemicals.

Finally, a list of 21 chemical elements that can be measured in biological matrices is provided in Table 5 (9). The inductively-coupled argon plasma/mass spectrometry (ICPMS) method is capable of concurrent measurement of 14 elements in a single urine sample.

Table 2 List of Nonpersistent Pesticides Monitored in Urine at the National Center for Environmental Health

Pesticide	Analyte	Urine volume (mL)	LOD (ng/mL)	References
Chlorpyrifos; Chlorpyrifos-methyl	3,5,6-Trichloro-2-pyridinol[a]	10	1.3	(37)
Diazinon	Oxypyrimidine	10	0.02	(36)
Malathion	Malathion diacid	10	0.3	(38)
Parathion; methyl parathion	4-Nitrophenol	3	0.1	(35b, Footnote 1)
Carbaryl	1-Naphthol[a]	10	1.4	(37)
Carbofuran	Carbofuranphenol[a]	10	1	(37)
Propoxur	2-Isopropoxyphenol[a]	10	1	(37)
Acetochlor	Acetochlor mercapturate	5	1	(35b, Footnote 2)
Alachlor	Alachlor mercapturate	10	15	(35b, Footnote 2)
Metolachlor	Metolachlor mercapturate	5	1	(35b, Footnote 2)
DEET	NN-Diethyltoluamide (DEET)	5	0.05	(35b, Footnote 2)
2,4-D, esters, salts	2,4-Dichlorophenoxyacetic acid (2,4-D)	10	0.3	(38)

2,4,5-T, esters, salts	2,4,5-Trichlorophenoxyacetic acid (2,4,5-T)	10	0.3	(35b, Footnote 2)
Dicamba	Dicamba[a]	10	0.5	(39)
Pentachlorophenol	Pentachlorophenol[a]	5	1	(37)
o-Phenylphenol	o-Phenylphenol	5	2	(35b, Footnote 2)
Synthetic pyrethroids	3-Phenoxybenzoic acid	10	0.5	(36)
Deltamethrin	cis-3-(2,2-Dibromovinyl)-2,2-dimethylcyclopropane-carboxylic acid	2.5	0.5	(35b, Footnote 3)
Permethrin	cis/trans-3-(2,2-Dichlorovinyl)-2,2-dimethylcyclopropane-carboxylic acid	2.5	0.5	(35b, Footnote 3)
Naphthalene	1-Naphthol; 2-Naphthol[a]	10	1.4	(37)
1,4-Dichlorobenzene	2,5-Dichlorophenol			(35b, Footnote 2 and 36)
Atrazine	Atrazine mercapturate	10	0.3	(38)

[a]Measured by gas chromatography/mass spectrometry/mass spectrometry (GC/MS/MS); all others by liquid chromatography/MS/MS.
Abbreviation: LOD, limit of detection.
Source: From Refs. 9, 35b.

Table 3 List of Other Groups of Nonpersistent Toxicants Measured at the National Center for Environmental Health

Toxicant group	Analytes (number)	Matrix	Volume (mL)	LOD (ng/mL)	References
Phthalates	Monocarboxylic acids (8)[a]	U	1	1	(40)
Phytoestrogens	Phytoestrogens/ metabolites (7)[a]	U, S	1	0.2–4 (U)	(41)
Volatile organic compounds	VOCs (32)[a]	WB	5	0.005–0.07	(29)
Selected VOCs; e.g., ethylene oxide, vinyl chloride	N-acetyl-S-(2-hydroxyethyl)-L-cysteine	U	1	0.68	(42)
Environmental tobacco smoke	Cotinine	S, U, Sa	1	0.05	(42,43)
	Nicotine/metabolites (6)[a]	U	1	0.01	(35c), Footnote 1
	4-Methylnitrosoamino-1-(3-pyridyl)-1-butanol (NNAL)	U	5	6×10⁻⁴	(35c), Footnote 2

[a]Values in parentheses are the number of analytes measured.
Abbreviations: LOD, limit of detection; U, urine; S, serum; WB, whole blood; Sa, saliva.
Source: From Refs. 9, 35c.

Table 4 List of Persistent Organic Pollutants by Class Measured in Serum at the National Center for Environmental Health

Toxicant (by class)	Serum volume (mL)	LOD (approximate) (ng/mL)	References
Polychlorodibenzo-p-dioxins (7 congeners)	10	$(15-430) \times 10^{-6}$	(45)
Polychlorodibenzo-furans (10 congeners)	10	15×10^{-6}	(45)
Coplanar PCBs (4 congeners)	10	65×10^{-6}	(45)
PCBs (37 isomers)	1	0.05–0.32	(45)
Organochlorine pesticides (12 compounds)	1	0.07–0.26	(45)

Abbreviations: LOD, limit of detection, PCBs, polychlorinated biphenyls.
Source: From Ref. 9.

USES OF EXPOSURE BIOMARKERS

There are seven major uses of exposure biomarkers in the context of protecting public health (1,25):

1. *Checking the Validity of Traditional Exposure Models.* Biologic markers can serve as a "reality check" on conventional exposure models. Models typically estimate exposure by combining information about chemical concentrations in air, water, food, dust, or soil with data on people's activities and behaviors. Then, using assumptions about intake and uptake, the internal dose is estimated. Because biomarkers are quantitative measures of body burden and represent integrated exposure, they can be compared to model outputs to verify the validity of predictions (7,25,57).

2. *Identifying Priority Exposures.* Because people are exposed to literally thousands of chemicals as part of their everyday lives, it is important to identify those that present the highest comparative risk to individuals and populations. Generally, substances that have a greater potential for toxicity and that also accumulate in the body are of greatest concern. Biomarkers can be used to identify chemicals whose concentrations exceed health-related benchmarks or are much higher than average so that follow-up actions can be initiated (25,26).

3. *Identifying At-Risk Populations.* Biomarkers can be used to distinguish differences in exposure between groups of people

Table 5 List of Elements Measured at the National Center for Environmental Health

Toxicant	Matrix	Amount (mL)	LOD (ng/mL)	Method	References
Lead[a]	WB	0.1	4.0	AAS	(46)
Cadmium[a]	WB	0.1	0.3	AAS	(47)
Mercury (total)	WB	0.1	0.14	AAS	(48)
Mercury (inorg)	WB	0.1	0.45	AAS	(48)
Selenium	S	0.05	2.0	AAS	(49)
Arsenic	U	0.10	4.0	AAS	(50)
Mercury	U	0.10	0.2	AAS	(51)
Nickel	U	0.10	0.4	AAS	(52)
Chromium	U	0.10	0.4	AAS	(53)
Barium[b]	U	0.10	0.12	ICP/MS	(54)
Beryllium[b]	U	0.10	0.13	ICP/MS	(54)
Cadmium[b]	U	0.10	0.06	ICP/MS	(54)
Cobalt[b]	U	0.10	0.07	ICP/MS	(54)
Cesium[b]	U	0.10	0.14	ICP/MS	(54)
Lead[b]	U	0.10	0.10	ICP/MS	(54)
Molybdenum[b]	U	0.10	0.80	ICP/MS	(54)
Platinum[b]	U	0.10	0.04	ICP/MS	(54)
Antimony[b]	U	0.10	0.04	ICP/MS	(54)
Thallium[b]	U	0.10	0.02	ICP/MS	(54)
Tungsten[b]	U	0.10	0.04	ICP/MS	(54)
Thorium[b]	U	0.10	0.006	ICP/MS	(54)
Uranium[b]	U	0.10	0.004	ICP/MS	(54)
Iodine	U	0.10	3.0	ICP/MS	(56)

[a]Measured simultaneously in 0.1 mL of whole blood.
[b]Measured simultaneously in 0.1 mL of urine.
Abbreviations: AAS, atomic absorption spectroscopy; ICP/MS, inductively coupled plasma/ mass spectrometry; S, serum; U, urine; WB, whole blood.
Source: From Ref. 9.

defined by demographic, geographic, or socioeconomic variables. For example, information on blood or urine concentrations of selected chemicals could help public health officials focus their efforts on groups that are more exposed because of differences in personal habits (smoking), occupation (working with toxic chemicals), proximity to emission sources (living near a freeway), cultural practices (eating fish as part of tribal heritage), and other factors (21,28,30,32).

4. *Providing Integrated Dose Measurements.* Biomarker measurements give exposure assessors an unequivocal indicator that uptake has occurred. Moreover, exposure biomarkers provide a

direct assay of body burden that integrates exposure from all sources and pathways, even ones that are hard to measure (10–15).

5. *Recognizing Time Trends in Population Exposures.* It is important to understand which chemicals are accumulating in people's bodies and how levels are changing over time. Periodically measuring biomarkers in a probability sample of the population can provide scientific evidence of how body burdens of toxic chemicals vary from season to season, year to year, or decade to decade (2,14,21).

6. *Establishing Reference Ranges for Comparison.* Because it is generally time consuming and expensive to select a random sample of people from whom to collect samples, most biomarker studies choose a sample based on convenience and practicality (e.g., workers in a particular factory, people living near a power plant, women and their children visiting a certain clinic). But, it is usually difficult to interpret the significance of biomonitoring results when samples are not part of a population-based statistical design. Biomarker measurements from a population of similar people with no known (or only minimal) exposure to the toxic chemicals of interest (i.e., reference ranges) provide a basis for comparison that helps to put measured biomarker values from a particular study into perspective (17–20).

7. *Evaluating Exposure Reduction and Prevention Activities.* Governmental agencies routinely take action to prevent or reduce exposures to toxic chemicals. It is important to assess the effectiveness of such actions by determining whether, in fact, exposures have been reduced and, if so, by how much and over what time period. This can be accomplished by taking biomarker samples from relevant populations before and after government intervention or by examining temporal changes in body burdens based on population-based probability samples (2,14,25).

Examples of the Value of Exposure Biomarkers

There are numerous cases demonstrating that traditional exposure estimators (questionnaires, proximity to sources, environmental concentrations, constructed scenarios) are not correlated with exposure biomarkers. For example, from 1962 to 1971, the U.S. Air Force sprayed the defoliant known as "Agent Orange" in Vietnam. Service members who were involved in that operation or who later came into contact with the herbicide were potentially exposed to high levels of dioxin (2,3,7,8-TCDD). Exposures were first estimated using a scenario approach, which involved average dioxin concentrations in the Agent Orange, the number of gallons used during a serviceman's tour of duty, and the frequency and duration of contact based on job description. However, when these estimates were compared with biomarker measurements of dioxin (2,3,7,8-TCDD) in blood serum, there was no correlation. A subsequent investigation of those with highest measured dioxin levels in their blood did identify some activities that contributed to exposure—such as cleaning contaminated chemical tanks (1,7,57).

There are also many cases illustrating that traditional exposure estimators are correlated with exposure biomarkers in certain situations. For example, in 1979 residents living downstream of a defunct DDT manufacturing plant in Alabama were thought to be at potential risk from ingestion of contaminated fish caught out of a nearby stream. A scenario evaluation based on concentrations in fish and the amount of fish eaten per week found correlations with levels of DDT and its metabolites DDE and DDD in the residents' blood serum. Similarly, in the late 1980s, chemical plant workers in New Jersey and Missouri became aware that they had been exposed to dioxin-contaminated compounds through inhalation, ingestion, and dermal contact. Despite the time interval that had occurred since the exposures ended in the late 1970s and the complexities of workers' contact with the chemical, a scenario method using occupational records to calculate duration of potential exposure was able to estimate internal doses accurately, as confirmed by measurements of dioxin in blood serum (1,7,57).

The U.S. decision to phase out lead in gasoline is the classic example of the value of biological monitoring (1,7,25,26). Prior to the decision, traditional exposure models suggested that eliminating lead in gasoline would have only a slight effect on levels of lead in blood. However, data from NHANES II revealed that from 1976 to 1980, as unleaded fuel was introduced for the first time and lead in gasoline decreased (by approximately 55%), there was a parallel decline in average blood lead levels in the U.S. population. Overall, average blood lead concentrations decreased from 16 to $<10\,\mu g/dL$, a reduction of about 37%. These data demonstrated the effectiveness, in terms of reduced exposures, of removing lead from gasoline and were a dominant factor in the Environmental Protection Agency's decision to phase out leaded gasoline in the United States. The average blood lead level in the U.S. population today is $<2\,\mu g/dL$ (1,7,25,26).

National Report on Human Exposure to Environmental Chemicals

The U.S. Centers for Disease Control and Prevention (CDC) released the first National Report on Human Exposure to Environmental Chemicals (the Report) in March 2001, and the second Report in January 2003 (1,58,59). The Report uses biomonitoring data to provide an ongoing assessment of exposure to more than 100 toxic chemicals for the U.S. population. Results are for chemicals or their metabolites measured in blood and urine specimens from selected participants in the 1999–2000 NHANES. For many chemicals, the Report provides first-time data on national exposures because these compounds have not been measured before in a nationally representative sample (1,58,59).

In the second Report (58,59), biomonitoring data are provided for 116 different chemicals, including: lead, mercury, cadmium, and other metals; organophosphate and organochlorine pesticides; carbamate pesticides; herbicides; pest repellents and disinfectants; cotinine (tobacco metabolite); phthalates; polycyclic aromatic hydrocarbons (PAHs); dioxins; furans; PCBs; and phytoestrogens. Tables of descriptive statistics, including geometric means and percentiles with confidence intervals, are presented in the Report for each chemical. Results are shown for the general population and also by age group, gender, and ethnicity/race (non-Hispanic black, Mexican American, non-Hispanic white) (58,59).

The Report is intended to provide new and unique information about people's actual exposure to toxic environmental chemicals (58,59). The public health uses of the Report include the following: determining which environmental chemicals get into people's bodies and at what concentrations; ascertaining the number (percentage) of people with body burdens above established health benchmarks or levels of concern; establishing reference ranges for individual chemicals that provide a baseline for comparison so that physicians and scientists can know whether a person or group has an above average or unusually high exposure; assessing the effectiveness of public health efforts to reduce people's exposure to toxic environmental chemicals; determining whether exposure levels are higher among children, women of childbearing age, minorities, and other potentially vulnerable groups; tracking trends over time in body burden levels of toxic environmental chemicals; and setting priorities for research on the effects of toxic environmental chemicals on human health (58,59).

Data from the Report have already shown some interesting trends in exposures. For example, NHANES data collected during 1991–1994 show that 4.4% of children aged one to five years had blood lead levels greater than or equal to $10\,\mu g/dL$ (the U.S. federal action level), while the geometric mean for this age group was $2.7\,\mu g/dL$. Data from NHANES collected during 1999–2000 reveal that only 2.2% of children aged one to five years had blood lead levels greater than or equal to $10\,\mu g/dL$, and the geometric mean decreased to $2.2\,\mu g/dL$. This finding suggests that public health actions continue to reduce lead exposure for children living in the United States, although special populations of children, such as those living in homes with lead-based paint or lead-contaminated dust, remain at unacceptably high risk (58,59).

Similarly, the Report indicates a hopeful trend in serum cotinine levels, which provide a biomarker (in nonsmokers) for exposure to environmental tobacco smoke. Median levels of serum cotinine decreased more than 70% (from 0.20 to $0.059\,ng/mL$) based on a comparison of NHANES data collected in 1988–1994 to similar data from 1999 to 2000. Although the drop in average cotinine levels provides objective evidence of reduced exposure to environmental tobacco smoke for the general U.S. population, more than half of American youth continue to be exposed to environmental tobacco smoke (58,59).

The CDC currently plans to release future Reports every two years, and will include findings from CDC studies of special-exposure populations, such as pesticide applicators, people living near hazardous waste sites, and workers in lead smelters, which are likely to have higher-than-average exposures to certain environmental chemicals (58,59).

CONCLUSIONS

Biomarkers are now considered the "gold standard" for exposure assessment because they provide unequivocal evidence that both exposure and uptake into the body have occurred. There is, nonetheless, an ongoing need to collect complementary exposure-related data on pollutant emissions, environmental concentrations, individual exposures, and human activities and behaviors in order to understand how, when, where, why, and for whom elevated exposures are likely to occur. In the future, technological advances will continue to improve biomarker detection methods so that investigators can measure lower and lower concentrations of more and more chemicals in smaller and smaller samples at less and less cost. Although biomarkers will continue to be a standard fixture in the exposure assessor's toolbox, further biomedical research on relevant pharmacokinetics, pharmacodynamics, and genetic susceptibility is needed to interpret the health significance of exposure biomarkers for most environmental chemicals.

REFERENCES

1. Sexton K, Needham LL, Pirkle JL. Human biomonitoring of environmental chemicals. Am Sci 2004; 92:36–45.
2. Sexton K, Callahan MA, Bryan EF, Saint CG, Wood WP. Informed decisions about protecting and promoting public health: rationale for a national human exposure assessment survey. J Exp Anal Environ Epidemiol 1995; 5(3):233–256.
3. National Research Council (NRC). Frontiers in Assessing Human Exposures to Environmental Toxicants. Washington, DC: National Academy Press, 1991.
4. National Research Council (NRC). Human Exposure Assessment for Airborne Pollutants, Advances and Opportunities. Washington, DC: National Academy Press, 1991.
5. Sexton K, Ryan PB. Assessment of human exposure to air pollution: methods, measurements, and models. In: Watson AY, Bates RR, Kennedy D, eds. Air Pollution, the Automobile, and Public Health. Washington, DC: National Academy Press, 1988:207–238.

6. Sexton K, Selevan SG, Wagener DK, Lybarger JA. Estimating human exposures to environmental pollutants: availability and utility of existing databases. Arch Environ Health 1992; 47(6):398–407.

7. Sexton K, Callahan MA, Byran EF. Estimating exposure and dose to characterize health risks: the role of human tissue monitoring in exposure assessment. Environ Health Perspect 1995; 103(Suppl 3):13–29.

8. Mukerjee D. Assessment of risk from multimedia exposures of children to environmental chemicals. J Air Waste Manage Assoc 1998; 48:483–501.

9. Needham LL, Sexton K. Assessing children's exposure to hazardous environmental chemicals: an overview of selected research challenges and complexities. J Exp Anal Environ Epidemiol 2000; 10(6):611–629.

10. DeCaprio AP. Biomarkers: coming of age for environmental health and risk assessment. Environ Sci Technol 1997; 31:1837–1848.

11. National Research Council (NRC). Biomarkers in Pulmonary Toxiciology. Washington, DC: National Academy Press, 1989.

12. National Research Council (NRC). Biomarkers in Reproductive Toxicology. Washington, DC: National Academy Press, 1989.

13. National Research Council (NRC). Biological Markers in Immunotoxicology. Washington, DC: National Academy Press, 1992.

14. National Research Council (NRC). Monitoring Human Tissues for Toxic Substances. Washington, DC: National Academy Press, 1991.

15. Hulka BS, Wilcosky TC, Griffith JD, eds. Biological Markers in Epidemiology. New York: Oxford University Press, 1990.

16. Fowle JR, Sexton K. EPA priorities for biologic markers research in environmental health. Environ Health Perspect 1992; 98:235–241.

17. Ashley DL, Bonin MA, Cardinali FL, McCraw JM, Wooten JV. Blood concentrations of volatile organic compounds in a nonoccupationally exposed US population and in groups with suspected exposure. Clin Chem 1994; 40:1401–1404.

18. Hill RH Jr, Head SL, Baker S, Gregg M, Needham LL. Pesticide residues in urine of adults living in the United States: reference range concentrations. Environ Res 1995; 71:99–108.

19. Needham LL, Patterson DG Jr, Burse VW, Paschal DC, Turner WE, Hill RH, Jr. Reference range data for assessing exposure to selected environmental toxicants. Toxicol Ind Health 1996; 12:507–513.

20. Paschal DC, Ting BG, Morrow JC, et al. Trace metals in urine of United States residents: reference range concentrations. Environ Res 1998; 76 A:53–59.

21. Sexton K, Adgate JL, Church TR, et al. Children's exposure to environmental tobacco smoke: using diverse exposure metrics to document ethnic/racial differences. Environ Health Perspect 2004; 112(3):392–397.

22. Silva MJ, Barr DB, Reidy JA, et al. Urinary levels of seven phthalates metabolites in the U.S. population from the National Health and Nutrition Examination Survey (NHANES) 1999–2000. Environ Health Perspect 2004; 112(3):331–338.

23. Wilcosky TC. Criteria for selecting and evaluating markers. In: Hulka BS, Wilcosky TC, Griffith JD, eds. Biological Markers in Epidemiology. New York: Oxford University Press, 1990.

24. Schulte PA. A conceptual framework for the validation and use of biologic markers. Environ Res 1989; 48:129–144.

25. Pirkle JL, Needham LL, Sexton K. Improving exposure assessment by monitoring human tissues for toxic chemicals as part of a National Human Exposure Assessment Survey. J Exp Anal Environ Epidemiol 1995; 5:403–422.

26. Pirkle JL, Sampson EJ, Needham LL, Patterson DG, Ashley DL. Using biological monitoring to assess human exposure to priority toxicants. Environ Health Perspect 1995; 103(suppl 3):45–48.

27. Patterson DG Jr, Needham LL, Pirkle JL, et al. Correlation between serum and adipose levels of 2,3,7,8-TCDD in 50 persons from Missouri. Arch Environ Contam Toxicol 1988; 17:139–143.

28. Cline RE, Hill RH Jr, Phillips DL, Needham LL. Pentachlorophenol measurements in body fluids of people in log homes and workplaces. Arch Environ Contam Toxicol 1989; 18:475–481.

29. Ashley DL, Bonin MA, Cardinali FL, et al. Determining volatile organic compounds in human blood from a large sample population by using purge and trap gas chromatography/mass spectrometry. Anal Chem 1992; 64:1021–1029.

30. Brugnone F, Perbellini L, Faccini GB, Pasini F, Maranelli G, Romeo L. Breath and blood levels of benzene, toluene, cumene, and styrene in nonoccupational exposure. Int Arch Occup Environ Health 1989; 61:303–311.

31. Environmental Protection Agency (EPA). Protein adduct forming chemicals for exposure monitoring: chemicals selected for further study. EPA Report, EPA/600/4-89/035, Washington, DC, 1989.

32. Mooney LA, Santella RM, Covey L, et al. Decline of DNA damage and other biomarkers in peripheral blood following smoking cessation. Cancer Epidemiol Biomed Prev 1995; 4:627–634.

33. Shuker DEG, Farmer PB. Relevance of urinary DNA adducts as markers of carcinogen exposure. Chem Res Toxicol 1992; 5:450–460.

34. Poirier MC, Santella RM, Weston A. Carcinogen macromolecular adducts and their measurement. Carcinogenesis 2000; 21:353–359.

35a. Book of Analytical Procedures. Toxicology Branch, DLS, CDC: Volume II, Chapter 4.

35b. Book of Analytical Procedures. Toxicology Branch, DLS, CDC: Volume II, Chapter 3, 5, 6.

35c. Book of Analytical Procedures. Air Toxicant Branch, DLS, CDC: Volume I, Chapters 5, 6.

36. Baker SE, Barr DB, Driskell WJ, Beeson MD, Needham LL. Quantification of selected pesticide metabolites in human urine using isotope dilution high-performance liquid chromatography/tandem mass spectrometry. J Exp Anal Environ Epidemiol 2000; 10(6):789–798.

37. Hill RH Jr, Shealy DB, Head SL, et al. Determination of pesticide metabolites in human urine using isotope dilution technique and tandem mass spectrometry. J Anal Toxicol 1995; 19:323–329.

38. Beeson MD, Driskell WJ, Barr DB. Isotope dilution high performance liquid chromatography/tandem mass spectrometry method for quantifying urinary metabolites of atrazine, malathion, and 2,4-dichlorophenoxyacetic acid. Anal Chem 1999; 71:3526–3530.

39. Shealy DB, Bonin MA, Wooten JV, Ashley DL, Needham LL, Bond A. Application of an improved method for the analysis of pesticides and their metabolites

in the urine of farmer applicators and their families. Environ Int 1996; 22(6): 661–675.

40. Blount BC, Milgram KE, Silva M, et al. Quantitative detection of eight phthalate metabolites in human urine using HPLC-APCIMS/MS. Anal Chem 2000; 72:4127–4134.

41. Valentin-Blasini L, Blount BC, Rogers HS, Needham L. HPLC-MS/MS for the measurement of seven phytoestrogens in human serum and urine. J Exp Anal Environ Epidemiol 2000; 10(6):799–807.

42. Barr DB, Ashley DL. A rapid, sensitive method for the quantification of N-acetyl-S-(2-hydroxyethyl)-L-cysteine in human urine using isotope-dilution HPLC-MS/MS. J Anal Toxicol 1998; 22:96–104.

43. Bernert JT, Turner WE, Pirkle, JL, et al. Development and validation of a sensitive measurement of serum cotinine in both smokers and nonsmokers by liquid chromatography/atmospheric pressure ionization tandem mass spectrometry. Clin Chem 1997; 43:2281–2291.

44. Bernert JT, McGuffey JE, Morrison MA, Pirkle JL. Comparison of serum and salivary cotinine measurements by a sensitive high-performance liquid chromatography/tandem mass spectrometry method as an indicator of exposure to tobacco smoke among nonsmokers and nonsmokers. J Anal Toxicol 2000; 24:333–339.

45. DiPietro ES, Lapeza CR Jr, Cash TP, et al. A fast universal automated cleanup system for the isotope-dilution high-resolution mass spectrometric analysis of PCDDs, PCDFs, coplanar-PCBs, PCB congeners, and persistent pesticides from the serum sample. Organohalogen Comp 1997; 31:26–31.

46. Miller DT, Paschal DC, Gunter EW, Stroud PE, D'Angelo J. Determination of lead using electrothermal atomization atomic absorption spectrometry with a L'vov platform and matrix modifier. Analyst 1987; 112:1701–1704.

47. Stoeppler M, Brandt K. Determination of cadmium in whole blood and urine by electrothermal atomic-absorption spectrophotometry. Fresenius Z Anal Chem 1980; 300:372–380.

48. Greenwood MR, Shahir P, Clarkston TW, Farant JP, Chartrand A, Khayat A. Epidemiological experience with the Magos' reagents in the determination of different forms of mercury in biological samples by flameless atomic absorption. J Anal Toxicol 1977; 1:265–269.

49. Lewis SA, Hardison NW, Veillon C. Comparison of isotope dilution mass spectrometry and graphite furnace atomic absorption spectrometry with Zeeman background correction for determination of plasma selenium. Anal Chem 1986; 58:1272–1273.

50. Paschal DC, Kimberly MM, Bailey GG. Determination of urinary arsenic by electrothermal atomic absorption spectrometry with the L'vov platform and matrix modification. Anal Chem Acta 1986; 181:179–186.

51. Littlejohn D, Fell GS, Ottaway JM. Modified determination of total and inorganic mercury mercury in urine by cold vapor atomic absorption spectroscopy. Clin Chem 1976; 22:1719–1723.

52. Paschal DC, Bailey GG. Determination of nickel in urine with graphite furnace atomic absorption spectroscopy using Zeeman correction. Sci Total Environ 1989; 89:305–310.

53. Paschal DC, Bailey GG. Determination of chromium in urine with graphite furnace atomic absorption spectroscsopy using Zeeman correction. Atomic Spectroscopy 1991; 12:151–154.
54. Paschal DC, DiPietro ES, Phillips DL. Age dependence of metals in hair in a selected U.S. population. Environ Res 1998; 48:17–28.
55. Ting BG, Paschal DC, Caldwell KL. Determination of Thorium and Uranium in urine with inductively coupled argon plasma mass spectrometry. J Anal Atomic Spectr 1996; 11:339–342.
56. Fecher PA, Goldmann I, Nagengast A. Determination of iodine in food samples by inductively coupled plasma mass spectrometry after alkaline extraction. J Anal Atomic Spectr 1998; 13:977–982.
57. Needham LL, Pirkle JL, Burse VW, Patterson DG, Holler JS. Case studies of relationship between external dose and internal dose. J Exp Anal Environ Epidemiol 1992; 2(suppl 1):209—221.
58. Centers for Disease Control and Prevention (CDC). Second national report on human exposure to environmental chemicals. National Center for Environmental Health, NCEH pub. no. 03–0022, Atlanta, GA, 2003.
59. National Report on Human Exposure to Environmental Chemicals at www.cdc.gov/exposurereport/.

4

Biomarkers in Environmental Epidemiology

Christopher P. Wild

*Molecular Epidemiology Unit, Centre for Epidemiology and Biostatistics,
Leeds Institute of Genetics, Health and Therapeutics,
University of Leeds, Leeds, U.K.*

INTRODUCTION

The environment plays a key role in determining risk for the majority of chronic diseases worldwide. In the case of cancer, significant risk factors include tobacco, diet, infectious agents, chemicals, and radiation. Much of the data implicating environmental risk factors comes from epidemiological observations. Geographic variations in cancer incidence are striking, with some differences between regions reaching two orders of magnitude (1,2). Hepatocellular carcinoma in West Africa is so prevalent that it accounts for about 10% of all adult male deaths and incidence rates in men are in excess of 40 per 100,000 per annum. In contrast, in northern Europe rates are around one to two per 100,000 per year. A changing environment can bring with it marked alterations in cancer risk, with incidences differing up to 10-fold in the same location within a few decades. Examples include the increase in lung cancer in the United Kingdom following the widespread introduction of cigarette smoking or the increasing incidence of esophageal adenocarcinoma in the Western world for as yet unknown reasons. Finally, as people migrate to new environments they tend to exhibit the cancer incidence patterns of the indigenous population within one or two generations (1).

The evidence described previously persuasively points to the importance of the environment in influencing cancer risk. The differences are too marked and too temporally variable to be explained by genetic variation. At the same time, individual response to the environment will be altered by genetic background, as well as other variables such as age, sex, socioeconomic, nutritional, and immune status. These factors affect which individuals within the population are susceptible to the prevalent environmental exposures. The scale and importance of the interplay between genes and environment will vary from one malignancy to another, and the effects may also vary throughout the natural history of the disease.

The place of environmental and genetic factors in the etiopathogenesis of cancer parallels other common chronic diseases such as cardiovascular and neurological disorders and diabetes as well as responses to more acute incidences of toxicity. Although this chapter focuses on cancer, the principles are more broadly applicable to studies of environmental epidemiology.

DISEASE MECHANISMS

The last two decades have seen rapid advances in understanding the complex molecular mechanisms underlying carcinogenesis. The sequencing and mapping of the human genome provides a foundation for the elucidation of protein function. Future studies will provide further opportunities to identify the genes and biochemical pathways implicated in cancer development. Such knowledge may offer opportunities for more effective treatment and management of cancer patients. While there has been significant progress in treatment in specific cases, such as childhood leukemia, for many cancers there remains much to be achieved; in Europe, the majority of common cancers still have five-year survival rates below 50% (3).

In addition to therapy, advances in elucidating gene and protein function carry the potential to improve understanding of cancer etiology and subsequently to develop better disease prevention strategies. In this area, some past successes can also be pointed out. For example, in Western Europe at least, the lung cancer epidemic has started to rescind in men, as individuals and governments have sought to reduce cigarette smoking (4). High rates of hepatocellular carcinoma should also be reduced by vaccination against hepatitis B virus (HBV) (5). As with therapy, however, the progress is patchy and for a significant proportion of many common cancers, knowledge of the causative factors remains limited.

Can the undoubted advances of the last two decades in understanding molecular disease mechanisms be translated to future reductions in cancer morbidity and mortality? Is it possible to use this fundamental knowledge to improve understanding of etiology, and specifically the complex interactions of environmental and genetic risk factors? Central to this type of investigation is the need to reliably measure at an individual level the environmental exposure of interest, the relevant genetic heterogeneity, and the disease status. Additional advances in statistical analysis of large datasets are also of critical importance. Biomarkers promise improvements in each of the former three areas; this is the domain of molecular epidemiology.

THE PROMISES OF MOLECULAR CANCER EPIDEMIOLOGY— EXPOSURE, SUSCEPTIBILITY, AND DISEASE

Deciding upon the precise birth date of molecular cancer epidemiology is difficult. Among the earliest examples in this field are the measurement of chemical carcinogen–DNA adducts in human tissues (6,7) and the determination of metabolic phenotype with respect to aromatic amine metabolism (8). These early studies highlight two of the promises of molecular cancer epidemiology, namely, to improve exposure assessment and to identify susceptible individuals.

One outstanding and largely unmet challenge is that of accurately assessing environmental exposure. Determining genetic polymorphisms became technically trivial with the introduction of the polymerase chain reaction (PCR). There remain limitations in interpreting genetic data, as discussed later, but analytically the methodology is largely reliable and simple to perform. The advent of genotyping therefore gave more precision to the measurement of genetic susceptibility compared to recording family history of cancer occurrence. This technical advance led to a shift in emphasis within the molecular cancer epidemiology field away from efforts to develop accurate biomarkers of environmental exposures towards the conduct of gene–disease association studies. This type of study, often involving a single polymorphism in a single gene, has formed a significant part of the molecular cancer epidemiology literature over the last decade. Although difficult to quantify, this has undoubtedly drawn resources away from the more technically challenging area of developing exposure biomarkers. However, the absence of an accurate definition of exposure is clearly a major handicap in understanding the impact of the majority of genetic polymorphisms on diseases of complex etiology. There is a desperate need for the same type of precision with regard to the environmental exposure as we have with regard to the individual's genome. We need tools that will permit definition of an individual's exposure history; we need an "exposome" to match the "genome."

Precision in measurement of environmental exposure is critical for putative risk factors where the associated disease risk is modest. Where the risk associated with an exposure is high, e.g., cigarette smoke and lung cancer, or where the cancer involved is rare, e.g., malignant mesothelioma and asbestos, a degree of imprecision in exposure assessment does not necessarily preclude the assignment of increased risk. However, where the exposures are associated with more modest increases in risk, errors in measurement may blur or completely obscure any underlying causal associations through misclassification of exposure status. It was in response to this need for improved exposure assessment, especially at low levels and/or where questionnaire approaches do not have the necessary resolution, that biochemical or molecular exposure markers were developed. Examples covered here include chemical metabolites as well as DNA or protein adducts in various body fluids.

The combination of measures of environmental exposure and genetic variation may reveal environment–disease associations in subgroups within the population that would be otherwise obscured by interindividual variation. In analogous fashion, the effect of a particular genotype–disease association can be examined in the presence or absence of exposure. These studies then permit the more formal statistical analysis of gene–environment interactions.

In parallel to the development of biomarkers to address exposure and genetic susceptibility, the tumor itself has become a potential source of etiologic information consequent to advances in molecular cancer biology. This follows the recognition that a histologically uniform set of tumors might be divided into subsets on the basis of their molecular alterations in key genes. Different underlying changes might identify tumors with different etiologies (9). Other categories of biomarker may occur in advance of clinical symptoms and so bring forward the diagnosis of the disease. Still others may provide information as to the most effective therapy for an individual tumor, in effect identifying the genetic susceptibility of the tumor to specific therapeutic agents.

Molecular cancer epidemiology therefore promised not only to better classify exposure and susceptibility, but also to better classify disease, and the field was launched on the basis of this trinity of biomarker categories. It is relevant, therefore, to ask how far these promises have been fulfilled and where future progress is likely to occur in the area of environmental epidemiology.

EXPOSURE ASSESSMENT

Major challenges to cancer epidemiology in the 21st century include the low levels and ubiquitous nature of many environmental exposures, the modest associated increases in risk, and the fact that many exposures occur as complex mixtures. All of these mean that the questionnaire approach may be insufficiently sensitive or precise. Biomarkers may address some of these limitations, but there are a number of key questions to be considered in regard to their application. Among these are what to measure, where to measure it, and when to measure it. These are considered in turn below.

WHAT TO MEASURE

Biologically Effective Dose and Internal Dose Markers

In the 1980s, significant advances were made in technologies to measure exposure to environmental chemicals (10). The formation of carcinogen–DNA and protein adducts, reflecting covalent binding of the chemical carcinogen to a cellular macromolecule, was established in human beings for a range of exposures by chromatography, mass spectrometry, immunoassays, or ^{32}P-postlabeling. These studies established for the first time that environmental levels of chemical carcinogen exposures were absorbed, distributed, and metabolized in similar ways to animals treated experimentally at much higher doses.

Initial pilot studies were able to demonstrate the presence of adducts in human biological samples and associate these with self-reported exposure measures. An example was the dose–response seen between polycyclic aromatic hydrocarbon (PAH)–DNA adducts, measured by ^{32}P-postlabeling, in human lung tissue and cigarette smoking (11). Such studies established the adequate sensitivity of the analytical methods and began the process of validating the biomarkers as reliable measures of exposure.

Throughout the 1980s and early 1990s, progress in the area of exposure biomarkers was made. A considerable number of different carcinogen DNA and protein adducts were measured including nitrosamines, PAH, aromatic amines, heterocyclic amines (HA), mycotoxins, etc. (10) Based on the mechanistic role of DNA adducts in chemical carcinogenesis, these adducts were referred to as biomarkers of biologically effective dose, i.e., a measure of the amount of the carcinogen reaching the critical cellular target. Protein adducts were, by virtue of sharing bioactivation pathways with DNA adducts, also classified as measures of biologically effective dose. However, it is important to bear in mind that DNA or protein adducts reflect not only exogenous exposure, but other processes such as absorption, distribution, metabolism, and DNA repair. As a result, the measured adduct level will be a composite of exposure and these other variables that will differ between individuals.

Both DNA and protein adducts have been successfully applied for different chemicals and in different study designs such that neither can be said to be inherently better than the other. A pragmatic approach to selection of biomarkers is needed in light of the chemical and its binding properties, the stability of adducts both in vivo and during analysis, and the availability of appropriate technology for sensitive and specific measurement. Sample availability has often been more of a limitation with DNA than with protein when blood samples are being used.

In addition to DNA and protein adducts, the parent chemicals or their metabolites have been used to measure exposure. An example is the use of 1-hydroxypyrene-glucuronide as a measure of PAH exposure from charbroiled beef (12). Similarly, the presence of HA metabolites in urine has been correlated to the level of these carcinogens in cooked meat (13). In this case, the chemicals are not bound to a critical target in the cell and hence are not markers of biologically effective dose but rather are termed markers of internal dose.

Despite the analytical advances that have permitted measurement of DNA and protein adducts as well as chemicals and their metabolites in human samples over the last 20 years, the number of chemicals for which reliable data are available to demonstrate that the biomarker reflects "true" intake is few. Correlations were established between dietary intakes of aflatoxins and the levels of urinary aflatoxin metabolites and DNA adducts (14) or aflatoxin–albumin adducts in blood (15) by conducting careful comparisons of plate food levels of the carcinogen, amounts eaten by each individual, and biomarker. Similar studies have been conducted with HA and polycyclic aromatic amines as mentioned above (12,13) where urinary metabolites were measured in relation to precise intakes in controlled feeding studies. In many instances, exposure markers are unfortunately applied to human studies without evidence in humans that the markers are a true reflection of exposure.

The above type of validation study is essential because there are instances where measurement of a carcinogen in body fluids does not reflect intake. For example, urinary aflatoxin P1, a metabolite of the dietary carcinogen aflatoxin B1, is not a good indicator of exposure (16), probably because the clearance is not only via the urine but the feces, and the balance between excretion pathways may differ between individuals. Similarly, ochratoxin A in plasma was shown not to be a good indicator of exposure to this dietary mycotoxin at the individual level, while urine levels did reflect exposure in a duplicate diet study (17). As discussed earlier, a perfect linear response between exposure and biomarker will not be expected because of the complexities of metabolism. The deviation from a simple linear association will reflect both measurement error and this source of interindividual variation in metabolism and excretion pathways.

Biomarker Specificity

A further consideration in selecting a biomarker as a measure of exposure is that of specificity. DNA and protein adducts involve measuring a specific bound chemical and by definition this measure will be specific for the target chemical. However, while some chemicals will equate to the exposure of interest, some may not. For example, urinary aflatoxin–DNA adducts are a specific measure for dietary exposure to aflatoxins. However, with benzo[a] pyrene (B[a]P)–DNA adducts, the B[a]P may originate from tobacco smoke, diet, urban air pollution, or certain occupational exposures. While the marker is chemical-specific, giving an accurate reflection of B[a]P exposure, it is not environmental exposure–specific. It is often the environmental exposure, e.g., urban air pollution, that is the focus of the epidemiological study, not one specific chemical from multiple sources. This point is well made in a study of PAH–DNA adducts in peripheral blood lymphocytes in firefighters (18). While there was no association between adducts and occupational smoke exposure (the main hypothesis of the study), there was a significant correlation with the number of barbecued meals the individuals had consumed. Here the dietary source of PAH was more significant than smoke.

Other categories of assay are less chemical–specific than adducts or metabolites and provide a more general measure of DNA damage. Among the most commonly used assays are "bulky" aromatic DNA adducts by ^{32}P-postlabeling, DNA strand breaks in the single cell gel electrophoresis ("comet") assay, and various measures of chromosomal damage (e.g., micronuclei, chromosomal aberrations, sister chromatid exchanges). These assays measure a composite of DNA damage that may reflect a category of genotoxic agent. In studies of patients with the precancerous condition of Barrett's esophagus, strand breaks in DNA from esophageal biopsies as measured in the comet assay were increased in those patients who were smokers (19). For such complex mixtures, these assays may provide an index of global genotoxic insult and the relative lack of chemical specificity can be used to advantage. However, ultimately the absence of chemical and structural identification of the source of the damage limits interpretation. In addition, there are analytical difficulties in, for example, assessing variations in recovery because there are no appropriate internal standards. Ultimately more chemical-specific assays are required for a full understanding of the important components of a given exposure.

WHERE TO MEASURE

Biomarkers of exposure have been measured in a number of different biological media, including urine, feces, saliva, plasma, serum, exfoliated cells, white blood cells, biopsies, and other tissue samples. Each of these sources of material may give different qualitative and quantitative information. It is important to bear in mind the information being sought when different biological materials are used for biomarker analysis.

A DNA adduct is believed to be on the pathway from exposure to cancer, hence the interest in measuring these events as biomarkers of exposure and disease risk. The critical DNA lesion, however, is defined at the tissue, cell, gene, and even DNA sequence level. Other exposure biomarkers such as protein adducts or internal dose markers have the additional caveat of not being on the disease pathway. These layers of complexity need to be considered when interpreting the information gained from biomarker measurements.

Many carcinogens in animals induce different levels of DNA adducts in different tissues. The level of adduct in a given organ is one determinant of the susceptibility of that tissue to carcinogenesis. In practice, of course, DNA or protein adducts can rarely be measured in the target organ in epidemiological studies. Consequently, measurements are made in more easily available material, typically plasma or serum, white blood cells, or urine.

Often the relationship of the adduct level in peripheral blood cells and internal organs is unknown, even in experimental studies. One study examined a series of four carcinogenic methylating agents, each with a differing primary target organ, namely the colon, esophagus, liver, and lung. DNA adducts were measured in the target organ, the liver, and the peripheral white blood cells. While adducts in the latter cells showed a relatively consistent relationship with adducts in the liver with all four agents, the relationship with the target organ varied markedly (20). Thus, measuring lymphocyte DNA adducts as a biomarker would not necessarily have revealed the critical level of exposure in the target organ for each of these carcinogens. The correlation between biomarkers in body fluids and internal organs has rarely been addressed in human studies, although opportunities do exist, e.g., in cases of bronchoalveolar lavage, colonoscopy, or upper gastrointestinal endoscopy.

If a biomarker, e.g., aflatoxin–albumin adducts in peripheral blood, has been validated in relation to external exposure, then the lack of knowledge concerning the relationship with the levels of chemical binding in cellular targets in internal organs does not invalidate that biomarker in terms of exposure assessment. However, the limited understanding of that relationship should be borne in mind in the interpretation of the data, particularly in relation to extrapolation to disease risk. Experimental models could provide valuable information in further understanding these relationships. Additionally, taking opportunities to make comparisons in humans between target organs and biological material from other sites is important and there are some valuable examples in the literature (21,22).

WHEN TO MEASURE

Environmental exposures will most often vary during an individual's life-course due to changes in lifestyle, place of residence, etc., and the exposure may have a greater or lesser impact on disease risk at different times of life. Exposures in childhood may be particularly relevant to disease many decades later (23,24). Yu et al. (25) suggested that risk of nasopharyngeal carcinoma was particularly linked to salted fish intake in the weaning period and early childhood rather than exposure in adult life. Age at HBV infection is a critical determinant of risk of becoming a chronic HBV carrier and therefore of developing hepatocellular carcinoma (26). The temporal variation in exposure and the varying significance of that exposure poses particular challenges to biomarkers that are by their biological nature transient.

The question of when to measure a biomarker of exposure in relation to the natural history of the disease is clearly a critical one. This requires some notion of when the critical exposure period occurred, the temporal variation of exposure, and the inherent stability of the biomarker being measured. With viruses, serum antibodies to viral antigens often persist and indicate past exposure. For chemical exposures, the ability to measure long-term past exposure is difficult to achieve. There are exceptions, for example, certain pesticide residues in plasma and adipose tissue (27). Nevertheless, in the majority of instances the biomarker will be of relatively short half-life and provide information only from a few days to a few months prior to sampling. One counterpoint is that in certain circumstances a biomarker responding rapidly to changes in exposure is advantageous. Examples include monitoring the impact of intervention strategies, e.g., antismoking programs (28) or chemoprevention (29) or in ascribing exposure to specific occupations during a working shift (30).

One attempt to reconstruct past exposures has been to seek longer-lived adducts by examining binding of chemicals to proteins that persist through cell division, such as histones (31). Alternatively, the analysis of mutation spectra in tumor DNA may be informative (9). In the case of aflatoxin, a G to T transversion in the third nucleotide of codon 249 in the *TP53* tumor suppressor gene has been geographically correlated with dietary exposure (32). More recently, the same mutation has been detected in plasma DNA from individuals in high aflatoxin exposure regions including West Africa (33) and China (34). It remains to be seen whether the mutation is an indication of early hepatocellular carcinoma or a marker of high aflatoxin exposure. Development of a highly sensitive mutation assay applied to nontumor material in ulcerative colitis cases showed a high frequency of G to A transitions in an area of inflamed tissue compared to noninflamed; this type of mutation is consistent with free radical-induced DNA damage (35). Quantitative mutation assays of this type applicable to human biopsies may permit longer-term exposure assessments to be made.

The issue of past exposure is most pressing in conditions such as cancer or cardiovascular disease where disease development spans many years or decades. In instances where the disease is related more closely in time to the exposure, such as in cases of acute toxicity, this limitation is far less evident. However, for cancer, the inherent short-term nature of most biomarkers means that careful consideration is needed in relation to study design.

EXPOSURE BIOMARKERS AND APPROPRIATE STUDY DESIGN

The most common epidemiological design to assess cancer etiology has been the case–control study. Genotype analyses are well suited to this design, as disease will not influence this parameter. However, as we have seen, current exposure may not reflect what has occurred in the past. In addition, the presence of disease could potentially influence the measure of exposure, including any biomarkers. This may be because the patients change their lifestyle postdiagnosis or because the presence of disease alters their physiology such that the biomarker is affected. This would result in a biased picture of the difference between cases and controls due to reverse causation. In a study of hepatocellular carcinoma, for example, two measures of aflatoxin exposure were used, aflatoxin levels in household foods and serum aflatoxin–albumin levels (36). While there was a positive correlation between the two measures in controls, this was not so in cases, possibly reflecting a reduced food intake, altered hepatic metabolism (the site of albumin biosynthesis), or both, in people with late-stage liver cancer.

Despite the above limitations, DNA adducts have been applied in case–control studies with positive findings. Bulky DNA adducts resulting from exposure to aromatic hydrocarbons were higher in white blood cells of bladder cancer cases compared to controls (37). Skipper et al. (38) took a more chemical-specific approach by measuring 3- and 4-aminobiphenyl hemoglobin adducts in bladder cancer cases and controls. Higher adduct levels were associated with increased cancer risk among smokers and non-smokers, with evidence of a dose–response.

An alternative to case–control studies is to establish prospective cohorts. A nested case–control study within the cohort limits the resources needed for the analysis. As all individuals are healthy at entry to the study when biological samples are collected, the problems of reverse causation are avoided and the design provides a measure of exposure prior to disease onset. In practice, the periods of follow-up still tend to encompass a relatively short fraction of the carcinogenic process (a few years rather than decades) and often involve only a single time-point (most often recruitment) for biological sampling. Nevertheless this design is more adapted to the type of exposure biomarker currently available. It is within this design that the most successful examples of biomarkers and disease outcome have been in evidence.

DNA and protein adducts as well as urinary metabolites have provided key evidence in establishing an exposure–disease association between aflatoxins and hepatocellular carcinoma (32,39). As aflatoxins are heterogeneously distributed in foods, representative sampling and exposure estimation based on food analysis is inaccurate. Diets in many high exposure countries are relatively uniform and therefore dietary questionnaires using frequently contaminated foods as a surrogate for exposure are uninformative. Consequently, efforts were put into validating urinary and blood-based biomarkers of aflatoxin exposure. In a nested case–control study of hepatocellular carcinoma in China (16), a significant increase in relative risk was associated with the presence of urinary aflatoxins in samples collected at the time of recruitment. At the same time, there was no positive association between a dietary assessment of foods likely to be contaminated with aflatoxins and risk. A study of similar design in Taiwan (40) using biomarkers of urinary aflatoxin and aflatoxin–albumin adducts gave similar results, with both studies showing interactions between aflatoxins and HBV.

In a nested case–control study of lung cancer, aromatic DNA adducts were higher in cases than controls when only smokers were included in the analysis (41). Current smokers at the time of recruitment who had elevated adducts in white blood cells were approximately three times more likely to be diagnosed with lung cancer cases in the follow-up than were smokers with lower adduct levels. Further support for the value of biomarkers of DNA damage in prospective studies comes from chromosomal aberrations (42) which were elevated at recruitment in individuals who later developed cancer. In this case, there was no specific exposure under investigation and the risk was seen when all cancers were considered together. Nevertheless this study again illustrates the power of incorporating exposure biomarkers in the prospective cohort design.

TESTS AND QUESTIONS

Not every study needs a biomarker to assign an exposure to a cancer risk. The high penetrance of some environmental risk factors and the reliability of self-reported exposures mean that laboratory measures are not needed. For example, evidence identifying tobacco smoke as the most important cause of the rising incidence of lung cancer was obtained as early as the 1930s, without sophisticated exposure assessment (43,44). In respect to the remaining causes of cancer, epidemiologists need to deal with environmental exposures presenting the twin problems of low levels and low penetrance. These are difficult to investigate without precise measures.

A typical example is provided by the HA, a group of chemical mutagens and carcinogens formed during cooking of meat and fish. Some studies have shown an increased risk of colorectal cancer with degree of doneness of the meat (45). The level of HA is dependent on the type of meat used and the temperature and duration of cooking. Attempts have been made to estimate HA exposure by asking questions about meat consumption, cooking habits, "doneness" of meat, as well as using information in databases on HA levels after cooking. Despite these efforts, there are difficulties in obtaining accurate self-reported data on these parameters. The HA are therefore a prime example where a biomarker could improve exposure assessment, and several are being considered, including urinary measures of metabolites (13,46).

While biomarkers may improve exposure assessment in the case of low-level exposures, there are situations where the absence of biomarkers of past exposure may mean that a questionnaire approach is more appropriate than a biomarker. For example, in the case of nasopharyngeal cancer and salted fish intake mentioned earlier, a biomarker of current salted fish intake in a case–control study, or even a cohort study begun in adult life would not have been as revealing as the questions posed to the mothers of cases and controls about their children's exposure early in life (25).

From the above discussion, it is clear that both biomarkers and questionnaire approaches have their place in exposure assessment. In some cases the test is better than the question, in others the question is better than the test. In the majority of cases, a combination of both approaches will be valuable in ensuring accurate classification of exposure.

GENETIC SUSCEPTIBILITY

Some genetic polymorphisms with a high penetrance result in the at-risk allele conferring a risk that approaches 100% (e.g., BRCA1 and breast cancer). The availability of the human genome sequence will no doubt permit identification of more genes of high penetrance. However, these genes associated with recognized genetic syndromes and familial aggregation are the exception (2).

The more widespread promise of the genome project in understanding cancer etiology comes from the potential to identify large numbers of low-penetrance genes and to elucidate their interaction with other genes and environmental risk factors. It is this that is the driving force behind establishing large population-based sample collections such as the U.K. Biobank (47). Categories of these genes include those coding for carcinogen metabolizing and DNA repair enzymes, as well as cytokines, enzymes involved in sex hormone metabolism, and those playing a role in cell-cycle regulation. Despite low penetrance, the high prevalence of genetic polymorphism in these genes means that some can have significant population effects, even when increases in relative risk are modest (48).

A majority of work on low-penetrance alleles in cancer epidemiology has focused on the carcinogen metabolizing genes, both those implicated in carcinogen activation and detoxification. An example relates to the HA, which are metabolized by N-acetylation and N-oxidation (49) involving the N-acetyltransferases and cytochrome P450 (CYP)1A2, respectively. Studies combining analysis of individual variation in these metabolizing enzymes with estimates of red meat intake, including measures of the "doneness" of meat, have revealed associations consistent with the hypothesis that rapid acetylators and rapid CYP1A2 individuals would be at highest risk of colorectal cancer following red meat consumption (49).

The introduction to this chapter draws attention to the advances in measuring individual genetic susceptibility due to the facile application of PCR technology in many laboratories. This has led to a much better classification of inherited susceptibility than could be achieved by recording family history. Nevertheless, the explosion in gene-association studies has led to rather equivocal conclusions with respect to many low-penetrance genetic polymorphisms (50). Meta-analyses for low-penetrance alleles have typically shown weak effects, if any, on cancer risk (51). The availability of high throughput genotyping techniques to simultaneously examine thousands of single nucleotide polymorphisms (SNPs) and haplotypes will bring further opportunities to broaden the areas of the genome examined in relation to disease status. However, these studies will bring with them additional challenges including the major risk of false-positive associations.

Candidate Genes and Genome-wide Screening

Studies of genes and common diseases have in the past mainly followed a candidate gene approach. An a priori knowledge about the gene leads to a hypothesis regarding disease risk. In some cases there are additional data on the functional effect of the polymorphism. This deductive approach has the advantage of providing information on biologically plausible associations. However, by definition it relies on pre-existing information about known genes. In contrast, the rapidly expanding list of SNPs offers the possibility to use genome-wide screening to indicate novel gene–disease associations. This is an inductive approach where the hypothesis is generated from the data obtained in the screening experiment.

Estimates suggest some 10 million SNPs exist within the human genome (52). Of these, only perhaps 1% are within the coding region and over 60% are within intronic regions. With this number of variants, there is significant scope for false-positive associations. This will be of increasing concern as the technologies become cheaper and statistical analysis struggles to catch up with the laboratory data generation. A number of points, therefore, need to be considered as this area of molecular epidemiology evolves.

First, it is important that associations between genes and disease are demonstrated to be reproducible across studies. Reproducibility is a cornerstone of observational studies (53). This will require funding agencies and scientific journals to give priority to well-conducted studies that seek to replicate earlier findings. Boffetta (54) has highlighted the potential for publication bias with regard to negative studies.

Second, the biological basis for an association needs to be considered, either a priori in the case of candidate genes or in follow-up studies in the case of genome screening. Examining the effects of polymorphisms on gene expression or on protein stability and function will become increasingly important. In addition, consideration of combinations of genes and their polymorphisms within relevant biological pathways is needed in order to establish at-risk phenotypes.

Third, laboratory rigor will need to further develop as larger studies with multiple genes become common. This calls for quality control measures to avoid DNA contamination or degradation, errors in labeling or in the genotyping itself. In parallel, appropriate statistical approaches to examine complex interactions between genes and environmental factors are required.

An additional consideration in gene–disease association studies for common disorders is that often the gene may influence disease only in the presence of a given exposure. For example, a deletion in the *GSTM1* detoxification gene is associated with lung cancer but predominantly in smokers rather than nonsmokers, suggesting that the effect of the gene is restricted to smokers (55). Future studies, therefore, need to combine measures of exposure and genetic status in order to derive full benefit from advances in understanding the human genome.

BIOLOGICAL PLAUSIBILITY

One of the Bradford Hill criteria for establishing a causal association between an exposure and disease is biological plausibility. This is one area, possibly undervalued, where biomarkers can contribute to cancer epidemiology.

If experimental studies have revealed something of the enzymes involved in the metabolism of the environmental chemical under investigation, then polymorphisms that affect the function of the relevant genes would be predicted to associate with the disease that is itself linked to exposure. If the association is in the hypothesized direction, this can provide support for the importance of the putative risk factor. For example, acute myeloid leukemia (AML) can occur as a result of cancer treatment. GSTP1 is involved in detoxification of some of the chemotherapeutic agents implicated in the risk of therapy-related AML. Polymorphisms in this gene were associated with altered risk in patients treated for their initial tumor with chemotherapy, but not radiotherapy, consistent with a role for these agents in cancer risk (56).

Biomarkers may help unravel some of the steps between exposure and disease. For example, if a particular genetic polymorphism in a DNA repair enzyme is thought to be associated with increased risk, then it may also be predicted to be associated with higher DNA adducts, an intermediate endpoint on the exposure-disease pathway. In a study of healthy individuals, "bulky" DNA adducts in lymphocytes, analyzed by the ^{32}P-postlabeling assay, were compared with polymorphisms in three different DNA repair enzymes (57). These authors found a dose–response relationship between the adduct level and the number of at-risk alleles. Similar correlations between CYP3A5 polymorphisms and aflatoxin–albumin adducts have been made (58). These studies strengthen the rationale for examining the relationship between polymorphisms and cancer risk precisely because they provide evidence that the former affect a significant step on the mechanistic pathway to cancer.

The availability of biomarkers makes the task of integrating human and experimental data easier when assessing the risks associated with environmental exposures. Aflatoxin serves as an example of how links can be made from experimental studies to human beings and how this body of evidence can contribute to assigning a compound as a human carcinogen (39).

The bioactivation, DNA adduct formation, and mutation induction with aflatoxin are known for a range of animal species. This knowledge formed a basis for developing the biomarkers of exposure mentioned earlier and in designing intervention studies (32). Equally, biomarkers have been key in exploring the synergy between HBV and aflatoxin observed in epidemiological studies. Evidence for a possible mechanism of interaction involving altered carcinogen metabolism in the presence of HBV infection has been provided by studies in exposed populations (59,60) and experimental studies in HBV transgenic mice (61).

BIOMARKER-BASED CLASSIFICATION OF DISEASE

Improved classification of individuals with respect to environmental and genetic exposures will improve the power of epidemiological studies to detect exposure–disease associations and interactions between risk factors. However, the heterogeneity of molecular alterations occurring in a given tumor type with similar clinical features is also recognized. Thus molecular characterization of tumors may permit more effective therapy based on the genetic susceptibility of the tumor. At the same time in epidemiological studies, cancer patients may be stratified on a molecular basis to permit examination of etiologic risk factors within these subgroups. This is consistent with observations from experimental studies that different chemical carcinogens induce different types of genetic change in the resultant tumors (9). In addition to the aflatoxin TP53 example, studies of the *TP53* tumor suppressor gene have also revealed characteristic mutation spectra in regard to UV light and skin cancer (C:C to T:T tandem mutation) and smoking and lung cancer among others (62).

In a case–control study of acute leukemia in adults, cytogenetic reports were collected for case subjects (63). Using these data, the individual cases were assigned to different groups. These case groups were shown to have distinct age profiles, potentially leading to epidemiologically useful distributions of heterogeneous disease. However, although initially promising, these groupings have not proven useful in relation to other risk factors (63). Newer technologies of microarrays for cDNA expression may also lead to possibilities for subdividing cases into meaningful groups (64).

Understanding the key genetic alterations occurring at early stages of the carcinogenic process can yield biomarkers that have the potential to refine surveillance approaches among high-risk groups. An example is Barrett's esophagus, a precancerous condition associated with an order of magnitude or more increased risk of adenocarcinoma (65). Despite this increased risk, the effectiveness of endoscopic surveillance has been questioned because of the high prevalence of Barrett's esophagus in the population and the relative rarity of cancer detection in absolute terms. In a prospective cohort study of Barrett's patients, those with overexpression of cyclin D1 at recruitment had a six- to sevenfold increased risk of progression to malignancy (66). The newer screening techniques in genomics, proteomics, and metabolomics may yield a new generation of candidate markers for application in this context and provide appropriate combinations of molecular markers to improve the sensitivity and specificity of this approach (see below).

WHITHER MOLECULAR EPIDEMIOLOGY?

A major promise of molecular cancer epidemiology is to unravel environmental and genetic cancer risk factors and their interactions. This is particularly relevant to the identification of thousands of SNPs and the large prospective cohort studies such as U.K. Biobank. In order to derive full benefit from high cost studies such as these, the advances in genetic research must be paralleled by developments in the assessment of environmental exposures. Only in this way will the large investments in collecting biological samples at recruitment be justified.

Genetic screening at the population level for low-penetrance alleles or those requiring a substantial environmental interaction is extremely unlikely to provide positive public health benefits (48). A more effective approach would be to reduce the level of exposure to the environmental risk factor(s), if these are identified. The ability to identify environmental risk factors through stratification of cases by genetic background will therefore be valuable. This may permit improved assignment of etiology, inform the setting of acceptable exposure levels based on knowledge of susceptible subgroups, and consequently provide a better rationale for minimizing exposure to harmful levels of environmental factors. In addition, assessing the effect of a genetic polymorphism implicated on a putative causal pathway can contribute to the establishment of the relevance of that pathway and hence add to the biological plausibility of an exposure–disease association.

The requirement to improve exposure assessment is just one area where effort and investment are required to take advantage of the benefits of genetic advances. Others are in statistical methodology and in bioinformatics, to meet the challenges of interpreting the vast amount of data generated by testing multiple genes and measuring multiple environmental exposures. This will need major methodological developments to produce a meaningful interpretation of data generated in epidemiological studies.

The screening of thousands of SNPs simultaneously on microarray chips will become increasingly common. Initially the cost may limit some applications to pooled DNA from cases and controls in order to identify candidate genes that could then be looked at in more detail on an individual basis. Haplotypes will also be constructed by examining SNPs in groups of genes on common pathways, e.g., carcinogen metabolism or signaling pathways within the cell.

Understanding the molecular characteristics of tumors promises to advance rapidly with the application of both genomic and proteomic technologies. Similarly, alterations in gene or protein expression between tumor cells or precancerous cells and normal cells may lead to identification of candidate genes involved in the carcinogenic pathway; some of these alterations may be translated to biomarkers of early cancer diagnosis. If validated in terms of their relationship to cancer, these would also be useful surrogate endpoints in prospective or intervention studies. Mass spectrometry is being used to yield patterns of serum proteins that segregate with disease state (67). Recent advances in the analysis of metabolite profiles in biofluids, termed metabolomics or metabonomics, offers a similar promise of identifying biomarkers that distinguish between healthy and diseased individuals (68).

Ultimately, multidisciplinary research using the new technologies in population-based studies requires the skills of laboratory scientists, epidemiologists, biostatisticians, and experts in bioinformatics. Potter (53) has pointed out succinctly that comparisons of gene or protein expression in human samples, perhaps between tumor and normal tissue from the same person or between sera from cancer cases and controls, are observational and not experimental studies. As such, the studies need to draw on the tools of epidemiology. The warning to account for confounding and bias and to seek reproducibility is one that needs heeding if progress in this area is not to be hampered by spurious findings. Similarly, appropriate statistical methodologies and criteria of reproducibility are needed to deliver confidence in the observations being made. This need to merge approaches is a continuation of the process begun with the introduction of biomarkers of exposure and susceptibility to cancer epidemiology some 20 years ago. It is one that constantly needs to be acknowledged if public health benefits are to flow from the exciting technological advances on offer.

ACKNOWLEDGMENTS

CPW was supported by a grant from the NIEHS USA No. ES06052.

REFERENCES

1. IARC. In: Stewart B, Kleihues P, eds. World Cancer Report. Lyon: IARC Press, 2003.
2. Peto J. Cancer epidemiology in the last century and the next decade. Nature 2001; 411:390–395.
3. Berrino F, Esteve J, Coleman MP. Basic Issues in Estimating and Comparing the Survival of Cancer Patients. Lyon: IARC Scientific Publications No 132, 1995:1–14.
4. Tyczynski JE, Bray F, Parkin DM. Lung cancer in Europe in 2000: epidemiology, prevention, and early detection. Lancet Oncol 2003; 4(1):45–55.

5. Hall AJ, Wild CP. Liver cancer in low and middle income countries—Prevention should target vaccination, contaminated needles, and aflatoxins. Br Med J 2003; 326:994–995.
6. Perera FP, Poirier MC, Yuspa SH, et al. A pilot project in molecular cancer-epidemiology—determination of benzo[A]pyrene DNA adducts in animal and human-tissues by immunoassays. Carcinogenesis 1982; 3(12):1405–1410.
7. Umbenhauer D, Wild CP, Montesano R, et al. O-6-Methyldeoxyguanosine in esophageal DNA among individuals at high-risk of esophageal cancer. Int J Cancer 1985; 36(6):661–665.
8. Cartwright RA, Rogers HJ, Barhamhall D, et al. Role of N-acetyltransferase phenotypes in bladder carcinogenesis—A pharmacogenetic epidemiological approach to bladder-cancer. Lancet 1982; 2:842–846.
9. Greenblatt MS, Bennett WP, Hollstein M, Harris CC. Mutations in the p53 tumor suppressor gene: clues to cancer etiology and molecular pathogenesis. Cancer Res 1994; 54:4855–4878.
10. Poirier MC. Chemical-induced DNA damage and human cancer risk. Nat Rev Cancer 2004; 4(8):630–637.
11. Phillips DH, Hewer A, Martin CN, Garner RC, King MM. Correlation of DNA adduct levels in human lung with cigarette smoking. Nature 1988; 336:790–792.
12. Kang DH, Rothman N, Poirier MC, et al. Interindividual differences in the concentration of 1-hydroxypyrene-glucuronide in urine and polycyclic aromatic hydrocarbon–DNA adducts in peripheral white blood-cells after charbroiled beef consumption. Carcinogenesis 1995; 16(5):1079–1085.
13. Strickland PT, Qian Z, Friesen MD, Rothman N, Sinha R. Metabolites of 2-amino-1-methyl-6-phenylimidazo(4,5-b)pyridine (PhIP) in human urine after consumption of charbroiled or fried beef. Mutat Res Fund Molec Mech Mutager 2002; 506:163–173.
14. Groopman JD, Hall AJ, Whittle H, et al. Molecular dosimetry of aflatoxin-N7-guanine in human urine obtained in the Gambia, West Africa. Cancer Epidemiol Bio Prev 1992; 1(3):221–227.
15. Wild CP, Hudson GJ, Sabbioni G, et al. Dietary intake of aflatoxins and the level of albumin-bound aflatoxin in peripheral blood in The Gambia, West Africa. Cancer Epidemiol Bio Prev 1992; 1:229–234.
16. Qian GS, Ross RK, Yu MC, et al. A follow-up study of urinary markers of aflatoxin exposure and liver cancer risk in Shanghai, People's Republic of China. Cancer Epidemiol Bio Prev 1994; 3:3–10.
17. Gilbert J, Brereton P, MacDonald S. Assessment of dietary exposure to ochratoxin A in the UK using a duplicate diet approach and analysis of urine and plasma samples. Food Addit Contam 2001; 18(12):1088–1093.
18. Rothman N, Correavillasenor A, Ford DP, et al. Contribution of occupation and diet to white blood-cell polycyclic aromatic hydrocarbon–DNA adducts in wildland firefighters. Cancer Epidemiol Biol Prev 1993; 2(4):341–347.
19. Olliver JR, Hardie LJ, Gong YY, et al. Risk factors, DNA damage and disease progression in Barrett's esophagus. Cancer Epidemiol Bio Prev. 2005; 14(3):620–625.
20. Bianchini F, Wild CP. Comparison of 7-Medg formation in white blood-cells, liver and target organs in rats treated with methylating carcinogens. Carcinogenesis 1994; 15(6):1137–1141.

21. Godschalk RWL, Maas LM, Van Zandwijk N, et al. Differences in aromatic–DNA adduct levels between alveolar macrophages and subpopulations of white blood cells from smokers. Carcinogenesis 1998; 19(5):819–825.
22. Nia AB, Maas LM, Brouwer EMC, Kleinjans JCS, Van Schooten FJ. Comparison between smoking-related DNA adduct analysis in induced sputum and peripheral blood lymphocytes. Carcinogenesis 2000; 21(7):1335–1340.
23. Anderson LM, Diwan BA, Fear NT, Roman E. Critical windows of exposure for children's health: cancer in human epidemiological studies and neoplasms in experimental animal models. Environ Health Perspect 2000; 108:573–594.
24. Wild CP, Kleinjans J. Children and increased susceptibility to environmental carcinogens: evidence or empathy?. Cancer Epidemiol Bio Prev 2003; 12(12): 1389–1394.
25. Yu MC, Mo CC, Chong WX, Yeh FS, Henderson BE. Preserved foods and nasopharyngeal carcinoma—a case–control study in Guangxi, China. Cancer Res 1988; 48(7):1954–1959.
26. Wild CP, Hall AJ. Hepatitis B virus and liver cancer: unanswered questions. Cancer Surveys 1999; 33:35–54.
27. Stellman SD, Djordjevic MV, Muscat JE, et al. Relative abundance of organochlorine pesticides and polychlorinated biphenyls in adipose tissue and serum of women in Long Island, New York. Cancer Epidemiol Bio Prev 1998; 7(6):489–496.
28. Maclure M, Bryant MS, Skipper PL, Tannenbaum SR. Decline of the hemoglobin adduct of 4-aminobiphenyl during withdrawal from smoking. Cancer Res 1990; 50:181–184.
29. Wang JS, Shen XN, He X, et al. Protective alterations in phase 1 and 2 metabolism of aflatoxin B-1 by oltipraz in residents of Qidong, People's Republic of China. J Natl Cancer Inst 1999; 91(4):347–354.
30. Ward EM, Sabbioni G, Debord DG, et al. Monitoring of aromatic amine exposures in workers at a chemical plant with a known bladder cancer excess. J Natl Cancer Inst 1996; 88(15):1046–1052.
31. Ozbal CC, Dasari RR, Tannenbaum SR. Stability of histone adducts in murine models: Implications for long-term molecular dosimetry. Abstr Papers Am Chem Soc 1998; 216:053-TOXI.
32. Wild CP, Turner PC. The toxicology of aflatoxins as a basis for public health decisions. Mutagenesis 2002; 17(6):471–481.
33. Szymanska K, Lesi OA, Kirk GD, et al. Ser-249 TP53 mutation in tumour and plasma DNA of hepatocellular carcinoma patients from a high incidence area in The Gambia, West Africa. Int J Cancer 2004; 110(3):374–379.
34. Jackson PE, Kuang SY, Wang JB, et al. Prospective detection of codon 249 mutations in plasma of hepatocellular carcinoma patients. Carcinogenesis 2003; 24(10):1657–1663.
35. Hussain SP, Amstad P, Raja K, et al. Increased p53 mutation load in noncancerous colon tissue from ulcerative colitis: a cancer-prone chronic inflammatory disease. Cancer Res 2000; 60(13):3333–3337.
36. Hall AJ, Wild CP. Epidemiology of aflatoxin-related disease. In: Eaton DA, Groopman JD, eds. Human Health, Veterinary and Agricultural Significance. New York: Academic Press, 1994:233–258.

37. Peluso M, Airoldi L, Magagnotti C, et al. White blood cell DNA adducts and fruit and vegetable consumption in bladder cancer. Carcinogenesis 2000; 21(2):183–187.

38. Skipper PL, Tannenbaum SR, Ross RK, Yu MC. Nonsmoking-related arylamine exposure and bladder cancer risk. Cancer Epidemiol Biol Prev 2003; 12(6):503–507.

39. IARC. Some Traditional Herbal Medicines, Some Mycotoxins, Naphthalene and Styrene. Lyon: IARC Monograph no. 56, 2002.

40. Wang LY, Hatch M, Chen CJ, et al. Aflatoxin exposure and risk of hepatocellular carcinoma in Taiwan. Int J Cancer 1996; 67(5):620–625.

41. Tang DL, Phillips DH, Stampfer M, et al. Association between carcinogen–DNA adducts in white blood cells and lung cancer risk in the Physicians Health Study. Cancer Res 2001; 61(18):6708–6712.

42. Bonassi S, Hagmar L, Stromberg U, et al. Chromosomal aberrations in lymphocytes predict human cancer independently of exposure to carcinogens. European Study Group on Cytogenetic Biomarkers and Health. Cancer Res 2000; 60(6):1619–1625.

43. Muller FH. Tabakmissbrauch und Lungencarcinom. Zeitschrift fur Krebsforschung 1939; 49:57–85.

44. Schairer E, Schoniger E. Lungenkrebs und Tabakverbruch. Zeitschrift fur Krebsforschung 1943; 54:261–269.

45. Cross AJ, Sinha R. Meat-related mutagens/carcinogens in the etiology of colorectal cancer. Environ Mol Mutagen 2004; 44(1):44–55.

46. Stillwell WG, Kidd LCR, Wishnok JS, Tannenbaum SR, Sinha R. Urinary excretion of unmetabolized and phase II conjugates of 2-amino-1-methyl-6-phenylimidazo[4,5-b]pyridine and 2-amino- 3,8-dimethylimidazo[4,5-f]quinoxaline in humans: relationship to cytochrome P4501A2 and N-acetyltransferase activity. Cancer Res 1997; 57(16):3457–3464.

47. Luan JA, Wong MY, Day NE, Wareham NJ. Sample size determination for studies of gene–environment interaction. Int J Epidemiol 2001; 30(5):1035–1040.

48. Vineis P, Schulte P, McMichael AJ. Misconceptions about the use of genetic tests in populations. Lancet 2001; 357:709–712.

49. Ishibe N, Sinha R, Hein DW, et al. Genetic polymorphisms in heterocyclic amine metabolism and risk of colorectal adenomas. Pharmacogenetics 2002; 12(2):145–150.

50. Rebbeck TR, Ambrosone CB, Bell DA, et al. SNPs, haplotypes, and cancer: applications in molecular epidemiology. Cancer Epidemiol Bio Prev 2004; 13(5):681–687.

51. Hashibe M, Brennan P, Strange RC, et al. Meta- and pooled analyses of GSTM1, GSTT1, GSTP1, anti CYP1A1 genotypes and risk of head and neck cancer. Cancer Epidemiol Bio Prev 2003; 12(12):1509–1517.

52. Cargill M, Altshuler D, Ireland J, et al. Characterization of single-nucleotide polymorphisms in coding regions of human genes. Nature Genet 1999; 22(3): 231–238.

53. Potter JD. Epidemiology, cancer genetics and microarrays: making correct inferences, using appropriate designs. Trends Genet 2003; 19(12):690–695.

54. Boffetta P. Molecular epidemiology. J Intern Med 2000; 248(6):447–454.
55. Kihara M, Noda K. Lung cancer risk of GSTM1 null genotype is dependent on the extent of tobacco smoke exposure. Carcinogenesis 1994; 15:415–418.
56. Allan JM, Wild CP, Rollinson S, et al. Polymorphism in glutathione S-transferase P1 is associated with susceptibility to chemotherapy-induced leukemia. Proc Natl Acad Sci USA 2001; 98(20):11592–11597.
57. Matullo G, Peluso M, Polidoro S, et al. Combination of DNA repair gene single nucleotide polymorphisms and increased levels of DNA adducts in a population-based study. Cancer Epidemiol Bio Prev 2003; 12(7):674–677.
58. Wojnowski L, Turner PC, Pendersen B, et al. Increased levels of aflatoxin-albumin adducts are associated with CYP3A5 polymorphisms in The Gambia, West Africa. Pharmacogenetics 2004; 14(10):691–700.
59. Wild CP, Fortuin M, Donato F, et al. Aflatoxin, liver enzymes, and hepatitis B virus infection in Gambian children. Cancer Epidemiol Bio Prev 1993; 2:555–561.
60. Turner PC, Mendy M, Whittle H, Fortuin M, Hall AJ, Wild CP. Hepatitis B infection and aflatoxin biomarker levels in Gambian children. Trop Med Int Health 2000; 5(12):837–841.
61. Chemin I, Ohgaki H, Chisari FV, Wild CP. Altered expression of hepatic carcinogen metabolizing enzymes with liver injury in HBV transgenic mouse lineages expressing various amounts of hepatitis B surface antigen. Liver 1999; 19(2):81–87.
62. Olivier M, Hussain SP, Caron de Fromentel C, Hainaut P, Harris CC. *TP53* mutation spectra and load: a tool for generating hypotheses on the etiology of cancer. In: Buffler P, Rice J, Baan R, Bird M, Boffetta P, eds. Mechanisms of Carcinogenesis: Contributions of Molecular Epidemiology. Lyon: IARC Scientific Publications No. 157, 2004:247–270.
63. Moorman AV, Roman E, Willett EV, Dovey GJ, Cartwright RA, Morgan GJ. Karyotype and age in acute myeloid leukemia. Are they linked? Cancer Genet Cytogenet 2001; 126(2):155–161.
64. Quackenbush J. Computational analysis of microarray data. Nat Rev Genet 2001; 2(6):418–427.
65. Wild CP, Hardie LJ. Reflux, Barrett's oesophagus and adenocarcinoma: burning questions. Nat Rev Cancer 2003; 3(9):676–684.
66. Bani-Hani K, Martin IG, Hardie LJ, et al. Prospective study of cyclin D1 over-expression in Barrett's esophagus: Association with increased risk of adenocarcinoma. J Natl Cancer Inst 2000; 92(16):1316–1321.
67. Wulfkuhle JD, Liotta LA, Petricoin EF. Proteomic applications for the early detection of cancer. Nat Rev Cancer 2003; 3(4):267–275.
68. Nicholson JK, Wilson ID. Understanding 'global' systems biology: metabonomics and the continuum of metabolism. Nat Rev Drug Discov 2003; 2(8):668–676.

5

Use of Biomarkers in Health Risk Assessment

Annette Santamaria
Environ International Corporation, Houston, Texas, U.S.A.

Laura Ferriby and Mark Harris
ChemRisk, Houston, Texas, U.S.A.

Dennis Paustenbach
ChemRisk, San Francisco, California, U.S.A.

INTRODUCTION

The aim of risk assessment is to provide society with estimates of the likelihood of illnesses and injury as a consequence of exposure to various hazards (1). It is a means to evaluate potential hazards associated with exposure to chemicals, mixtures, or processes; ascertain the likelihood that exposed individuals will be adversely affected; and characterize the nature of the effects they may experience. Risk assessment involves the systematic evaluation of scientific information comprising four components: (i) hazard identification—the determination of whether a particular substance is or is not causally linked to particular health effect(s), (ii) dose–response assessment—the ascertainment of the relationship between the magnitude of exposure and the probability of occurrence of the health effects in question, (iii) exposure assessment—the determination of the extent of human exposure, and (iv) risk characterization—the description of the nature and the magnitude of human risk, including uncertainties (2). Risk assessments of chemicals require the incorporation of scientific information about the level of exposure, absorption, metabolism, toxicology, mechanism of action, dose–response, and health effects associated with the exposure of interest. It is essential to have adequate dose–concentration–response data to conduct a quantitative risk assessment.

Much of the information for the hazard identification section comes from studies conducted in laboratory animals and typically requires the use of assumptions about the mechanism of action in animals to extrapolate the findings to humans. An understanding about the dose–response curve and whether there are threshold levels below which adverse effects do not occur may also be obtained from animal studies. Because the doses that are used in toxicology studies are typically much higher than the exposure levels that humans will likely encounter, high- to low-dose extrapolation is usually required. There are various mathematical models that are employed to extrapolate from high to low doses; however, these models can introduce additional sources of uncertainties and error and necessitate the use of safety factors to account for inter-species differences. Exposure parameters and estimates of absorbed doses must also be determined to estimate the magnitude of exposure in the population of interest. This typically involves estimating the exposure levels of the substance being investigated, modeling how much may be bioavailable ("dose"), and evaluating whether the dose is high enough to potentially cause the health outcome of concern (e.g., cancer, reproductive effects, cardiovascular effects) in a particular population (3). Further, exposure estimates in a human population are fraught with uncertainties and require the use of assumptions (e.g., duration of exposure, magnitude of exposure, inhalation, oral, and/or dermal absorption parameters, and amount of water, food, and soil ingested containing the substance of concern). Default assumptions are typically required in the absence of actual data and specific knowledge about the parameter of interest. The default position is one of being protective of public health, and typically results in overestimating the true health risks.

Indirect estimates of exposure are frequently used (e.g., models) along with the use of animal data for hazard identification and dose response modeling, hence the incorporation of several uncertainty factors into the risk assessment process is required. These uncertainties include: (i) species to species extrapolation, (ii) high-to low-dose extrapolation, (iii) mechanism of action responsible for the effects, (iv) interindividual differences in susceptibility, and (v) inadequate exposure data for estimating the actual health risks (4). The greatest uncertainties in risk assessments almost always result from inadequate exposure data, lack of knowledge about the mechanisms of toxicity, and insufficient understanding of the dose–response relationships (5).

These uncertainties, which are inherent in the risk-assessment process, have resulted in an increasing movement toward the development and use of biomarkers to reduce the number of assumptions used. High-quality biomarkers should improve the accuracy of risk assessment, making it predictive of actual risks rather than protective of theoretical risks (6).

BIOMARKERS AND THE RISK-ASSESSMENT PROCESS

A biomarker is any substance, structure, or process that can be measured in the body to evaluate exposure, predict an outcome or disease, or identify sensitive or genetically susceptible individuals (1,6). Biomarkers are biological and observable endpoints in a continuum of events leading from exposure to toxic agents to diseases resulting from exposure. Because many significant diseases develop over long periods of time, methods for detecting early events that can predict risk are important for prevention and should be incorporated into the risk-assessment process.

Currently, there are three main classes of biomarkers—biomarkers of exposure, effect, and host susceptibility—which are typically used for research purposes. While susceptibility factors, such as the presence of a specific genetic polymorphism, are increasingly being discovered, evaluated, and applied in studies (7), there are several epidemiological and occupational studies that have utilized various exposure and effect biomarkers (8). Tables 1 and 2 describe the effect of different chemical and metal exposures on levels of biomarkers of exposure and effect in occupationally and environmentally exposed groups, respectively. The integration of biomarker data from these types of studies into the risk-assessment process is anticipated to produce more accurate estimates of risk compared to current methods that typically require a number of assumptions and data extrapolations. Acceptance of the use of biological markers in the risk-assessment process appears to be increasing among researchers and will likely be further facilitated by the National Children's Study Biomarkers Database created by Lobdell and Mendola (10). The database, developed to identify both routine or standardized biomarkers as well as new and emerging biomarkers, will be instrumental in encouraging researchers to utilize biomarker data as the basis for more accurate risk assessments. This database is accessible to the general public and can be found online at http://cfpub.epa.gov/ncea/cfm/recordisplay.cfm?deid=85844.

When used in risk assessments, information provided by biological markers may replace default assumptions when specific information regarding exposure, absorption, and/or toxicokinetics is unavailable or limited (11). This has developed as a result of the availability of sensitive scientific methods to measure a variety of chemicals, metabolites, DNA adducts, and other molecular parameters in human tissues in an effort to assess internal dose and/or subclinical effects following exposure to a variety of substances. However, in order to use biomarkers to evaluate environmental or occupational health risks, it is imperative that they are both relevant and valid. Relevance refers to the appropriateness of biomarkers to provide information on questions of interest and importance to public and environmental health authorities and other decision-makers. Validity refers to a range of characteristics that provides the best approximation of the true exposure

Table 1 Effect of Exposure on Biomarkers of Exposure and Effect in Occupationally Exposed Groups

Group/sample size	Exposure type		Effect of exposure on biomarkers							
		Urinc[a]	DNA adducts[b]	Protein adducts[c]	Comet	CAs	SCEs	MN	HPRT	p^{53}/p^{21} proteins
Coke oven workers										
Exp = 68; C = 56	PAHs	—	E	—	—	—	—	—	—	—
Exp = 65; C = 34	PAHs	—	—	—	—	E	E	—	—	—
Exp = 24; C = 28	PAHs	—	—	—	No E	—	—	—	—	—
Exp = 80	PAHs	E	—	—	—	—	—	—	—	—
Exp = 75; C = 24	PAHs	E	No E	—	—	—	—	—	—	E
Exp = 59; C = 48	PAHs	—	—	No E	—	—	—	—	—	—
Exp = 50; C = 50	PAHs	E	—	—	No E	No E	E	E	—	—
Foundry workers										
Exp = 95	PAHs	—	E	—	—	—	—	—	—	—
Graphite-electrode workers										
Exp = 29; C = 32	PAHs	—	—	—	E	—	—	—	—	—
Soldiers										
Exp = 20; C = 33	Oil well fires, PAHs	No E	No E	—	—	—	—	—	—	—
Gasoline station attendants										
Exp = 12; C = 12	Benzene	—	—	—	—	—	—	No E	—	—

Exp = 12; C = 12	Benzene	—	—	—	E	—	—	—	—
Exp = 22; C = 19	Benzene	—	—	—	—	No E	—	E	—
Exp = 45; C = 45	Benzene	—	—	—	—	No E	—	—	—
Workers									
Exp = 43; C = 42	Benzene	—	E	—	—	—	—	—	—
Exp = 43; C = 44	Benzene	—	—	E	—	—	—	—	—
Exp = 43; C = 44	Benzene	—	—	E	—	—	—	—	—
Exp = 35; C = 13	Benzene	—	—	—	—	—	No E	—	—
Workers									
Exp = 19; C = 19	1,3-Butadiene	—	—	No E	E	E	No E	—	—
Exp = 15; C = 11	1,3-Butadiene	E	—	—	—	—	—	—	—
Exp = 24; C = 19	1,3-Butadiene	—	—	—	E[d]	—	—	—	—
Exp = 14; C = 14	Epichlorohy-drin	—	No E	—	—	E	No E	No E	No E
Exp = 8; C = 8	Propylene oxide	—	E	E	—	E	—	—	—
Shipbuilding workers									
Exp = 181; C = 27	PAHs	E	M	—	—	—	—	—	—

[a]Metabolites in urine.
[b]By ^{32}P-postlabeling or ELISA.
[c]Hemoglobin or albumin adducts.
[d]Effect on CAs only using challenge assay.

Abbreviations: —, biomarker not analyzed; C, number of subjects in control group; CA, chromosomal aberrations; Comet, Comet assay; E, statistically significant effect of exposure on biomarkers of exposure and effect; Exp, number of subjects in exposed group; HPRT, mutations in the hypoxanthine–guanine phosphoribosyltransferase gene; M, moderately significant; MN, micronuclei; PAHs, polycyclic aromatic hydrocarbons; p53/p21, activation of oncogenes coding for p53 or p21 proteins; SCEs, sister chromatid exchanges.
Source: From Ref. 9 with modifications.

Table 2 Effect of Exposure on Biomarkers of Exposure and Effect in Environmentally Exposed Groups

Group/sample size	Exposurer type	Urine[a]	DNA adducts[b]	Protein adducts[c]	Comet	CAs	SCEs	MN	HPRT
Bus drivers									
Exp = 57	VOCs	–	E	–	–	–	–	–	–
Rural population									
Exp = 31; C = 27	Arsenic	–	–	–	–	E	–	E	–
Exp = 32; C = 18	Arsenic	–	–	–	–	E	–	E	–
Exp = 113; C = 30	Arsenic	E	–	–	–	–	–	–	–
General populations									
Exp = 65	Pyrene	No E	–	No E	–	–	–	–	–
Women									
Exp = 51	PAHs	E	No E	–	–	–	–	–	–
Traffic police									
Exp = 34; C = 36	B[a]P	–	E	–	–	–	–	–	–

Exp = 54; C = 35	PAHs	—	—	—	—	—	No E	—
Exp = 82; C = 34	PAHs	—	—	—	—	—	—	No E
Exp = 94; C = 52	PAHs	No E	—	—	—	—	—	—
Children								
Exp = 87; C = 12	Ozone	—	E	—	E	—	—	—
Students								
Exp = 42	Ozone	—	—	—	E	—	—	—
Men								
Exp = 34; C = 26, 28	Simazine	—	—	—	—	—	No E	No E

[a]Metabolites in urine.
[b]By ^{32}P-postlabeling or ELISA.
[c]Hemoglobin or albumin adducts.
[d]Effect on CAs only using challenge assay.
Abbreviations: —, biomarker not analyzed; C, number of subjects in control group; CA, chromosomal aberrations; Comet, Comet assay; E, statistically significant effect of exposure on biomarkers of exposure and effect; Exp, number of subjects in exposed group; HPRT, mutations in the hypoxanthine–guanine phosphoribosyltransferase gene; MN, micronuclei; SCEs, sister chromatid exchanges.
Source: From Ref. 9 with modifications.

or health effect of interest. The validation process includes a laboratory phase and a population phase (12).

Ultimately, validation requires the use of epidemiological study designs to assess at least one of three types of relationships: exposure–dose, biological effects–disease, and susceptibility influencing an exposure–disease relationship (1). Studies that contribute to these types of validation and bridge the gap between laboratory experimentation and population-based epidemiology have been referred to as "transitional" studies (13–15). They may be designed to evaluate exposures, health effects, or susceptibility, and some may have the characteristics of pilot or developmental studies (16). After a biomarker is developed in the laboratory, it may be incorporated into the design of an epidemiological study to serve as a measure of exposure and/or effect in the cohort. Most of the data on the validation of biomarkers have come from "molecular"*Molecular epidemiology studies that evaluate the relationship between exposure to environmental pollutants and the quantification of effect biomarkers that predict clinical disease. There are three categories of validity: measurement validity, internal-study validity, and external validity (18). Measurement validity is the degree to which a biomarker indicates what it is intended to measure, internal-study validity is the degree to which inferences drawn from a study actually pertain to study subjects and are true, and external validity is the extent to which findings of a study may be generalized to other populations (18). The use of invalid biomarkers can result in misleading inferences and generalizations and ultimately, risk assessments with erroneous conclusions (1).

The use of biomarkers of exposure, effect, and susceptibility offer the opportunity to reduce uncertainties inherent in the risk-assessment process in several ways. However, one caveat regarding the use of biomarkers in risk assessments is the fact that there are only a few exposure, effect, and susceptibility biomarkers currently available, and only a limited number have been validated for use in large population studies. Others that have not been validated are of questionable significance for predicting the risk of adverse health effects in a population.

Biomarkers of exposure indicate whether exposure to and absorption of an agent has taken place, and include the measurement of specific metabolites and/or adducts formed by the reaction of the compound or its metabolites with macromolecules (1). These biomarkers are only available for those substances that have a reasonable half-life and can be measured as the parent compound or metabolite in biological tissues. Table 3 shows many of the chemicals that have been proven to be useful biomarkers of exposure. In addition,

---

*Molecular epidemiology studies are defined by the use of biomarkers, including biochemical, molecular, genetic, immunologic, or physiologic signals of exposure or effects in biological systems in their protocol (17).

biomarkers of exposure can be used as indicators of dose, which can then be assessed against classic measures of morbidity or mortality. Measuring a chemical or metabolite in biological fluids or tissues allows for the scientific estimation of external exposure levels that are necessary for characterizing risks. Biomarkers of exposure may, therefore, also reduce the uncertainty associated with external-dose measurements necessary for developing the dose–response analysis as well as characterizing risks. Further, the uncertainties regarding extrapolation from the administered doses in an animal study are reduced when the target tissue doses in the population of interest are known.

The second type of biomarkers, called biomarkers of effect, provides an indication of early events in the development of toxicity, carcinogenesis, and disease. These markers can reduce uncertainty in the risk-assessment process in several ways: (i) they can increase the sensitivity of risk assessments because such markers typically measure subclinical effects rather than the traditional endpoints of morbidity, mortality, tumors, and tissue pathology; (ii) the current risk-assessment process uses uncertainty factors to extrapolate across levels of effect severity (e.g., predict clinical effects from biochemical or early changes in cells or tissues), so the use of biomarkers of effect may

Table 3 Half-Lives of Various Biomarkers of Exposure

Half-life		Chemical	Indicator	Sample
Very short	2.5 h	Benzene	Benzene	Blood and exhaled air
	3.5 h		Phenol	Urine
	5 h	Carbon monoxide	Carboxyhemo-globin	Blood
Short	5 h	Styrene	Mandelic acid	Urine
	14 h	*n*-Hexane	2,5-Hexanedione	Urine
	18 h	Polycyclic hydrocarbons	Pyrenol	Urine
	96 h	Tetrachloroe-thylene	Tetrachloroe-thylene	Blood and exhaled air
Long	18 days	Mercury	Mercury	Blood and urine
	30 days	Lead	Lead	Blood
	100 days	Cadmium	Cadmium	Blood
Very long	2 years	Hexachloro-benzene	Hexachloro-benzene	Serum
	5 years	Lead	Lead	Bones
	7 years	2,3,7,8-TCDD	2,3,7,8-TCDD	Blood
	>10 years	Cadmium	Cadmium	Urine

Source: From Ref. 19 with modifications.

reduce the need for these uncertainty factors and the need for other safety factors; (iii) biomarkers of effect may provide useful information for deriving chemical-specific adjustment factors that replace default uncertainty factor values for toxicodynamics, and (iv) biomarkers of effect can reduce uncertainty in the choice of low-dose extrapolation models, where the underlying mechanism for induction of the early effect is unknown and presumptions about the likely shape of the dose–response curve are made (20).

Biomarkers of effect are often used in epidemiological studies to relate the occurrence of adverse health effects to exposure to a substance in a study population. These data contribute to the validation of the biomarker if the individuals that have elevated levels of effect biomarkers develop the disease or health outcome of interest. In addition, data from the workplace, where exposure biomonitoring for a variety of potentially harmful substances may be conducted to determine whether additional exposure-reducing controls are necessary, may also help identify relevant and valid biomarkers. The data obtained on biomarkers of effect from epidemiological and occupational studies may be useful for integration into certain chemical risk assessments.

Biomarkers of susceptibility, the third type of marker, are essential because some individuals in the population may be more vulnerable to the toxic effects of certain chemicals by virtue of their genetics. For example, some individuals biotransform absorbed chemicals into toxicologically effective doses even at the low exposure levels encountered by the vast majority of the population who do not exhibit any adverse effects (21). Risk assessments traditionally take "susceptible populations" into consideration by applying additional safety factors to the dose–response evaluation process. There is a growing body of research on biomarkers of susceptibility, which provide a means to identify those individuals that may be at an increased risk. This information may also help identify previously unknown susceptible populations that may not be protected under current risk assessments. By understanding the mechanisms involved with the increased susceptibility for adverse effects, more realistic factors may be incorporated into the risk-assessment process to protect all members of the population.

Use of Biomarkers in Hazard Identification

Hazard identification involves the analysis of available experimental data on the chemical of interest to determine what health effects are of concern for the risk assessment. The way that biomarkers may contribute to the hazard identification step of a risk assessment is in understanding the mechanism of toxicity and to identify potential thresholds of effect. Specifically, if the substance is or is not a carcinogen will significantly impact the risk-assessment process. EPA guidelines require a weight-of-evidence approach, integrating all relevant human, animal, and mechanistic data into a coherent picture of a compound's carcinogenic potential in humans (22).

Carcinogens are assumed, for regulatory purposes, not to have thresholds; however, biochemical and molecular information obtained from biomarker studies may provide valuable information on the mechanism of action and may permit the identification of a threshold. For example, several studies involving workers occupationally exposed to benzene at high doses have documented increases in chromosome aberrations, genetic mutations, and DNA oxidative damage in cells by measuring different biomarkers and in doing so have elucidated potentially important mechanisms for the induction of leukemia by benzene (23–31). Another example of the use of biomarkers in assessing mechanisms of carcinogenicity is the 1996 study conducted by Rothman et al. (32). In their work, these researchers measured urinary metabolites and mutagenicity and determined the genotypes and phenotypes for *N*-acetyl-transferase 2 (NAT2) and glutathione-*S*-transferase m1 (GSTM1) in workers exposed to benzidine and benzidine-based dyes to help assess a mechanism for the development of urinary bladder tumors in this population. Additionally, further analysis of DNA-adducts measured during this study revealed benzidine as a definitive hazard by demonstrating that exposed groups had adduct levels that were 12 times higher than controls.

Use of Biomarkers in Dose–Response Assessment

A key component of risk assessment is dose–response evaluation, which establishes the probability or degree of response that may be expected from different levels of exposure (33). Acceptable daily intake, environmental guidelines, and occupational exposure limits are most often extrapolated from experimental studies involving animals. If available, data on metabolism, pharmacokinetics, and DNA and protein biomarkers are useful for species-to-species extrapolation, high-to-low dose extrapolation, and physiologically based pharmacokinetic (PBPK) modeling (4). Understanding the mode of action also permits rational extrapolation across species and from high-to-low doses (22). Uncertainties in extrapolating thresholds across species and dose levels provide the justification for the use of safety factors. In a deterministic model (i.e., when a theoretical progression exists from exposure, through the absorption and distribution, to early effects and clinical disease), the use of experimental animal data is fully justified.

For new chemicals, there are limited alternatives to animal experiments because the evaluation of chemical-specific health risks should obviously precede human exposure. To reduce uncertainties of the extrapolation process, biomarkers may be used to assess dose as well as effects and susceptibility, thus deriving dose–effect and dose–response relationships in the target species, usually humans. In these studies, the concentration of the parent compound or its metabolites in accessible biological media or target molecules (biomarkers of internal dose) may be used as independent variables to assess their relationship with biomarkers of effect. Indeed, several studies have demonstrated that benzene-exposed workers experienced a dose- and time-dependent increase of chromosome aberrations (23,29,30,34,35) which appear to be predictive of cancer risk (36). In other investigations assessing the effects of benzene, significant dose-dependent increases of oxidative DNA adducts excreted into the urine of exposed workers were reported (24–27). Additionally, Nordberg et al. (37) used biomarkers of renal dysfunction to demonstrate a clear dose–response pattern in relation to cadmium and arsenic exposure of residents living in the Guizhou province of China (Fig. 1). In summary, epidemiological studies rely more and more on biomarkers as a consequence of exposure to environmental agents.

It is important to bear in mind that biomarkers are surrogate measurements of something that may be difficult or impossible to measure, is inaccessible, technically difficult, unacceptably disruptive, or unduly expensive (21). Although biomarkers are expected to increase the sensitivity of traditional approaches based on crude measures of exposure (e.g., job titles) and outcome (e.g., death certificates), their validation is a real challenge due to the intimate nature of surrogate indicators of something difficult or impossible to measure.

Use of Biomarkers in Exposure Assessment

Biomarkers of exposure are used to obtain more realistic estimates of exposure for use in risk assessments primarily because the exposure-assessment component has generally been considered the weakest link in the risk-assessment process. The use of biomarkers in exposure assessment may: (i) provide unequivocal data to establish the occurrence of exposure in

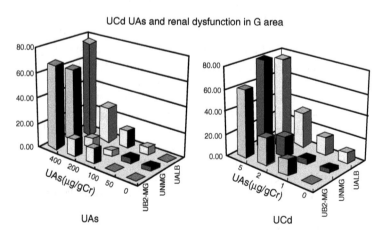

Figure 1 Prevalence (%) of elevated urinary excretion (above cut off level) of biomarker proteins by urinary arsenic (UAs) and urinary cadmium (UCd) in G-area. *Abbreviations*: Uh2MG, urinary beta-2-microglobulin; UNAG, urinary *N*-acetyl-glucosaminidase; UALB, urinary albumin. *Source*: From Ref. 37.

population studies; (ii) reduce misclassification in epidemiological studies, and (iii) model internal dose, i.e., that occurring at the critical organ, cell, or molecule. Whatever the aim, biomarkers of exposure focus on the body burden or on the total dose absorbed, integrating multiple sources of exposure and routes of intake, the pattern of exposure over time, and inter-individual differences in history, habits, and behaviors (1).

It is important to be able to ensure representativeness of exposure measurements for a population, differences in exposures within and between individuals, individual differences in uptake and biotransformation, identification of factors that control or modify exposures, exposure estimation methods applicable in the absence of direct measurements, and identification of the most relevant dose metric (the most relevant measure of dose) for the agent under consideration (12). Biomarkers of exposure may reduce many of the uncertainties associated with all of these parameters in the risk-assessment process.

Epidemiological studies designed to evaluate environmental or occupational exposures typically utilize exposure surrogates rather than direct measurements. For example, surrogates might include geographical location such as residence for a drinking water or air pollution study, age of housing in studies of lead-based paint exposures, or proximity of residence to electrical power lines. Occupational studies often use surrogates such as job title or job group, years worked at a plant, amount of substance produced or applied, airborne concentration of the contaminant, and tasks performed when direct measurements are not available or are limited (38). Biomarkers may serve to evaluate the completeness of exposure-assessment information by associating environmental or source information, exposure measurements, and epidemiological and human activity data with internal dose (39). For example, the 1996 study by Rothman et al. mentioned previously utilized benzidine–DNA adduct biomarkers to assess the exposure of workers to benzidine and to determine the relationship between internal dose and markers of biologically effective doses. As with hazard identification, urinary metabolites have been utilized as biomarkers for exposure to butadiene. Boogaard et al. (40) measured 1,2-dihydroxybutyl mercapturic acid (DHBMA) and 1- and 2-monohydroxy-3-butenyl mercapturic acid (MHBMA) due to their sensitivity as biomarkers for butadiene in an effort to evaluate exposure and establish a basis for cancer risk assessment in exposed workers (Fig. 2). The use of quantified direct measurements of personal exposures can lower uncertainty in the risk-assessment process considerably compared to the use of such exposure surrogates (12).

Regulatory Agencies and Biomarkers

Regulatory agencies have recognized the potential value of using biomarker data in human health risk assessments for deriving inhalation reference concentrations (41), cancer risk assessments (42), and in deriving biological exposure indices for occupational exposures (43). EPA's cancer risk-assessment

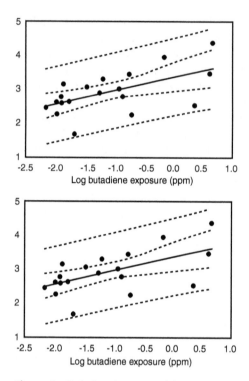

Figure 2 Relation between airborne butadiene and MHBMA (upper panel) and DHBMA (lower panel) levels in end-of-shift urine (21 workers). The regression line with 95% confidence intervals for individual (outer dashed line) and group values (inner dashed line) is shown. *Source*: From Ref. 40.

guidelines currently require that the probable effects of carcinogens in humans be estimated from results of animal bioassays. However, estimates of risk are derived from mathematical models that fit data of tumor incidence at high doses and require the extrapolation to probable human exposures that may be orders of magnitude lower, demonstrating a clear need for additional methods with which to assess exposures and outcomes.

The concepts and principles supporting the use of biomarkers in the assessment of human health risks from exposure to chemicals have been reviewed by the International Program on Chemical Safety (1). Monographs were prepared on the methodology for the assessment of human health risks, which includes the use of biomarkers (44,45).

LIMITATIONS OF BIOMARKERS

Like other classic measures of exposure and effect, there are limitations to the use of biomarkers for the risk-assessment process. A major limitation of exposure biomarkers is the general inability to describe historic exposures. For example, exposure biomarkers may only indicate recent exposure and may have narrow windows of time in which they can provide useful information depending on the half-lives of the substance being measured (e.g., parent compound, metabolite) (Table 3). Additionally, the potential for multiple sources of exposure to the same substance (e.g., diet, ambient air, workplace) may introduce confounding due to inappropriate allocation of the responsible source. There are many questions about markers of exposure—do they relate to an exposure dose, an internal dose, a target organ dose, or a biologically effective dose? To what types of effects, such as early biological effects and disease endpoints, can the biomarker be linked? Additionally, what does this mean in terms of quantifying risk of an adverse effect or in identifying susceptible groups, or even in terms of identifying early disease stages?

Limitations of biomarkers of effect include questions about the significance of the measured parameter in relation to human health risk or outcome of disease, that is, how predictive of future disease is the parameter that is being measured. There is also a lack of specificity for many biomarkers of effect, such as DNA damage, enzyme induction or inhibition, metabolic changes, or generation of reactive oxygen species, which may be caused by a variety of substances. Because many of the biomarkers of effect are not specific for the chemical substance of concern, they may provide misleading information about the responsible agent. Moreover, biomarkers of susceptibility present many questions about the specificity of effect and implications for future health effects. Biomarkers of effect or susceptibility may also present ethical concerns about confidentiality because they may represent intrusion in one's personal life, possibly resulting in discrimination or stigmatization.

Two important impediments to the development of biomarkers of value in the risk-assessment process were presented by Goldstein in 1996 (1). The first is the over-reliance on mathematical models to the exclusion of exposure monitoring data. This occurs because regulators have a need to make a decision and, for expedience, use models until better approaches are developed. Once locked into a regulation, the existence of the model serves as a major inhibition to the development of more reliable methods of indicating exposure and effect, including biomarkers. The second impediment is that medical review boards may not permit research designed to validate the biomarker because this would involve exposing subjects to levels of a substance they would not normally be exposed to in the general environment or at work. Therefore, it is at times difficult to obtain pharmacokinetic data to validate the biomarker in humans for use in the risk-assessment process.

While use of biomarkers can reduce misclassification, it is also possible that measurement error in the marker itself may introduce some degree of bias in the measure of association in a risk assessment (46). Such error can be evaluated and its impact adjusted for, but it is better to avoid or minimize it with good laboratory and epidemiological practices. While biomarkers are another tool for improving the risk-assessment process and should be utilized to contribute to the estimation of actual or "true" risks, they should not replace traditional measures such as exposure assessment, medical record reviews, job exposure matrices, and questionnaires.

Inappropriate Use of Biomarkers in Risk Assessment—A Case Study Involving Chromium

While the use of biomarkers in human health risk assessment is promising, there are already many examples that illustrate the potential for inappropriate use of biomarkers. One such example is the attempted use of biomarkers as a surrogate for exposure to hexavalent chromium in a residential setting in New Jersey. Three chromate chemical manufacturing facilities were at one time located in Hudson County, New Jersey, and produced several million tons of chromite ore processing residue (COPR) from the early 1900s through 1971. Throughout the time COPR was generated, it was used as a source of fill at over 200 residential and commercial properties in Hudson County. Because of the widespread distribution of COPR in Hudson County and concern regarding environmental exposure to hexavalent chromium by local residents and workers, a number of environmental investigations were initiated (47). Regulatory agencies and local universities attempted to utilize several biomarkers to evaluate exposure of the general population to hexavalent chromium.

The Community Medical Surveillance Project

In 1994, the New Jersey Department of Health (NJDOH) released the results of the Community Medical Surveillance Project (CMSP) (48). The researchers collected 1712 urine samples from residents and workers in Hudson County and reported limited evidence of chromium (Cr) exposure in a small number of people. Table 4 presents a summary of the results from the CMSP. Based on these results, the NJDOH and New Jersey Department of Environmental Protection (NJDEP) referred 158 adults and children for additional medical follow-up.

Understanding the Usefulness of the CMSP Data

As discussed previously, for an endpoint to be considered a biomarker, it must be both relevant and valid. In the case of urinary chromium, use of a relevant and valid biomarker in an occupational setting had been demonstrated; however, this is not the situation in environmental settings. In response to the initiation of the CMSP by NJDOH/NJDEP, several studies were conducted that were designed to determine the validity of the chromium biomarker of exposure in an environmental setting and to provide information on how to interpret the likely results of the study.

Table 4 Summary of Urinary Chromium Results for Residents and Workers in Hudson County as Determined in the CMSP

Population characteristic	N	Mean	Median	90th Percentile
All	1712	0.22	0.20	0.72
Age (years)				
1–5	52	0.35	0.37	1.14
6–18	185	0.26	0.25	0.78
19–60	1311	0.21	< 0.20	0.69
61+	164	0.23	0.23	0.74
Sex				
Male	669	0.23	0.21	0.89
Female	1043	0.21	0.20	0.66
Race				
NonWhite	990	0.23	0.21	0.76
White	722	0.21	<0.20	0.64

Source: From Ref. 49.

In an effort to understand whether the ingestion of COPR-impacted soil or household dust could be determined by measuring urinary chromium, six human volunteers ingested 400 mg of COPR per day for three days (low-dose group), and two other human volunteers ingested 2000 mg of COPR per day for the same amount of time (high-dose group). The study design and results are described in detail elsewhere (50,51). The COPR ingested by the low- and high-dose group contained 103 ± 20 mg/kg of total chromium and 9.3 ± 3.8 mg/kg of Cr(VI). These exposures were greatly in excess of any conceivable dose that residents of Hudson County could absorb from household dust. The study lasted a total of six days, with the first day's urine voiding (prior to the ingestion of the COPR) providing background urinary chromium values for each individual. On the second, third, and fourth days of the study, the volunteers ingested capsules containing the prescribed amounts of COPR. Urine was collected by each volunteer at each voiding over a six-day period during the study and analyzed for chromium content. Over 220 samples were analyzed for chromium as part of this study.

The results of the study were as follows:

1. The ingested COPR did not influence the urinary chromium concentrations of the human volunteers compared to each individual's background concentrations. For the low-dose group, background urinary chromium concentrations averaged 0.14 ± 0.20 µg Cr/g creatinine and urinary chromium concentrations following ingestion of COPR ranged from 0.11 ± 0.10 to 0.19 ± 0.35 µg Cr/g creatinine; these results were not statistically different from

the background value. Similar results were observed for the high-dose group.

2. Background concentrations of urinary chromium fluctuated within a large range for the volunteers. Specifically, background urinary chromium values ranged from 0.2 to 2.9 μg Cr/L of urine. The urinary chromium concentrations reported in the CMSP for individuals living and working in Hudson County were well within the background concentrations reported in these studies (Table 4).

It is clear from these results that the ingestion of COPR had no influence on urinary chromium concentrations. Consequently, these outcomes provide evidence that urinary chromium is not a suitable biomarker for measuring exposure to hexavalent chromium at the low doses often found in settings involving environmental contamination.

Ingestion of Safe Doses of Cr(VI)

While the ingestion of COPR-containing chromium concentrations similar to that in household dust in Hudson County homes provided data that suggested the agencies were simply measuring background variations in urinary chromium, there was concern regarding how to interpret the upper end of the background range of urinary chromium. Indeed, the first series of studies demonstrated that inter- and intra-personal variability was significant (0.2–2.9 μg Cr/L of urine). For example, on day 1, which was used to determine an individual's background urinary chromium value, one individual had a spot urine chromium concentration of 2.9 μg/L. Because the NJDOH and NJDEP had not adequately validated this potential biomarker, such a value would have been interpreted by these agencies as evidence of excessive exposure to COPR, when in reality, none had occurred. Furthermore, NJDOH and NJDEP would have referred this individual for further medical follow-up.

To address this concern, a second study was conducted. In this study, human volunteers ingested "safe" doses of Cr(VI) and Cr(III) in pure form (not in COPR) and urinary chromium concentrations were measured. A "safe" dose was defined as the USEPA reference dose (RfD) of Cr(VI) and Cr(III) (at that time, 0.005 and 1.0 mg/kg-day, respectively). Potassium chromate was the source of Cr(VI) used in the study, and chromic oxide was used as the Cr(III) compound because these are the forms likely to be found in COPR and are also the forms in the toxicity studies used to derive the RfDs. Ingestion of Cr(VI) at the RfD resulted in urinary chromium concentrations ranging from <0.2 to 97 μg Cr/L, while ingestion of Cr(III) at the RfD resulted in urinary chromium concentrations ranging from <0.2 to 6.3 μg Cr/L. These results demonstrate that the urinary chromium concentrations measured by NJDOH and NJDEP were well below the urinary chromium values that would be expected if an individual ingested the

USEPA defined "safe" oral dose (Table 4). These data clearly provide information on how to interpret the study results associated with this biomarker. The results of this study are described in detail elsewhere (52).

Use of Urinary Chromium as a Biomarker of Environmental Exposure in Hudson County, New Jersey—Lessons Learned

Clearly, the NJDEP/NJDOH initiated the CMSP prior to understanding whether or not urinary chromium was a suitable biomarker for environmental exposure to chromium. However, the results of Finely et al. (52) help to interpret the results of the CMSP and confirm that at the time of sample collection, residents participating in the study were not being exposed to hexavalent chromium at levels exceeding the USEPA reference dose. Thus, based on the results of Gargas et al. (50), urinary chromium levels are unlikely to be useful biomarkers of exposure for evaluating typical low level environmental exposure to chromium.

DNA Protein Crosslinks as a Biomarker of Exposure to COPR in Hudson County, New Jersey

DNA–protein crosslinks are macromolecules that are created when a substance (e.g., protein, chemical) becomes covalently bound to DNA. Biologically relevant proteins that have been shown to be crosslinked to DNA in vivo include actin, lectin, aminoglycoside nucleotidyl transferase, histones, heat shock protein GRP78, vimentin, protein disulfide isomerase, and transcription factors/co-factors. The formation of these molecules can occur subsequent to the exposure of cells to a variety of agents, including ultraviolet light and ionizing radiation, metals, metalloids, chemicals, and some chemotherapeutic drugs (53). In 1995, Taioli et al. (54) published an article that suggested DNA–protein crosslinks were elevated in some residents in Hudson County. The authors reported that the level of DNA–protein crosslinks in leukocytes of the residents of Hudson County ($n = 33$) was $1.3 \pm 0.5\%$, whereas the control group had $0.8 \pm 0.4\%$ ($p < 0.001$). Residents were permitted to take part in the study if they had a urinary chromium value $>0.5\,\mu g/L$ as determined by the NJDOH during the CMSP. Taioli et al. (54) concluded that further studies were necessary to confirm the possible association between high levels of DNA–protein crosslinks and exposure to chromium.

Three studies were conducted following the publication of Taioli et al. (54) that served to show that this potential biomarker was also not useful for measuring environmental exposure to chromium. First, Costa et al. (55) reported on an interlaboratory validation of the DNA–protein crosslink assay that had been used in Hudson County. Specifically, six independent laboratories tested a number of compounds in the DNA–protein crosslink assay and the results were compared. The laboratories found that

DNA–protein crosslinks could not be induced by a number of compounds, including potassium permanganate, mercury chloride, magnesium perchlorate, aluminum chloride, and cadmium chloride. However, copper sulfate, arsenic trioxide, and potassium chromate were found to induce DNA–protein crosslinks in the assay but only at cytotoxic doses.

The second experiment, conducted by Costa et al. (56), investigated the formation of DNA–protein crosslinks by various industrial chemicals in cultured human lymphoma cells. Chemicals investigated included acetaldehyde, acrolein, diepoxybutane, paraformaldehyde, 2-furaldehyde, propionaldehyde, chloroacteldehyde, sodium arsenite, and a deodorant tablet named Mega-Blue (hazardous component listed as tris[hydroxymethyl]nitromethane). In this series of studies, DNA–protein crosslink formation was investigated at two washing temperatures (45 and 65°C). A number of compounds were found to cause the formation of DNA–protein crosslinks at both temperatures, including acrolein, diepoxybutane, paraformaldehyde, and Mega-Blue. In contrast, 2-furaldehyde, acetaldehyde, and proprionaldehyde only produced DNA–protein crosslinks at 45°C. With the exception of two compounds (2-furaldehyde and paraformaldehyde), DNA–protein crosslinks were only observed at concentrations that caused cell death within four days of dosing, suggesting that this biomarker is not suitable for use in environmental exposure scenarios.

In the third study, Kuykendall et al. (57) investigated the potential formation of DNA–protein crosslinks in leukocytes in humans following ingestion of hexavalent chromium and trivalent chromium. Four human volunteers ingested 5000 µg of hexavalent chromium dissolved in 0.5 L water and blood samples were collected 0, 60, 120, 180, and 240 minutes postexposure. Elevated chromium concentrations were detected in both red blood cells and urine of each study participant. Despite this, DNA–protein crosslinks were not elevated in any of these study participants.

The results of Costa et al. (55,56) and Kuykendall et al. (57) indicate that the use of DNA–protein crosslinks is also not a suitable biomarker for evaluating environmental exposure to hexavalent chromium. Studies such as these should have been performed before utilizing the DNA–protein crosslink assay to evaluate a potentially impacted population. Had these studies been performed in the proper sequence, the DNA–protein crosslink assay would not have been deemed useful for evaluating the potentially exposed population in Hudson County.

CONCLUSIONS

The field of risk assessment is a relatively new discipline that was launched professionally in the mid-1970s. In recent years, the methodology has been accepted by virtually every industrialized country. While the underlying principle of human risk assessment relies on these ideals to promote assessment methods that reveal "true" risks to public health, determining actual risks associated with exposures is much more difficult due to ambiguities in the risk-assessment process. Extrapolation of experimental results in rodents to humans has many uncertainties and may not be adequate in determining risks associated with low-level chemical exposures. Furthermore, exposure estimates in human populations often require the use of default assumptions due to the absence of actual data and specific knowledge about the parameter of interest. These concerns and others, including lack of knowledge about the mechanisms of toxicity and insufficient understanding of dose–response relationships, have clearly demonstrated a need for more research to further develop a biological basis for risk assessment.

As the development of molecular techniques has progressed rapidly over the past few years, there has been an increasing movement toward the development and use of biomarkers to (i) reduce the number of uncertainties in the risk-assessment process, and (ii) to improve the accuracy of risk assessment to make it predictive of actual risks rather than protective of theoretical risks. Three primary categories of biomarkers have been utilized in epidemiological studies designed to facilitate the risk-assessment process: biomarkers of exposure, biomarkers of effect, and biomarkers of susceptibility. The application of these biomarkers to the different components of the risk-assessment process, including hazard identification, dose–response modeling, and exposure assessment, has demonstrated their usefulness in reducing uncertainties and providing more precise estimates of risk.

While it is likely that such biomarkers will prove to be sufficiently accurate tools for the risk-assessment process, it is essential that these biomarkers be both relevant and valid in order to avoid misleading inferences and generalizations. Additionally, it is important to consider the limitations of biomarkers in risk assessments. These biomarkers will not be able to indicate historical exposure or differentiate between multiple sources of exposure to the same substance, and many biomarkers, particularly biomarkers of effect, lack specificity. Other impediments to the use of biomarkers include established governmental policies, and ethical concerns regarding confidentiality and validation research study designs. Lastly, the potential for misuse of biomarkers in the risk-assessment process should be noted. As demonstrated in the case of hexavalent chromium in Hudson County, NJ, the use of biomarkers may not be applicable to the risk assessment of all chemicals in specific environmental exposure situations. It is incumbent upon the researchers to validate the biomarker prior to utilizing it on potentially impacted populations.

REFERENCES

1. International Programme on Chemical Safety (IPCS). Environmental Health Criteria 222: Biomarkers in risk assessment: validity and validation. Geneva: World Health Organization, 2001.

2. National Research Council (NRC). Risk Assessment in the Federal Government: Managing the Process. Washington: National Academy of Sciences, 1983.
3. Paustenbach DJ, ed. Human and Ecological Risk Assessment: Theory and Practice. New York: Wiley-Interscience, 2002.
4. Swenberg JA, Gorgeiva N, Ham A, et al. Linking pharmacokinetics and biomarker data to mechanism of action in risk assessment. Human Ecol Risk Assess 2002; 8:1315–1338.
5. McClellan RO. Risk assessment and biological mechanisms: lessons learned, future opportunities. Toxicology 1995; 102:239–258.
6. Paustenbach DJ, Galbraith D. Biomonitoring: Is body burden relevant to public health? Reg Toxicol Pharmacol 2006. In press.
7. Norppa H. Cytogenetic biomarkers and genetic polymorphisms. Toxicol Lett 2004; 149:309–334.
8. Au WW, Lee E, Christiani DC. Biomarker research in occupational health. J Occup Environ Med 2005; 47:145–153.
9. Sram RJ, Binkova B. Molecular epidemiology studies on occupational and environmental exposure to mutagens and carcinogens 1997–1999. Environ Health Perspect 2000; 108(Suppl 1):57–70.
10. Lobdell DT, Mendola P. Development of a biomarkers database for the National Children's Study. Toxicol Appl Pharmacol 2005; 206(2):269–273.
11. Ponce RA, Bartell SM, Kavanagh TJ, et al. Uncertainty analysis methods for comparing predictive models and biomarkers: A case study of dietary methyl mercury exposure. Regul Toxicol Pharmacol 1998; 28:96–105.
12. Schulte PA, Waters M. Using molecular epidemiology in assessing exposure for risk assessment. Ann NY Acad Sci 1999; 895:101–111.
13. Hulka BS. ASPO Distinguished Achievement Award Lecture. Epidemiological studies using biological markers: issues for epidemiologists. Cancer Epidemiol Biomarkers Prev 1991; 1:13–19.
14. Schulte PA, Rothman N, Perera FP, Talaska G. Biomarkers of exposure in cancer epidemiology. Epidemiology 1995; 6:637–638.
15. Rothman N, Stewart WF, Schulte PA. Incorporating biomarkers into cancer epidemiology: a matrix of biomarker and study design categories. Cancer Epidemiol Biomarkers Prev 1995; 4:301–311.
16. Hulka BS, Margolin BH. Methodological issues in epidemiologic studies using biologic markers. Am J Epidemiol 1992; 135:200–209.
17. Schulte PA. Use of biological markers in occupational health research and practice. Toxicol Environ Health 1993; 40:359–366.
18. Schulte PA, Perera FP. Transitional studies. IARC Sci Publ 1997; 142:19–29.
19. Bernard AM. Biokinetics and stability aspects of biomarkers: recommendations in population studies. Toxicology 1995; 101:65–71.
20. Maier A, Savage RE Jr, Haber LT. Assessing biomarker use in risk assessment—a survey of practitioners. J Toxicol Environ Health A 2004; 67:687–695.
21. Mutti A. Biological monitoring in occupational and environmental toxicology. Toxicol Lett 1999; 108:77–89.
22. Albertini R, Clewell H, Himmelstein W, et al. The use of non-tumor data in cancer risk assessment: reflections on butadiene, vinyl chloride, and benzene. Regul Toxicol Pharmacol 2003; 37:105–132.

23. Carere A, Antoccia, A, Cimini D, et al. Genetic effects of petroleum fuels: II. Analysis of chromosome loss and hyperploidy in peripheral lymphocytes of gasoline station attendants. Environ Mol Mutagen 1998; 32:130–138.
24. Liu L, Zhang Q, Feng J. Urine level of trans, trans-muconic acid used as an index internal dose of exposure to benzene [Chinese]. Zhonghua Yu Fang Yi Xue Za Zhi 1996; 30:148–150.
25. Liu L, Zhang Q, Feng J, et al. The study of DNA oxidative damage in benzene-exposed workers. Mutat Res 1996; 370:145–150.
26. Liu ZT, Wang LS, Chen SP, Li W, Yu HX. Analysis and prediction of structure–reactive toxicity relationships of substituted aromatic compounds. Bull Environ Contam Toxicol 1996; 57:421–425.
27. Nilsson RI, Nordlinder RG, Tagesson C, Walles S, Jarvholm BG. Genotoxic effects in workers exposed to low levels of benzene from gasoline. Am J Ind Med 1996; 30:317–324.
28. O'Connor SR, Farmer PB, Lauder I. Benzene and non-Hodgkin's lymphoma. J Pathol 1999; 189:448–453.
29. Rothman N, Haas R, Hayes RB, et al. Benzene induces gene-duplicating but not gene-inactivating mutations at the glycophorin A locus in exposed humans. Proc Natl Acad Sci USA 1995; 92:4069–4073.
30. Smith MT, Rothman N. Biomarkers in the molecular epidemiology of benzene-exposed workers. J Toxicol Environ Health A 2000; 61:439–445.
31. Smith MT, Zhang L, Wang Y, et al. Increased translocations and aneusomy in chromosomes 8 and 21 among workers exposed to benzene. Cancer Res 1998; 58:2176–2181.
32. Rothman N, Bhatnagar VK, Hayes RB, et al. The impact of interindividual variation in NAT2 activity on benzidine urinary metabolites and urothelial DNA adducts in exposed workers. Proc Natl Acad Sci USA 1996; 93:5084–5089.
33. National Research Council (NRC). Pharmacokinetics in Risk Assessment: Drinking Water and Health. Washington: National Academy of Sciences, 1987.
34. Tompa A, Major J, Jakab MG. Monitoring of benzene-exposed workers for genotoxic effects of benzene: improved-working-condition-related decrease in the frequencies of chromosomal aberrations in peripheral blood lymphocytes. Mutat Res 1994; 304:159–165.
35. Zhang L, Rothman N, Wang Y, et al. Benzene increases aneuploidy in the lymphocytes of exposed workers: a comparison of data obtained by fluorescence in situ hybridization in interphase and metaphase cells. Environ Mol Mutagen 1999; 34:260–268.
36. Forni A. Benzene-induced chromosome aberrations: a follow-up study. Environ Health Perspect 1996; 104:1309–1312.
37. Nordberg GF, Jin T, Hong F, Zhang A, Buchet JP, Bernard A. Biomarkers of cadmium and arsenic interactions. Toxicol Appl Pharmacol 2005; 206:191–197.
38. Goldberg M, Hemon D. Occupational epidemiology and assessment of exposure. Int J Epidemiol 1993; 22(Suppl 2):S5–S9.
39. Dary CC, Quackenboss JJ, Nauman CH, Hern SC. Relationship of biomarkers of exposure to risk assessment and risk management. In: Blancato JN, Brown RN, Dary CC, Saleh MA, eds. Biomarkers for Agrochemicals and Toxic Substances; ACS Symposium Series 643. Washington: American Chemical Society, 1996:2–23.

40. Boogaard PJ, van Sittert NJ, Megens HJ. Urinary metabolites and heamo-globin adducts as biomarkers of exposure to 1,3-butadiene: a basis for 1,3-buta-diene cancer risk assessment. Chem–Biol Interact 2001; 135–136:695–701.
41. Environmental Protection Agency (EPA). Methods for derivation of inhalation reference concentrations and application of inhalation dosimetry. EPA/600/8-90-066F, Washington: Office of Health and Environmental Assessment, 1994.
42. Environmental Protection Agency (EPA). Guidelines for Carcinogenic Risk Assessment. EPA/630/P-03/001F, Washington: Office of Research and Development, 2005.
43. American Conference of Governmental Industrial Hygienists (ACGIH). Threshold Limit Values for Chemical Substances and Physical Agents and Biological Exposure Indices. Cincinnati: ACGIH, 2001.
44. International Programme on Chemical Safety (IPCS). Environmental Health Criteria 170: Assessing human health risks of chemicals: derivation of guidance values for health-based exposure limits. Geneva: World Health Organization, 1994.
45. International Programme on Chemical Safety (IPCS). Environmental Health Criteria 210: Principles for the assessment of risks to human health from exposure to chemicals. Geneva: World Health Organization, 1999.
46. Saracci R. Comparing measurements of biomarkers with other measurements of exposure. IARC Sci Publ 1997; 142:303–312.
47. Proctor D, Harris M, Rabbe D. Risk assessment of chromium-contaminated soils: twelve years of research to characterize the health hazards. In: Paustenbach DJ, ed. Human and Ecological Risk Assessment: Theory and Practice. New York: Wiley-Interscience, 2002:513–583.
48. New Jersey Department of Health (NJDOH). Chromium Medical Surveillance Project: Summary of Final Technical Report. NJDOH, Trenton: Environmental Health Services. 1994.
49. Fagliano JA, Savrin J, Udasin I, Gochfeld M. Community exposure and medical screening near chromium waste sites in New Jersey. Regul Tox Pharmacol 1997; 26:S13–S22.
50. Gargas ML, Norton RL, Harris MA, Paustenbach DJ, Finley BL. Urinary excretion of chromium following ingestion of chromite-ore processing residues in humans: implications for biomonitoring. Risk Anal 1994; 14:1019–1024.
51. Gargas ML, Norton RL, Paustenbach DJ, Finley BL. Urinary excretion of chromium by humans following ingestion of chromium picolinate. Drug Metab Disp 1994; 22:522–529.
52. Finley B, Scott P, Norton RL, Gargas ML, Paustenbach DJ. Urinary chromium concentrations in humans following ingestion of safe doses of hexavalent chromium and trivalent chromium: implications for biomonitoring. J Toxicol Environ Health 1996; 48:479–499.
53. Barker S, Weinfeld M, Murray D. DNA–protein crosslinks: their induction, repair, and biological consequences. Mutat Res 2005; 598:111–135.
54. Taioli E, Zhitkovich A, Kinney A, Udasin I, Toniolo P, Costa M. Increased DNA–protein crosslinks in lymphocytes of residents living in chromium contaminated areas. Biol Trace Elem Res 1995; 50:175–180.
55. Costa M, Zhitkovich A, Gargas M, et al. Interlaboratory validation of a new assay for DNA–protein crosslinks. Mutat Res 1996; 369:13–21.

56. Costa M, Zhitkovich A, Harris M, Paustenbach D, Gargas M. DNA–protein cross-links produced by various chemicals in cultured human lymphoma cells. J Toxicol Environ Health 1997; 50:433–449.
57. Kuykendall JR, Kerger BD, Jarvi EJ, et al. Measurement of DNA–protein cross-links in human leukocytes following acute ingestion of chromium in drinking water. Carcinogenesis 1996; 17:1971–1977.

6

Biomarkers of Toxicant Susceptibility

Sofia Pavanello

Occupational Health Section, Department of Environmental Medicine and Public Health, University of Padova, Padova, Italy

INTRODUCTION

Considerably varying responses to toxicant exposure exist in humans. Variations in absorption, distribution, metabolism, DNA repair, and cell turnover processes can modify the risk for adverse effects and the levels of biomarkers after exposure to toxic agents. Some of these differences are ascribed to heritable traits, which modify the effects of exposure to toxicants. Individual susceptibility to the hazardous action of chemicals may have a genetic basis, and gene–exposure interactions also exist. Responses/effects may be distinguished as short-term, (e.g., adverse drug side-effects) and long-term (e.g., genotoxic carcinogen-induced neoplasia). The former are easier to study and follow as regards effects than the latter. In this chapter, metabolic and DNA repair variations are considered for their importance in detecting the impact of genotype on biological indicators of genotoxic risk and on adverse drug side-effects.

GENETIC POLYMORPHISM

Brief History of Genetic Toxicology

That genetic constitution influences an individual's sensitivity towards exogenous substances was first observed in cases of pharmacological treatment. Nearly 50 years ago, the inherited impairment of a phase I reaction, hydrolysis of the muscle relaxant succinylcholine by butyrylcholinesterase (pseudocholinesterase), served as an early stimulus for the development of pharmacogenetics. It was shown that about one in 3500 Caucasian subjects is homozygous for a gene encoding an atypical form of butyrylcholinesterase and is relatively unable to hydrolyze succinylcholine, thus prolonging drug-induced muscle paralysis and consequent apnea (1). At almost the same time, it was observed that a common genetic variation in a phase II pathway of drug metabolism, N-acetylation, could result in striking differences in the half-life and plasma concentrations of drugs metabolized by *N*-acetyltransferase. Such drugs included the antituberculosis agent isoniazid, the antihypertensive agent hydralazine, and the antiarrhythmic drug procainamide, and this variation had clinical consequences in all cases. The bimodal distribution of plasma isoniazid concentrations in subjects with genetically determined fast or slow rates of acetylation in one of those early studies strikingly illustrates the consequences of inherited variations in this pathway for drug metabolism (2).

It was in the 1970s that bimodal distribution in the ability to metabolize the antihypertensive drug debrisoquine to its 4-OH metabolite, linked to the polymorphic expression of a CYP active in its metabolism, CYP2D6, was also shown. Approximately 5% to 10% of Caucasian subjects were found to have a relative deficiency in their ability to oxidize debrisoquine. Subjects with poor metabolism of these two drugs had lower urinary concentrations of metabolites and higher plasma concentrations of the parent drug than did subjects with extensive metabolism. Furthermore, the drugs had an exaggerated effect in the former subjects, and family studies demonstrated that poor oxidation of debrisoquine and sparteine was inherited as an autosomal recessive trait, that is, subjects with poor metabolism had inherited two copies of a gene or genes that encoded either an enzyme with decreased CYP2D6 activity or one with no activity (3). Subsequent studies have confirmed that phenotypic variation in the metabolism of many clinical drugs is the consequence of genetically determined differences (i.e., polymorphisms) in the activities of several human drug-metabolizing enzymes, some of which are also involved in the metabolism of genotoxic carcinogens.

Genetic Toxicology in Cancer Research

Until about 20 years ago, cancer susceptibility was mainly attributed to the level and length of exposure to carcinogens. Classic epidemiological research had identified a number of populations at risk (i.e., smokers and high occupationally exposed workers), demonstrating a precise association between exposure to some mixtures of compounds and tumor development. Although this relationship is still true for most of the human population, it has now been shown that the multistep carcinogenic process, which leads from carcinogen exposure to cancer, can be modulated in individuals.

However, these individual susceptibility factors are not equal. There is a rare group of individuals (1–2%) in whom a tumor suppressor gene (for example, P53 in the Li-Fraumeni syndrome) is altered and who display a dramatic increase in cancer susceptibility, in terms of both incidence and age of tumor incidence, the number of steps required for cancer development decreasing by at least one. Besides these very marked predispositions, there is also the more subtle one of low-penetrance genes, involving different stages of the cancer process (i.e., metabolism, DNA repair) in a large portion of the population, the consequences of which are far from being severe.

Metabolism of Xenobiotics

Xenobiotic metabolism in humans occurs in two distinct phases; phase I, or activation, creates a reactive center in the molecule while phase II, or detoxification, is responsible for the conjugation reactions involving the incorporation of a moiety, mostly glutathione or glucuronic acid, into the molecule (Table 1). Most carcinogens and many noncarcinogenic xenobiotics are electrophilic compounds able to bind to nucleophilic sites of DNA (or protein) only after metabolic activation. Exposure to genotoxic carcinogens causes a chemical modification of the genome as a result of covalent DNA adduct formation which, if not recognized by the DNA repair process, may initiate the multistep process of carcinogenesis (4). Genetic polymorphisms exist for a number of activating/detoxifying enzymes as well as for DNA repair proteins, and their connection, especially with the carcinogenic process, has been extensively studied (5,6). To date, many genetic bases of polymorphic enzymes, which influence drug metabolism, have been identified. The newly discovered polymorphisms affecting DNA repair are considered to be of special importance in conferring differing sensitivity to the carcinogenic action of endogenous and exogenous compounds. Genetic polymorphisms are thus considered to play a primary role in individual responses to carcinogen-induced disease and have been indicated as biomarkers of susceptibility. Currently, there is great interest in polymorphisms in environmental and occupational medicine, mainly concerning their role in modulating individual responses to exposure to genotoxic carcinogens. These responses may be measured in exposed populations by detecting the levels of markers of genotoxic risk (biological monitoring studies) (7).

Biological Indicators of Genotoxic Risk

Methods for evaluating exposure and/or biological effects to genotoxic compounds are listed in Table 2. Biological indicators (biomarkers) of genotoxic risk are subdivided into indicators of internal dose, biologically effective dose, and early biological effects. According to this classification, it is possible to identify a biological indicator at every step of the pathway of a genotoxic substance within the organism, from absorption to nucleophilic

Table 1   Enzymes Involved in Drug Metabolism in Humans

Phase I	Phase II

Microsomal mono-oxygenation
FAD-containing mono-oxygenases:
add oxygen to amines, sulfur
compounds, and organophosphorus
compounds
P450 cytochromes:
"Mixed-function oxygenases" (MFO)—
"mixed function"=1/2 used to
oxidize xenobiotic, 1/2 reduced to
water
Nonmicrosomal oxidation (in cytosol or
mitochondria)
Dehydrogenases (cytosolic)
  Alcohols → Aldehydes
  Aldehydes → Acids
Amine oxidases (mitochondrial)
  Endogenous nervous system
    function—neurotransmitter
    turnover
  Other tissues—deamination of
    aliphatic amines to aldehydes
  Byproduct formation of hydrogen
    peroxide (toxic)
Reduction (cytosolic)
  Addition of $H^+ + e^-$
Hydrolysis (microsomal and cytosolic)
  Carboxyl esterases and amidases
    e.g., ACHase (normal nervous
    system function)
Epoxide hydration (microsomal and
  cytosolic)
  Epoxide hydrolases
Dichloro-diphenyl-trichloro-ethane-
  dechlorinase (and other
  dechlorinating enzymes)
Dichloro-diphenyl-trichloro-ethane-
  type dechlorinases (cytosolic)
Other dechlorinases can be P450
  mediated (microsomal)
Quinone reduction (cytosolic)
  Reduction of quinone group to
    hydroxyl
	Glycoside conjugation—conjugation
	  with glucuronic acid. Enzyme: UDP
	  glucuronosyl transferase
	Sulfate conjugation—formation of
	  sulfate esters. Enzymes:
	  sulfotransferases
	Methylation—addition of methyl group.
	  Enzymes: methyltransferases
	Glutathione conjugation—Enzymes:
	  glutathion S-transferase
	Acylation-Enzymes: acyltransferase

(*Continued*)

Table 1 Genetic Polymorphisms of *BchE* (*Continued*)

Phase I	Phase II
Important role in detoxifying quinones Oxidative stress Redox cycling production of superoxide anion and hydrogen peroxide Alternative name: DT-diaphorase	

attack, damage fixation, and excretion. In biological monitoring, a distinction must be made between indicators of exposure and of effect. The former (concentration of the substance or its metabolites in biological fluids; mutagenicity of excreted substances; attack by metabolites on hemoglobin and DNA) aim at highlighting the absorption of the compound in question and, if possible, at measuring its internal dose and biologically effective dose. The latter [chromosome aberrations (CA), sister chromatid exchanges (SCE), micronuclei (MN), hypoxanthine-guanine phosphoribosyl transferase (*HPRT*) mutants, simple cell gel electrophoresis (also called COMET assay), etc.] measure alterations in important genetic targets (i.e., chromosomes, chromatids, gene sequences, etc.). The link between the measured parameter and the development of tumors is very probably closer in the case of indicators of effect. In particular, elevated CA levels have clearly been associated with higher incidence of cancer (8).

Molecular Basis of Polymorphisms

Polymorphisms are sequence variations such as nucleotide substitutions, deletions/insertions, and gene duplications/deletions. By definition,

Table 2 Indicators of Genotoxic Risk

Indicators of internal dose	Indicators of biologically effective dose	Indicators of early biological effects
Substance or its metabolites in biological fluids	Protein adducts (hemoglobin and plasma protein adducts)	Chromosome aberrations
Urinary mutagenicity	DNA adducts	Sister chromatid exchanges Micronuclei COMET assay *HPRT* mutants Glycophorin variants A in erythrocytes

polymorphisms occur at a population frequency of at least 1%, although this arbitrary value is loosely interpreted in practice. These variations may or may not cause alterations in protein function and phenotype; the resulting changes in protein activity range from slight to significant. Some of the principal ways in which genetic polymorphisms affect the expression of gene products or the catalytic activity of the respective enzymes may be summarized as follows: (i) nucleotide variations in the coding region of the gene result in amino acid substitution and alter enzyme activity or substrate binding (e.g., CYP2D6); (ii) deletions in/of the coding region lead to an inactive enzyme or lack of protein synthesis (e.g., CYP2A6, CYP2D6, GSTM1); (iii) polymorphisms in the noncoding region affect transcriptional control elements involved in basal enzyme expression and induction (e.g., CYP1A1); (iv) variations in the polyadenylation signal of a gene affect transcript half-life and thus the quantity of enzyme (e.g., NAT1); (v) gene amplification increases the quantity of enzyme (e.g., CYP2D6); and (vi) complex interactions of polymorphic genes and/or their enzyme catalysis products (e.g., GSTM1-deficient subjects or cells have greater induction of CYP1A1 and 1A2, probably because of the greater bioavailability of inducer compounds). Single nucleotide polymorphisms (SNPs), which cause amino acid substitution, are either defined as synonymous SNP (replacement of one amino acid by a similar one) and tend to produce minimal mutation effects on a protein, or as nonsynonymous SNP (replacement of an amino acid having substantially different chemical properties), which may have detrimental effects.

Characteristics of Genetic Polymorphisms of Metabolic Enzymes

The most studied genetic polymorphisms of enzymes involved in the metabolism of xenobiotics are the following: *ALDH2* (aldehyde dehydrogenase), *CYP1A1, CYP1A2, CYP2C, CYP2D6* (P450 cytochromes), *EPHX* (epoxide hydrolase), *GSTM1, GSTM3, GSTP1, GSTT1* (glutathione S-transferase), *NAT2, NAT1* (N-acetyltransferase), *NQO1* [NAD(P)H quinone oxidoreductase], and *PON1* (paraoxonase). The newly discovered polymorphisms of some DNA repair genes have also been considered in studies dealing with biomonitoring of genotoxic risk: *ERCC1* (excision repair cross-complementing 1), *ERCC2* (excision repair cross-complementing 2), or *XPD, XRCC1,* and *XRCC3* [X-ray repair cross-complementing groups 1 and 3 and *hOGG1* (human 8-OH-guanine glycosidase)]. The characteristics of these polymorphisms and their related biological activities are briefly reported (Tables 3 and 4).

Figures 1–4 show the main metabolic pathways, from the genotoxic point of view, of some of the most important classes of genotoxic carcinogens (BaP as an example of polycyclic aromatic compounds; aromatic amines; benzene).

Table 3 Polymorphisms of Metabolic Enzymes and Related Biological Activity

Gene (enzyme)	Allele	Mutation	Enzyme activity
ALDH2	*1	Wild-type	Normal
(aldehyde	*2	Glu487Lys	Decreased
dehydrogenase 2)			
EPHX	R or *1	Wild-type	Normal
(epoxide hydrolase)	H	Exon 3 −Tyr113His	Decreased
	Y	Exon 4 −His139Arg	Increased
NQO1	*1	Wild-type	Normal
[NAD(P)H quinone	*2	C609T exon 6	Null
oxidoreductase]			
PON1	A	192 Gln	Low
(paraoxonase)	B	192 Arg	High
NAT2	*4	Wild-type	Rapid
(N-acetyl	*5A	T341C; C481T	Slow
transferase)			
	*5B	T341C; C481T	Slow
	*5C	A803G	Slow
	*6A	T341C; A803G	Slow
	*7B	G590A C282T; G857A	Slow
NAT1	*4	Wild-type (T1088; A1095)	Normal
(N-acetyl	*10	T1088A	Rapid
transferase)			
CYP1A1[a]	*1	Wild-type	Normal
(cytochrome P450	*2 or Mspl	T6235 C	Increased
1A1)			
	*3 or Ile/Val	A4889 G	Increased
	*4	T5639 C	Increased
	*5	C4887 A	
CYP1A2[a]	*1	Wild-type	Normal
(cytochrome P450	*1C	-G3858 A	Decreased activity in smokers
1A2)			
	*1D	-T2464 delT	Increased activity in smokers
	*1F	-A163 C	Increased activity in smokers
CYP2E1[a]	*1 or C1	Wild-type	Normal
(cytochrome P450	*3 or C2 dra	C1019 T5′ flanking region	Increased
2E1)			
CYP2D6[a]	*1	Wild-type	Normal (EM)
(cytochrome P450	*3 or A	Base deletion	Null
2D6)			

(Continued)

Table 3 Indicators of Genotoxic Risk (*Continued*)

Gene (enzyme)	Allele	Mutation	Enzyme activity
	*4 or B	Base mutation	Null
	*5 or D	Gene deletion	Null
	*6 or E	Base deletion	Null
	*15 or T	Base insertion	Null
GSTM1	*1 or Active	Wild-type	Normal
(glutathione S-transferase)	*0	Deletion	Null
GSTM3	A	Wild-type	Normal
(glutathione S-transferase)	B	Deletion of 3 bp	Low
GSTT1	*1 or Active	Wild-type	Normal
(glutathione S-transferase)	*0	Deletion	Null
GSTP1	A	Wild-type	Normal
(glutathione S-transferase)	B	Iso104Val	Low
	C	Iso104Val; Val113Ala	Low

[a]see the Web site http://www.imm.ki.se/CYPalleles/ for an up-to-date nomenclature.
Abbreviation: EM, extensive metabolizer.

Table 4 DNA Repair Polymorphisms and Related Biological Activity

Gene (enzyme)	Mutation	Enzyme activity
ERCC1 (excision repair cross-complementing 1)	A→C 8092	Decreased
ERCC2 or XPD (excision repair cross-complementing group 2)	312 Asp→Asn 751 Lys→Gln	Decreased
hOGG1 (human 8-OH-guanine glycosidase)	326 Ser→Cys	Decreased
XRCC1 (X-ray repair cross-complementing group 1)	194 Arg→Trp 280 Arg→His 399Arg→Gln	Decreased
XRCC3 (X-ray repair cross-complementing group 3)	241 Thr→Met	Decreased

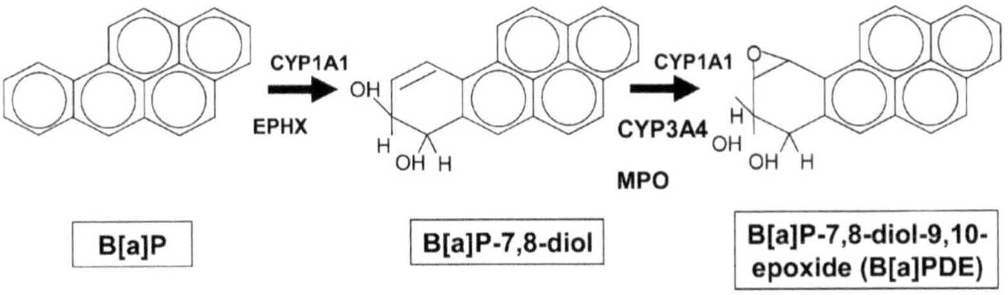

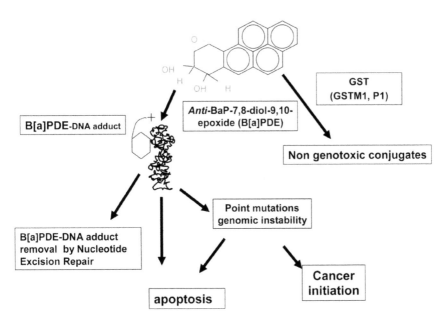

Figure 1 B[*a*]P genotoxic activation. *Abbreviations*: CYP, cytochrome; EPHX, epoxide hydrolase; B[*a*]P, benzo[*a*]pyrene.

Aldehyde Dehydrogenase

Aldehyde dehydrogenase 2 (ALDH2) is a mitochondrial enzyme and one of the two main isoenzymes of aldehyde dehydrogenase (ALDH1 with high K_m; ALDH2 with low K_m). Together with alcohol dehydrogenase, ALDH2 is the main metabolizer of ethyl alcohol. It is also involved in the metabolism of toluene (in particular, in the step from benzyl alcohol to benzoic acid) and also appears to be implicated in that of vinyl chloride monomer (VCM; ethylene oxide chloride→chloroacetaldehyde). About half the Japanese population lacks ALDH2 activity (9). This means that, after

Figure 2 Critical step in the carcinogenic pathway of B[*a*]P; formation of anti-B[*a*]PDE–DNA adduct. *Abbreviations*: GST, glutathione S-transferase; B[*a*]P, benzo[a]pyrene.

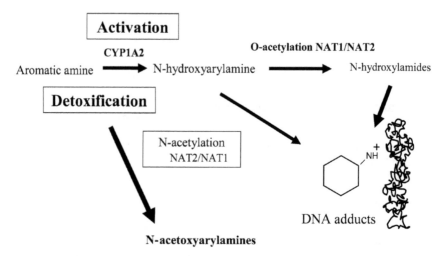

Figure 3 Genotoxic metabolism of aromatic amines. *Abbreviations*: CYP, cyto-chrome; NAT, N-acetyl transferases.

alcohol intake, the metabolism of acetaldehyde is inefficient and it accumu-lates in the organism, giving rise to nausea, hypotension, and tachycardia. This lack of catalytic activity results from a homozygous point mutation of the amino acid in position 487 (Glu > Lys; *ALDH2*2/*2*) of the wild allele of the *ALDH2* gene (*ALDH2*1*). The same mutation has also been

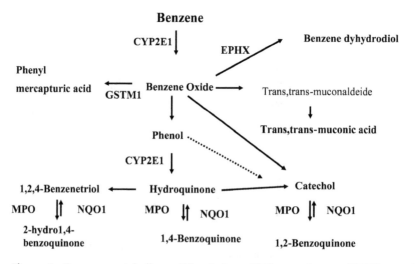

Figure 4 Benzene metabolism. *Abbreviations*: CYP, cytochrome; EPHX, epoxide hydrolase; GST, glutathione S-transferase; NQO1, NAD(P)H quinone oxidoreduc-tase 1.

found in American and Caucasian populations, but at much lower frequencies than in Asiatic ones. Subjects with *ALDH2*1/*2* genotype have reduced ALDH2 activity.

CYP1A1

Cytochromes P450 (CYP) are enzymes that catalyze the insertion of one atom of molecular oxygen into a substrate. This is a typical reaction of activation (phase I) that converts indirect carcinogens into active electrophiles capable of interacting with the biological macromolecules DNA, RNA, and protein. CYP are coded by genes of the *CYP* superfamily. In particular, the gene product of CYP1A1 is aryl hydrocarbon hydroxylase (AHH), which catalyzes the first step of the metabolism of polycyclic aromatic hydrocarbons (PAHs) to electrophilic compounds. The gene is induced by exposure to substances such as dioxin, benzo[*a*]pyrene B[*a*]P, and other PAHs. In recent years, some molecular mechanisms involved in gene induction have been clarified, linked to polymorphisms of the catalytic domains or regulators of CYP1A1, genes of the receptor of aryl hydrocarbon (AHR), or of the nuclear protein transporting the receptor (ARNT). At the present time, four main polymorphisms in gene *CYP1A1* are known, of which one is specific to African populations. These polymorphisms have been given numbers in order of publication, preceded by the symbol * (i.e., *CYP1A1*1* is the wild-type). The first mutation found (polymorphism *CYP1A1*2*) is a 6235 T > C transition in exon 7, causing a new cut site for the restriction enzyme Mspl. This mutation is overexpressed in the Japanese population (20%), less in the Caucasian, and is in incomplete linkage disequilibrium with another mutation of exon 7, 4889 A > G (polymorphism *CYP1A1*3* or Ile/Val). This point mutation confers an at least threefold increase in catalytic activity. The polymorphism specific to African populations (5639 T > C; allele *CYP1A1*4*) is located in intron 7, outside the coding region. More recently, another very rare polymorphism has been identified in exon 7, called *CYP1A1*5* (4887 C > A) (10).

CYP1A2

The P450 1A2 cytochrome (CYP1A2) has been identified as a key factor in the activation metabolism of many carcinogens (N-oxidation of the amine hexocyclic group) such as aflatoxin, aromatic and heterocyclic amines, and some nitro-aromatic compounds. CYP1A2 also contributes to the deactivation (deacetylation) of various constituents of diet and drugs (caffeine and acetaminophen). Its activity may be induced by exposure to cigarette smoke and to meat cooked at high temperature, or by exposure to PAH or aromatic amines. This enzyme was first detected only in liver, but it has also recently been found in brain and the endothelial cells of the umbilical cord. Ample interindividual variability has been found in the activity of CYP1A2, by means of in vivo tests for the phenotype (mainly the caffeine test). Some authors have thus distinguished CYP1A2 rapid subjects (about 40%) from others with slow or intermediate activity (the remaining 60%). Contributor to interindividual variability in CYP1A2 activity is the occurrence of polymorphisms in the *CYP1A2* gene (10). A number of CYP1A2 SNPs have been reported, four of which lie in the 5-noncoding promoter region. One of the known CYP1A2 SNPs, *CYP1A2 −G3860A (CYP1A2*1C)*, has been reported to cause decreased enzyme activity in smokers but seems to be rare. Another SNP, very common in Caucasians (~60%), *CYP1A2− A163C* polymorphism (*CYP1A2 *1F*), has also been associated with reduced activity in smokers and may contribute significantly to the substantial interindividual variation in CYP1A2 activity. Recently, another polymorphism, the *CYP1A2 1D - T2467delT,* has been suggested to be analyzed in the Caucasian population for routine assessment of *CYP1A2* genotype. In view of the great importance of CYP1A2 in the activation of many environmental carcinogens, it has been hypothesized that, although its expression (and thus xenobiotic activation) mainly occurs in liver, it may be a risk factor for the development of cancers in other tissues (lung, bladder, colon) (11).

CYP2E1

The P450 2E1 cytochrome (CYP2E1) metabolizes many indirect carcinogens such as nitrosoamines (N-nitrosodimethylamine and N-nitrosopyrrolidine), some components of tobacco smoke, and many chlorinated and nonchlorinated solvents, including benzene. CYP2E1 may be induced by ethanol, and thus alcohol intake may influence carcinogenesis by exposure to carcinogens activated by this enzyme. In man, it is mainly expressed in liver, with a high degree of variability. Gene *CYP2E1* reveals one of the most complex cases of polymorphism nomenclature. *CYP2E1*1* is the wild or normal type (10). Allele *CYP2E1*2* was attributed to the first polymorphism discovered in 1987 by McBride et al. (12), and consists of a $C > G$ mutation in intron 7, which creates a restriction site for enzyme Taq1. Two polymorphisms (*CYP2E1*3* and *CYP2E1*5*) are recognized by the restriction enzyme *Rsa1*. Unlike *5, *3 results from loss of the restriction site for *Rsa1*, and is in complete linkage disequilibrium with another restriction site recognized by *Pts1*. Two other polymorphisms also have been discovered, *CYP2E1 *4* and *6*, the former due to a mutation involving loss of the restriction site for enzyme *Dra1* and the latter recognized by restriction enzyme *Msp1*. All these polymorphisms are located in the noncoding region of *CYP2E1* and appear to act on the transcriptional regulation of the enzyme, increasing its activity.

CYP2C

The P450 2C cytochrome (CYP2C), a subfamily of CYP2, has four isoforms, CYP2C8, CYP2C9, CYP2C18, and CYP2C19. The genetic polymorphism of enzyme CYP2C19, the activity of which is associated with hydroxylation of S-mephenitoin, has been clearly characterized. Two enzymatic phenotypes are known, one a poor metabolizer (PM) and the other an extensive metabolizer (EM) of S-mephenitoin. The frequency of PM is higher in Japanese (20%) than in Caucasian populations (3%). Two mutated alleles, *CYP2C19*2* and *CYP2C19*3*, have been characterized, the latter occurring only in the Japanese, both leading to a reduction in enzyme activity. CYP2C9 metabolizes several drugs and is the main enzyme involved in the metabolism of S-warfarin, phenitoin, tolbutamide, and some nonsteroid anti-inflammatory drugs (e.g., acetyl salicylic acid, ibuprofen). Mutations in two different alleles have been identified in *CYP2C9*: 432 C>T for allele *CYP2C9*2* and 1077 A>C for allele *CYP2C9*3*. The frequencies of alleles *CYP2C9*1* (wild-type), *CYP2C9*2*, and *CYP2C9*3* in Caucasians are about 0.86, 0.08, and 0.06, respectively. These genetic polymorphisms generally enhance enzyme activity and the expression of mRNA. In contrast, the substrate specificity of CYP2C18 is not well characterized. This enzyme, like CYP2C9 and CYP2C19, can metabolize cyclophosphamide and isophosphamide, two alkylating agents used in chemotherapy. With cyclophosphamide as substrate, CYP2C19 has the lowest K_m, followed by K_m CYP2C9 $< K_m$ CYP2C18; with isophosphamide, the order is K_m CYP2C19 $< K_m$ CYP2C18 $< K_m$ CYP2C9. A mutation that changes a restriction site for enzyme *DdeI* has been identified in the 5'-region of gene *CYP2C18*. This allele, called *CYP2C18*2*, appears to cause lower enzyme activation for cyclophosphamide but greater catalytic activity for isophosphamide (13).

CYP2D6

Gene *CYP2D6*, of the *CYP2* gene family, encodes for the CYP2D6 enzyme. More than 80 compounds have been recognized as substrates of this cytochrome, including drugs acting on the cardiovascular system and the CNS. Loss of enzyme activity may have serious clinical effects and in some cases lead to death. Among representative substrates for CYP2D6 are the hypotensive drug debrisoquine and a component of tobacco smoke, nitrosamine NNK [4-methylnitrosoamine-1-(3-pyridyl)-1-butanone]. Most individuals (80–90%) have at least one normal allele of gene *CYP2D6*, called *CYP2D6*1*. These subjects, functionally classified as EM, present a wide range of variability (up to about 1000-fold) in drug metabolism, have subpopulations with intermediate activity (IM) due to a mutation of gene *CYP2D6*, and have ultra-rapid activity (UM), explained by the amplification either of a mutated gene or of a normal one. PM, the minority group (5–10% Caucasians, 2% Afro-Americans, 1% Japanese), are identified by loss of gene function and lack the hepatic protein.

One example of the very complex polymorphism of this enzyme is summarized in a recent work by Sachse et al. [(14), see also (10)], in which

15 alleles are listed, associated with low enzyme activity (*CYP2D6*2*, **9*, **10*) or its absence (*CYP2D6* **3*, **4*, **5*, **6*, **7*, **8*, **11*, **12*, **13*, **14*, **15*, **16*). Due to the nature of the substances metabolized by this enzyme, screening of PM subjects would seem to be more suitable in studies aimed at identifying subjects with anomalous responses to a given drug, rather than predicting subjects at risk of cancer.

Epoxide Hydrolase

Microsomal epoxide hydrolase (EPHX) catalyzes the addition of a molecule of H_2O to an epoxide to form dihydrodiol. This irreversible reaction produces metabolites, which are more water soluble, less reactive, but readily conjugated and excreted. Although EPHX is considered a detoxifying enzyme, the dihydrodiols deriving from PAHs may be further transformed by specific CYP into still more reactive species (i.e., dihydrodiol epoxides, the most mutagenic and carcinogenic of the PAH metabolites). Currently, three polymorphisms of gene *EPHX* are known: the wild-type R and two mutants. Replacement at codon 113 (Tyr > His) of exon 3 reduces enzyme activity (allele H), whereas codon 139 substitution (His > Arg) of exon 4 is associated with increased activity (allele Y). Thus, in the case of exposure to PAHs, increased activity caused by the mutation of exon 4 may be considered as an unfavorable genotype, unlike other substances for which increased EPHX activity involves enhanced detoxifying activity and, thus, a reduction of possible toxic or carcinogenic action (15).

Glutathione S-Transferases

Glutathione S-transferases (GST) are one of the major groups of detoxifying enzymes. Each GST has distinct catalytic properties, i.e., conjugation with glutathione, peroxidation, and isomerization. In humans, eight distinct gene families encode these soluble GST; α on chromosome 6, μ on chromosome 1, θ on chromosome 22, π on chromosome 11, z on chromosome 14, σ on chromosome 4, κ (chromosomal location not known; the enzyme, probably soluble, is expressed in mitochondria), and χ (also called ω) on chromosome 10. Polymorphism has been described in many genes in these families, although until now most attention has focused on allelism in the μ, θ, and π families (16).

GSTM1: The first GST polymorphisms to be determined were those of class μ. They were characterized both by measuring enzyme activity in relation to a given substrate (trans-stilbene oxide) and by isolating and identifying the isoenzymes. Class μ includes at least five genes coding for an equal number of enzymes (GSTM1, M2, M3, M4, M5). The gene coding for isoform *GSTM1* is polymorphic and has four allele variants *GSTM1*A*, **B*, **C*, and **0*. The first two do not have apparent differences with regard to type of substrate, and allele C is very rare. Individuals who are homozygous for the variant *0 lack the enzyme activity. About 50% of Caucasians lack GSTM1 activity. Lack of the isoenzymatic μ form is associated with reduced efficiency in binding genotoxic substrates, including epoxides deriving from PAH and aflatoxin. One of the consequences of inheriting a nonfunctional *GSTM1* allele appears to be an increased risk for cancer associated with these carcinogenic exposures, particularly of the bladder and lung. McLennan et al. (17) have described further allele variants, with ultrarapid enzyme activity as a result, having two *GSTM1* genes between *GSTM2* and *GSTM5*. Allelism has also been identified in *GSTM3*, with *GSTM3 *A* and *GSTM3 *B* differing in intron 6 by a 3 bp deletion in *GSTM3 *B*.

GSTP1: Polymorphisms of gene *GSTP1* were reported for the first time by Board et al. in 1989 (18). They consist of an A > G transition of nucleotide 313 in exon 5 (*GSTP1*B*) and a G > T transition to nucleotide 341 in exon 6 (*GSTP1*C*), involving substitution of two amino acids in the active enzyme sites (Ile > Val and Val > Ala). These allele variants appear to reduce GSTP1 activity. The presence of GSTP1 in many tissues, together with its capacity to inactivate important carcinogens like diol epoxides of PAH, indicate that this enzyme is also involved in susceptibility to cancers consequent to carcinogenic exposure (19).

GSTT1: In addition to the null polymorphism of locus *GSTM1*, another null polymorphism has been found in the class of θ transferases to locus T1 (wild normal allele *GSTT1*1*, null allele *GSTT1*0*). The frequency of homozygotic *GSTT1*0* (*0/*0*) varies in several populations, 16% in the British and 38% in Nigerians. It is difficult to predict the biological consequences of genotype *GSTT1* null, since this enzyme has both detoxifying and activating properties, which affect many environmental pollutants. From a genotoxic point of view, although GSTT1 detoxifies monohalomethanes (e.g., methyl bromide) and epoxides of the alkenes, ethylene and butadiene, it activates methylene chloride and some bifunctional alkylating agents. Human erythrocytes, unlike those of rodents, express GSTT1, and this activity allows red blood cells to sequester the reactive conjugates resulting from the "toxifying" activity of GSTT1, thus preventing their genotoxic attack on DNA (20).

NAT1 and NAT2

N-acetyl transferases (NAT) transfer an acetyl group to the nitrogen atom of aromatic amines and hydrazine or to the oxygen atom of hydroxylated aryl amines. In this way, they can catalyze both reactions of detoxification, such as N-acetylation, and of activation, producing metabolites reactive to DNA, such as O-acetylation of N-hydroxyaryl amines. In man, three NAT genes are known, one of which (*NATP*) is an unexpressed pseudogene [see (21) for a comprehensive literature review on *NAT1* and *NAT2* genes]. The two expressed genes, *NAT1* and *NAT2*, are located on chromosome 8 and present homology of about 85% in the coding region. While the alleles responsible for variations in NAT2 activity are well characterized in various ethnic populations, the molecular basis for the variation in NAT1 activity is still being revealed. About 26 different *NAT2* alleles have been identified. *NAT2*4* allele is considered the wild-type and those *NAT2* alleles containing the G191A, T341C, A434C, G590A, and/or G857A missense substitutions (low-activity mutant alleles) are associated with slow acetylator phenotype(s). *NAT2* slow acetylators vary between 10% and 80%, depending on ethnic group, and their reduced activity is due to either slight expression or instability or reduced catalytic activity of the enzyme synthesized. As recently described by Meyer and Zanger (22), the low-activity mutant alleles *NAT2*5A, B, C, NAT2*6A, NAT2*7B*, and *NAT2*13* identify more than 99% of slow acetylators in Caucasians. In Asian populations, such as Japanese, Chinese, Korean, and Thai, slow acetylators vary between 10% and 30%, while most populations of Europe and North America have frequencies between 40% and 70%. Slow acetylators are identified by the homozygotic presence of low-activity alleles; rapid acetylators are carriers of wild allele *NAT2*4* in hetero- or homozygotic form. The human gene *NAT2* is expressed at both hepatic and extrahepatic levels, and its activity is not inducible. Phenotyping studies also indicate considerable structural variations in the *NAT1* gene and the existence of high- and/or low-activity phenotypes. Genotyping studies have confirmed these findings and indicate that a polymorphism at position 1088 of the *NAT1* gene (*NAT1 *0* allele) is present in approximately 30% of populations with European ancestry. This mutation is believed to increase mRNA stability by altering the polyadenylation signal and thereby raising levels of NAT1 and consequently its activity.

Aromatic and heterocyclic amines are carcinogenic compounds found in cigarette smoke, panfried meat, and the work environment. The differing susceptibility to NAT2-dependent cancers in various tissues is the result of the different expression and complex metabolic pathways of aromatic and heterocyclic amines of NAT enzymes, enzymes of activation, conjugation, and deconjugation. The most important are, respectively, CYP1A2, UDP-glucuronosyl transferase, and β-glucuronidase (23).

NAD(P)H Quinone Oxidoreductase1

NAD(P)H quinone oxidoreductase 1 (NQO1) or diaphorase is a two-electron reductase involved in the activation/detoxification of quinones (e.g., mitomycin C) and similar active compounds, including benzene metabolites (hydrobenzoquinone, benzoquinone). Three alleles of gene *NQO1* have been identified in human populations: normal *NQO1*1* (Arg 139/Pro 187), nonfunctional *NQO1*2* (Arg 139/Ser 187), and *NQO1*3* (Trp 139/Pro 187), associated with reduced enzyme activity. The best-known polymorphism is *NQO1*2*. About 70% of Caucasians are wild-type homozygotic (*NQO1*1/*1*), 27% are heterozygotic (*NQO1*1/*2*) with reduced enzyme activity, and 3% to 4% homozygotic ($NQO1^*2/^*2$) with null enzyme activity. In contrast, in Chinese populations, the homozygote $NQO1^*2/^*2$ shows a frequency of 23% and, in workers severely exposed to benzene, has been shown to be a risk factor for hemotoxicity (24,25).

Paroxonase 1

Paroxonase 1 (PON1) is a Ca^2-dependent enzyme whose mechanism of action is still not completely known. *PON1* is a member of a family of at least three other associated genes. It was originally identified as responsible for the hydrolysis of paraoxon, a catabolite of the insecticide parathion, but it is also capable of hydrolyzing the active metabolites (oxons) of a number of organophosphorus (OP) insecticides such as parathion, diazinon, and chlorpyrifos. It is equally able to hydrolyze other substrates like phenyl acetate. *PON1* has two sequence polymorphisms, Gln 192 > Arg and Met 55 > Leu (called alleles B and C). Allele B has been shown to cause increased detoxifying activity of PON1 to parathion with respect to the lower activity of allele A wild-type (Gln 192) (26).

Genetic Polymorphisms of Enzymes Involved in DNA Repair Genes

DNA Repair Mechanisms

DNA lesions are of many different types, including single- and double-strand breaks (induced by X rays), inter- and intrastrand crosslinks (caused by chemical agents, such as the cytostatic cisplatin), and various kinds of base modifications. The consequences of these lesions are at both the cellular level [i.e., cell-cycle arrest, (programmed) cell death, and genomic instability (mutagenesis)] and at the organism level. DNA lesions have been implicated in genetically inherited diseases, carcinogenesis, and aging (27). DNA repair is usually specific for a class of damage; double-strand breaks are repaired by homologous recombination-dependent repair or in an end-joining reaction, and most small base modifications (base damage induced by ionizing radiations and monofunctional alkylating agents) are removed by base excision repair (BER). Nucleotide excision repair (NER) removes primarily bulky adducts, helix-distorting adducts (e.g., BaP, cyclobutane pyrimidine dimers, photoadducts). Mismatches or structural abnormalities at replication forks are repaired by the mismatch repair pathway. However, ample overlap exists in the substrate specificity of repair pathways, and certain proteins are used in more than one pathway (28). NER is one of the major and versatile cellular pathways for the removal of many bulky DNA adducts induced by agents such as UV, cisplatin, and 4-nitroquinoline-1-oxide. In eukaryotes, NER is complex and necessitates the co-ordinated action of about 20 proteins. NER involves: (i) damage recognition and incision, (ii) excision of damage as part of an oligonucleotide, (iii) repair resynthesis, and (iv) DNA ligation. The BER pathway uses three types of enzymes: (i) DNA glycosylases, which remove modified base(s) from DNA by hydrolysis of the N-glycosidic bond (e.g., 3-methyladenine DNA glycosylase), (ii) AP endonucleases, which excise the abasic sugar and replace it with a correct nucleotide (e.g., *Escherichia coli* endonuclease III), and (iii) enzymes which have both glycosylase and AP endonuclease activities (e.g., T4 endonuclease V) (29).

Polymorphisms of DNA Repair Genes

Apart from individuals with rare and recessive syndromes, i.e., ataxia-telangiectasia (A-T), Fanconi anemia, Bloom's syndrome, characterized by both chromosomal instability and high risk of cancer, and *xeroderma pigmentosum* [XP; a disease caused by a deficiency in NER and character-ized by extreme susceptibility to ultraviolet (UV) light-associated skin cancer], normal individuals differ widely in their capacity to repair DNA damage by both exogenous agents, such as tobacco smoke and exposure to sunlight, and endogenous reactions, such as oxidations. Such interindividual differences probably have a genetic origin. Unlike the syndromes men-tioned earlier, these genetic polymorphisms are highly prevalent in the general population and have been associated with a slight increase in cancer risk.

XRCC1 (X-ray repair cross-complementing) plays a role in the BER pathway, interacts with DNA polymerase β, poly-ADP-ribose polymerase (PARP), and DNA ligase III, and has a BCRT domain, characteristic of proteins involved in cycle checkpoint functions and response to DNA damage. Ionizing radiation and alkylating agents cause DNA base damage and strand breaks, which elicit the BER system. Shen et al. (30) identified three coding polymorphisms in the *XRCC1* gene at codons 194 (Arg → Trp), 280 (Arg → His), and 399 (Arg → Gln), coding for nonconservative amino acid changes (including the Arg 399Gln change in the PARP binding domain), which suggests potential functional importance, but their impact on phenotype is unknown. Genotype and allele frequencies for *XRCC1* polymorphisms 194Trp and 280His alleles are low in blacks (0.05 for 194Trp and 0.02 for 280His) and Caucasians (0.06 for 194Trp and 0.03 for 280His), but are significantly more prevalent in Taiwanese (0.27 for 194Trp and 0.11 for 280His). The 399Gln-allele frequency is significantly different among all three populations, with the frequency being highest in Caucasians (0.37), intermediate in Taiwanese (0.26), and lowest in blacks (0.17).

XRCC3 (X-ray repair cross-complementing) participates in DNA double-strand break recombination repair and is a member of an emerging family of Rad-51-related proteins which probably participate in homolo-gous recombination to maintain chromosome stability and repair DNA damage. Thr241Met substitution in *XRCC3* is a nonconservative change, but it does not reside in the ATP-binding domains, which are the only func-tional domains that have been identified in the protein at this time (30).

XPD/ERCC2 (excision repair cross-complementing) is involved in the NER pathway (29), which recognizes and repairs a wide range of structurally unrelated lesions such as bulky adducts and thymidine dimers. The XPD protein is an evolutionarily conserved helicase, a subunit of transcription factor IIH (TFIIH), that is essential for transcription and NER. Recently, the entire coding region of the DNA repair gene *XPD/ERCC2* was resequenced in 12 normal individuals, and six polymorphic variants were described (30). Rare XPD mutations, which prevent interaction with p44, another subunit of TFIIH, and reduce its helicase activity result in three distinct clinical genetic diseases: XP, trichothiodystrophy, and XP combined with Cockayne sydrome. The functional significance of these newly identified XPD variants is not known. Many *XPD* polymorphisms are identified, e.g., *C22541A* at codon 156 of exon 6, at codon 199 (Ile→Met), at codon 312 (Asp→Asn), and *A35931C* at codon 751 of exon 23 (Lys→Gln). Allele frequencies are higher than 25% in sample populations from North America, England, and Italy, but homozygous alleles are very rare. XPD-Lys751Gln polymorphism, a conservative substitution, is associated with reduced in vitro repair of X-ray-induced DNA damage.

ERCC1 is involved in the incision step of NER. DNA incision on both sides of the lesion occurs using two different endonucleases. It is believed that the 3′ incision is made first by the XPG protein followed by 5′ incision carried out by the complex formed by XPF and ERCC1 proteins. Therefore, ERCC1 is important in repairing DNA damage (e.g., removal of DNA adducts and rejoining of double-strand DNA breaks caused by X-ray irradiation). Recently, a polymorphism in the 3′-untranslated region of ERCC1, a subunit of the NER complex, has been discovered. This A/C polymorphism at 8092 of ERCC1 (30) affects mRNA stability and reduces protein activity.

The human *OGG1* gene (*hOGG1*) belongs to the *BER* gene family and encodes a DNA glycosylase/AP-lyase, specifically catalyzing the excision of 8-OH-dG:dC but is completely inactive against 8-OH-dG:dA (31). The gene *hOGG1* encoding for this activity has been cloned and described, and is expressed in seven major alternative splicing isoforms, but only one of them, Type la, has a nuclear translocation signal. A further splice variant Type 2a has been located on the inner membrane of mitochondria and is suggested to be responsible for the removal of 8-OH-dG in mitochondria. Expression of *hOGG1* has been shown in several different tissues, the highest amounts being found in both fetal and adult brain tissue. Relatively high expression has also been detected in human lung, kidney, thymus, testis, and ovary. Several variant *hOGGI* alleles have been described, some only in tumors. Whether these mutations represent polymorphisms has not been studied as yet. Kohno et al. (32) described a polymorphism in exon 7 causing an amino acid change 326 Ser→Cys. This polymorphism has been shown to be very common in the Japanese population (Cys allele frequency about 40%), but less common in Caucasians (about 25%). The 326Cys variant has been shown to have weaker 8-OH-dG repair capacity in complementation assays using an *E. coli* mutant strain deficient in 8-OH-dG repair (mutM/mutY). A very recent report (33) states that NO, an inflammatory mediator, directly inhibits this important BER enzyme.

INFLUENCE OF METABOLIC AND DNA REPAIR GENO(PHENO)-TYPES ON BIOLOGICAL INDICATORS OF GENOTOXIC RISK

In the last 10 years, several research groups have been involved in studying the influence of metabolic and DNA repair genotypes on biological indicators of genotoxic risk in environmental, occupational, or life-style types of exposure.

Internal Dose Indicators: Urinary Metabolites and Mutagens

Studies on the modulation of genetic polymorphisms on metabolites of gen-otoxic compounds are mainly limited to measuring the excretion of the rele-vant mercapturic acids or urinary metabolites. The former is greater in subjects with high GST activity, with a specificity that changes according to compound (e.g., 1,3-dichloroprene and styrene). In particular, styrene biomarkers are so greatly influenced by *GSTM1* genotype (excretion being fivefold greater in *GSTM*-positive subjects) that two different biological exposure indices (BEI) have been proposed specifically for mercapturic acid (34). Instead, in exposure to benzene, the alternative metabolic pathway is that of *trans–trans* muconic acid (*t,t*-MA), which is amplified in subjects with reduced GST activity (*GSTM1* and *T1* null) (35). In exposure to ben-zene, there is also an increase in *t,t*-MA with other genotypes, although further experimental verification is necessary.

As regards exposure to PAHs, according to some studies urinary 1-pyrenol and PAH metabolites are significantly influenced by genotypes *CYP1A1* or *GSTM1* null; in exposure to aromatic amines, the influence of NAT2 on exposure markers (levels of acetylated and nonacetylated meta-bolites) has been confirmed. Of interest is the recent report of the evident effect of reduced CYP2A6 activity (genotype *CYP2A6 *4/*4*) on the half-life of levels of urinary cotinine in the urine of smokers (36), revealing a limitation in the analysis of urinary cotinine in evaluating exposure to tobacco smoke.

In urinary mutagenicity, the effect of genotype *GSTM1* null, and of the same genotype combined with *NAT2* slow, in nonsmoker subjects highly exposed to PAH and in coke oven workers who are also smokers has been reported. As regards exposure to aromatic amines (primary and heterocyc-lic) due to smoking or dietary habits (after a meal of barbecued meat), a clearcut influence of CYP1A2- and NAT2-mediated metabolic activities

(EM and slow acetylators) on the excretion of mutagenic substances in urine after exposure has been observed (7).

Biologically Effective Dose Indicators: Protein and DNA Adducts

Only one study reports the effect of genotype *NAT2* in working exposure to aromatic amines. Many studies on tobacco smoking habits report an increase in the adduct specific to the hemoglobin of 4-aminobiphenyl (4-ABP) in subjects with geno–phenotype NAT2 slow, alone or in combination with high CYP1A2 activity. The influence of *GSTT1* null on the hydro-xyethylvaline/hemoglobin adduct (HEV) in exposure to ethylene oxide (hospital workers and smokers) and to acrylonitrile (smokers) has been reported (7). Most studies assessing the effects of genotypes in biological monitoring in exposure to genotoxic agents refer to DNA adducts and many to environmental exposure to PAHs, both in the workplace and due to life-style. The clearcut influence of genotype *GSTM1* null is evident on levels of DNA aromatic adducts in white blood cells or their lymphomonocyte fraction (generally determined with the ^{32}P postlabeling method), either alone or in combination with mutated genotypes *CYP1A1* (with greater activity). The involvement of the metabolic pathways of activation/detoxification of PAHs has also been confirmed, since the specific adduct benzo[*a*]pyrene diol epoxide (B[*a*]PDE)–DNA, determined by HPLC-fluorescence, is higher in coke oven workers with genotypes *GSTM1* null and *CYP1A1* *1/*2 or *2/*2 (37,38). The literature contains sporadic reports on the influence of two other polymorphic cytochrome genotypes, *CYP2D6* and *CYP3A*, on the level of DNA aromatic adducts. In exposure to tobacco smoke, other genotypes as well as *GSTM1* *0/*0 have been shown to be capable of modulating the level of DNA aromatic adducts: reduced GSTP1 activity, genotypes *NAT1* and *NAT2* slow acetylators, *ALDH2* *1/*2 or *2/*2 (with reduced ALDH2 activity), and *GSTT1* *0/*0, alone or together with geno-types *NAT2* and *NAT1* slow (7).

Some of the repair polymorphisms of DNA, only recently identified, have been related to the level of DNA adducts in working and/or life-style exposure to genotoxins. Even the presence of only one of the mutated alleles of DNA repair genes (*XRCC1* 399 Gln and/or *XPD* 751 Gln) can cause a significant increase in DNA damage in the general population (39–41). The specific aflatoxin–DNA adduct has also been found to be higher in the placenta of mothers with reduced repair capacity, due to the presence of the mutated allele *XRCC1 399 Gln* (42).

Oxidative damage to DNA, of both endogenous and exogenous origin, may be estimated from the levels of 8-hydroxy-deoxyguanosine (8-OH-dG) in urine or leucocyte DNA. Also reported is the significant influence of gen-otype *ALDH2* *2/*2 (reduced detoxifying enzyme activity) on increased levels of 8-OH-dG in the leucocytes of alcohol drinkers.

Indicators of Early Biological Effects: Exchanges Between Sister Chromatids, Chromosome Aberrations and Micronuclei, COMET, and Other Indicators of Genotoxic Damage

Many studies on the frequency of SCE in human lymphocytes indicate an interaction between this biomarker of genotoxic effect and genotypes. It should be noted that the baseline level of SCE is influenced both by the genetic characteristics of the individual and by the interaction between those characteristics and exposure to environmental or endogenous genotoxins (e.g., halomethanes, ethylene oxide, fatty acid peroxides). The baseline value of SCE in *GSTT1* active subjects is lower than that of *GSTT1* null subjects. Thus, identification of *GSTT1* subjects (of either type) must definitely be borne in mind when SCE are used as biomarkers to highlight genotoxic damage in man. Workplace studies have reported the influence of *GSTM1* null on SCE in exposure to epichloridrine and genotype *ALDH2* (with low detoxifying activity), alone or in combination with genotype *CYP2E1* with high metabolizing activity, and mutated *XRCC1* (43) in exposure to chloride vinyl monomer (CVM).

Increased frequency of CA in the lymphocytes of peripheral blood has been associated with a greater probability of developing tumors later, highlighting the importance of finding the increased frequency of this indicator in populations exposed to genotoxins. In two different studies on working exposure to styrene, genotype *EPHX* slow was found to be associated with increased CA (44,45). The same finding occurred in a case of exposure to a mixture of pesticides, due to the association of genotypes unfavorable to detoxification, i.e., *CYP2E1, GSTM1,* and *PON1,* and in one case of exposure to pollutants in an urban area, due to an association between *GSTM1* null and *NAT2* slow. In workers exposed to low concentrations of 1,3-butadiene, CA were more frequent in subjects with no *GSTT1* activity. There have been no studies until now on the effects of genetic polymorphisms on the frequency of MN, either in human lymphocytes or in other cell types.

Some studies assessing the influence of metabolic polymorphisms on genetic damage due to exposure to environmental xenobiotics applied the relatively new COMET method, instead of the more usual cytogenetic tests. Gel electrophoresis of DNA of single cells treated with alkali [single cell gel electrophoresis (SCGE) or COMET] is a very sensitive method for measuring DNA helix breaks caused by exposure to genotoxic substances. In working exposure to styrene, a significant increase in DNA damage measured by the COMET assay has been found, especially in subjects with high activating capacity (*CYP2E1*3*) (45). Some types of exposure have been studied according to their capacity to produce in vivo mutations in man. Mutation at the *HPRT* locus (resistence to thioguanine) of circulating lymphocytes has been assessed in occupational exposure to genotoxic agents, and is influenced by metabolic genotypes *CYP2E1*1/*3* and *GSTP1*A/*B* in exposure to styrene (45) and by genotypes *EPHX* with low activity, with and without null polymorphisms of GSTM1 and T1, in exposure to butadiene in the rubber industry (46). An increase in the somatic variants of glycophorin A in erythrocytes, reported in smokers, depends on reduced DNA repair activity of the mutated genotype *XRCC1* 399 Gln (42).

INFLUENCE OF METABOLIC GENO(PHENO)-TYPES ON ADVERSE DRUG SIDE EFFECTS

Butyrylcholinesterase

The plasma enzyme butyrylcholinesterase (BChE) is of clinical interest because it may give rise to genetic variants with decreased ability to hydrolyze, and therefore inactivate, muscle-relaxant drugs such as suxamethonium. Analysis of BChE involves identification of both enzyme activity and biochemical phenotypes, which are used to determine the risk of so-called "scoline apnea." Problems in analysis arise from both the lack of a universally accepted reference method and the variety of substrates and conditions employed for determining activity and phenotypes. The phenotype of BChE is identified by enzyme inhibitors that produce phenotype-specific patterns of "inhibitor numbers."

DNA analysis is now possible, and genotypes can be revealed. BChE is encoded by a single gene locus (*BCHE*), located on the long arm of chromosome 3 at 3q26.49. It is 73 kb long, with four exons separated by three introns. The gene product is the BChE subunit, four of which are needed to activate the enzyme. Exon 2 is large and codes for 83% of the subunit, including the active (esteratic) site at amino acid 198. Analysis of the gene for mutations/polymorphisms causing the observed biochemical phenotypes has isolated those responsible for all of the better-known variants. In particular, abnormal serum cholinesterase (response) phenotypes cause prolonged apnea following succinylcholine administration (called an atypical phenotype), linked to a single nucleotide difference within the triplet codon for amino acid 70 (*BchE D70G*). It is sufficient simply to change AA70 from aspartate to glycine in the atypical (dibucaine-resistant) BChE. This slight structural alteration reduces the binding affinity for choline ester substrates for the atypical enzyme and makes it almost completely ineffective as an esterase for hydrolyzing succinylcholine. About 95% of Caucasians in Canada have normal esterase activity, 3.8% have a mixture of the usual and atypical variants, and about 1 out of 2800 persons manifested only atypical esterase (47). Table 5 shows the identified genetic polymorphisms of *BchE* (48).

Acetylation Polymorphism

Nongenotoxic drugs, the metabolism of which is affected by acetylation, include isoniazid, hydralazine, procainamide, sulfonamides, aminoglutethimide,

Table 5 Genetic Polymorphisms of *BchE*

Variant name (Symbol)	Mutation	Amino acid change
Atypical (A)	nt 209 (GAT - > GGT)	D70G
Fluoride (F1)	nt 728 (ACG - > ATG)	T243M
Fluoride (F2)	nt 1169 (GGT - > GTT)	G390V
Kalow (K)	nt 1615 (GCA - > ACA)	A539T
James (J)	nt 1490 (GAA - > GTA)	E497V
Hammersmith (H)	nt 424 (GTG - > ATG)	V142M

Abbreviation: BchE, butyrylcholinesterase.

and dapsone, in addition to some drugs without free amino groups but with an amino group introduced via metabolism (e.g., caffeine, sulfasazine, nitrazepam, clonazepam). Individuals are identified as rapid or slow acetylators by determining the plasma concentration of a test drug (such as isoniazid) at a specified time after administering a fixed dose.

It has been recognized that a defect(s) in N-acetyltransferase ("slow acetylator" phenotype) may have several adverse drug side-effects, e.g., isoniazid neurotoxicity, drug-induced lupus erythematosus, sulfasazine-induced hemolytic anemia, and phenytoin toxicity from concomitant use of isoniazid. The first recognized case of drug toxicity linked to slow acetylator status was isoniazid neurotoxicity, associated with vitamin B6 (pyridoxine) deficiency, which causes peripheral neuropathy. Treatment with pyridoxine antagonizes the toxicity of isoniazid, which is also a potent central nervous system irritant. Slow acetylators also show a phenytoin–isoniazid interaction in which isoniazid noncompetitively inhibits phenytoin metabolism (hydroxylation), causing reduced renal excretion and enhanced accumulation. Increased phenytoin levels lead to toxic reactions.

The relationship between acetylator status and isoniazid-induced hepatitis in the literature is conflicting. A 20-year database of the occurrence of hepatitis with jaundice was summarized for 1757 slow and 1238 rapid acetylators treated with isoniazid alone or in combination with other anti-TB drugs. The overall incidence of liver damage measured in this way was 1.9% in slow and 1.2% in rapid acetylators. This difference was statistically insignificant, and it was concluded that the incidence of clinical hepatotoxicity with jaundice is unrelated to acetylator status (49). It is well established that isoniazid treatment is associated with hepatotoxicity more frequently in older individuals (over 35 years of age) than in younger patients. Liver damage measured in terms of transaminase elevation was found to be significantly greater among slow (46.6%) than rapid acetylators (13.3%), and the most severe signs of damage were confined to slow acetylators (50). These observations indicate that rapid acetylators are not predisposed to isoniazid-induced liver disease—in fact, the opposite appears to be true. They also indicate that the significance of acetylator status as a predictor of susceptibility to hepatitis depends on the criterion chosen to measure damage. If clinical jaundice is the criterion, liver damage is unrelated to acetylator status. If a biochemical index such as transaminase level is chosen, then there is a relationship. The prevalence of the slow acetylator phenotype in various gene pools is the following; Ethiopian, 90%; Causasian European, 50%; East/Central Asian, 10% to 20%; Canadian Eskimo, 5% (51).

Cytochrome P450 CYP2D6

Phenotype variations in CYP2D6 activity were first described as idiosyncratic adverse responses to debrisoquine, an antihypertensive drug, and included postural hypotension and dizziness. Variability was reflected in changed rates of debrisoquine hydroxylation, the major metabolic pathway for this drug (see section titled "Brief History of Genetic Toxicology"). Cytochrome P450 CYP2D6 is responsible for the metabolism of approximately 20% to 25% of prescription medicines, many of which are common central nervous system and cardiovascular drugs and include carvedilol, S-metoprolol, propafenone, timolol, tricyclic antidepressants, haloperidol, perphenazine, rispiradone, and thioridazine. Mutations in the *CYP2D6* gene may result in ultrarapid (UM), extensive (EM), intermediate (IM), or poor PM phenotypes. Clinically important phenotypes are UM and PM, because when the defect is present, less or more metabolically active forms of drugs occur, respectively, when inactive compounds are administered. On an average, 7% to 10% of Caucasians are PMs. Substantially fewer PMs have been found in Asian and African-American populations. The distribution of the PM phenotype varies according to ethnic group: 7% to 10% among Caucasians, < 1% among East Asians.

CYP2D6 is the primary enzyme that hydroxylates debrisoquine; it also metabolizes many other prescription drugs (~25% of all known drugs). Debrisoquine hydroxylase activity correlates with the presence of variant alleles of *CYP2D6*, at least 20 of which exist, different variants predominating in different ethnic groups (see Table 3 for genotypes). Variants include SNPs in the open reading frame, causing frame shifts or amino acid substitutions. SNPs at exon junctions cause splice variants, gene deletion, and multiple gene copies. The percentage of the EM phenotype also varies among ethnic groups; Northern Europeans (Sweden), 1% to 2%, Southern Europe (Spain, Sicily); 7% to 10%, and North Africa, Middle East (Ethiopia, Saudi Arabia), 20% to 30%. Variations in CYP2D6-dependent metabolic capacity may have major clinical implications and therefore rapid genotyping screening systems are being developed.

Other Metabolic Enzymes

Polymorphisms for other CYP forms also exist. An example is CYP2C19, responsible for the metabolism of the commonly prescribed anticoagulant warfarin. The PM phenotype occurs in 3% to 5% of Caucasians and 20% of ethnic Chinese. PMs are at risk of hemorrhage.

Paraoxonase (PON1) is an HDL-associated enzyme capable of hydrolyzing many substrates, including several organophosphorus (OP) insecticides and nerve agents, oxidized lipids, and a number of drugs or pro-drugs. Two polymorphisms in the *PON1* gene have been described to affect either the catalytic efficiency of hydrolysis or the expression level of PON1. Animal studies characterizing PON1 polymorphisms have demonstrated its importance in modulating OP toxicity and the existence individual PON1 status, i.e., genotype and phenotype taken together rather than genotyping alone. Nevertheless, direct confirmation in humans of the relevance of PON1 status in conferring susceptibility to OP toxicity is still elusive. Recent studies on PON1 status in determining OP susceptibility in, for instance, Gulf War veterans with decreased capacity for detoxifying OP substances resulting from low serum PON1 activity have been reported to have contributed to the development of the Gulf War Syndrome (52). This may represent a step in the right direction, but more studies are needed, with better documentation of both level and consequences of exposure.

More Recent Examples

It has been found that approximately 1 out of 300 pediatric cancer patients treated with thiopurine drugs is at risk of severe life-threatening myelosuppression, due to the complete lack of ability to methylate thiopurines. Metabolic deficiency due to two SNPs in the open reading frame of the thiopurine N-methyl transferase (*TPNMT*) gene results in an inactive enzyme. Additional variations in the 5′ flanking region (17 bp repeat element, repeated four to eight times) probably affect the level of enzyme expression. Routine phenotype screening on red blood cells of TPNMT activity is required, followed by genotying for confirmation.

Final Considerations

Several lines of evidence indicate the influence of genetic constitution on the individual's sensitivity towards drugs used in pharmacological treatment and towards genotoxic carcinogens.

The most recent findings on monitoring exposure to genotoxic agents also indicate that in the future, metabolic polymorphisms must be taken into due account on genetic bases. In particular, this concern applies to genotype *GSTM1* in identifying thioesters, metabolites of benzene, and pyrenol, and also, in the latter case, *CYP1A1*. The unfavorable association for the activation/detoxification metabolism of PAH seems to represent a risk factor, due to the formation of PAH–DNA adducts. The unfavorable combination of the metabolism of aromatic amines, i.e., high activity of CYP1A2/NAT2 slow, is a risk factor both for the formation of 4-ABP protein adducts and for increased excretion of urinary mutagens in smokers. In two studies on occupational exposure to styrene, genotype *EPHX* slow has been found to increase the number of CA, reliable predictive genotoxic markers of carcinogenic risk. The role played by genetic polymorphisms in DNA repair in modulating the genotoxic risk associated with environmental habits such as diet (aflatoxin, PAH) and life-style (smoking habits and general environment) must be studied in further depth.

Results published until now demonstrate that the effect of polymorphisms has mainly been identified in studies in which exposure was clearly defined, the exposure markers used were specific and sensitive, and the genotype(s) analyzed were appropriate for the type of exposure in question. Thus, future studies will require careful advance planning, in choosing both genotypes and the size of the study population, to ensure sufficient statistical power to evaluate genotype combinations, which are significant from the viewpoint of genotoxic risk but which are not frequently found in the general population.

Knowledge of genetic toxicology is becoming increasingly important. Its principal aim is determination of groups at risk, i.e., those subjects who are more susceptible to toxicants. The very fact of exposure is important to reveal individual susceptibility, without which many susceptibility factors cannot be determined. Individual susceptibility to toxicants exists and partly depends on heritable traits, which modify the effects of exposure. Responses/effects depend on the nature of chemical exposure: short-term effects, e.g., those linked to serum cholinesterase (response) geno(pheno) types and long-term, e.g., those linked to the metabolism of genotoxic carcinogens. The former are easier to study and follow as regards effects than the latter since the effect (tumor development) cannot occur.

Genetic toxicology is still a young discipline. Until now, only some of the relevant functions, from the toxicology standpoint, have been studied because of their genetic complexity. In view of the rapid development of molecular biology methods, for example, DNA microarrays are rapidly becoming one of the tools of choice for large-scale toxicogenomic studies— genetic toxicology is expected to become an important field of study.

Ethical Problems

Many studies have shown that genotoxic risk can be modulated by differences in genetic bases and indicate that the consequent risk of cancer can also be modified, suggesting that these markers of individual susceptibility should be evaluated in populations at risk of carcinogenic exposure (e.g., coke oven and aluminium workers occupationally highly exposed to PAHs, smokers) with the aim of identifying subjects who are more susceptible to developing tumors given exposure to carcinogens. The identification of subjects at higher risk, exposure being equal, forms part of biological monitoring and health surveillance of workers exposed to carcinogens. Its aim is precisely the same as that of screening smokers to identify subjects who are susceptible to developing lung cancer, who should then be screened for secondary prevention (early diagnosis). The case of tobacco smokers, in whom abolishing exposure can only be made according to the will of single individuals, is very different from that obtained in the workplace. This is because subjects who are highly susceptible (owing to their peculiar genetic characteristics) can be removed definitively from their at-risk working environment, as opposed to possible primary prevention measures, which aim at minimizing exposure to genotoxic substances in the working environment.

The application of genetic screening highlights several ethical, social, and scientific problems. In the absence of actual exposure to carcinogenic agents, individual susceptibility has little importance, so that the identification and protection of hypersusceptible people is not simply an alternative to reducing exposure to harmful substances in the environment or workplace. It is also true that excluding some types of workers from certain work on the basis of their characteristic and genetically-based hypersusceptiblity to genotoxicants is not without its problems, but it may represent an effective form of prevention. Genetic screening may allow us to estimate the risk associated with exposure to genotoxicants, and may be used as part of routine health surveillance. Therefore, it is only within the context of rigorous disease prevention (by means of more suitable working/ambient/behavioral conditions) and not in the context of the prediction of disease, with the potential for discrimination, that the use and application of genetic biomarkers can be considered as different from other diagnostic actions. Lastly, the practical usefulness of susceptibility tests must satisfy several strictly methodological requirements, such as the use of validated methods, the pertinence of tests based on scientific evidence, and the capacity to classify subjects correctly in relation to their metabolic genotype.

REFERENCES

1. Kalow W, Gunn DR. The relation between dose of succinylcholine and duration of apnea in man. J Pharmacol Exp Ther 1957; 120:203–214.
2. Price Evans DA, Manley KA, McKusick VA. Genetic control of isoniazid metabolism in man. BMJ 1960; 2:485–491.
3. Mahgoub A, Idle JR, Dring LG, Lancaster R, Smith RL. Polymorphic hydroxylation of debrisoquine in man. Lancet 1977; 2:584–586.
4. Hussain SP, Harris CC. Molecular epidemiology and carcinogenesis: endogenous and exogenous carcinogens. Mutat Res 2000; 462:311–322.
5. Bartsch H, Nair U, Risch A, Rojas M, Wikman H, Alexandrov KR. Genetic polymorphism of CYP genes, alone or in combination, as a risk modifier of tobacco-related cancers. Cancer Epidemiol Biomarkers Prev 2000; 9:3–28.
6. Goode EL, Ulrich CM, Potter JD. Polymorphisms in DNA repair genes and associations with cancer risk. Cancer Epidemiol Biomarkers Prev 2002; 11:1513–1530.

7. Pavanello S. Metabolic and DNA repair variations in susceptibility to genotoxins. Polycyclic Arom Comp 2003; 23:49–107.
8. Hagmar L, Stromberg U, Bonassi S, et al. Impact of types of lymphocyte chromosomal aberrations on human cancer risk: results from Nordic and Italian cohorts. Cancer Res 2004; 64:2258–2263.
9. Wong RH, Wang JD, Hsieh LL, Cheng TJ. XRCC1, CYP2E1 and ALDH2 genetic polymorphisms and sister chromatid exchange frequency alterations amongst vinyl chloride monomer-exposed polyvinyl chloride workers. Arch Toxicol 2003; 7:433–440.
10. http://www.imm.ki.se/CYPalleles.
11. Sachse C, Bhambra U, Smith G, et al. Colorectal Cancer Study Group. Polymorphisms in the cytochrome P450 CYP1A2 gene (CYP1A2) in colorectal cancer patients and controls: allele frequencies, linkage disequilibrium and influence on caffeine metabolism. Br J Clin Pharmacol 2003; 55:68–76.
12. McBride OW, Umeno M, Gelboin HV, Gonzalez FJ. A Taq I polymorphism in the human P450IIE1 gene on chromosome 10 (CYP2E). Nucleic Acids Res 1987; 15:10071.
13. Chang TK, Yu L, Goldstein JA, Waxman DJ. Identification of the polymorphically expressed CYP2C19 and the wild-type CYP2C9-ILE359 allele as low-Km catalysts of cyclophosphamide and ifosfamide activation. Pharmacogenetics 1997; 7:211–221.
14. Sachse C, Brockmoller J, Bauer S, Roots I. Cytochrome P450 2D6 variants in a Caucasian population: allele frequencies and phenotypic consequences. Am J Hum Genet 1997; 60:284–295.
15. Seidegard J, Ekstrom G. The role of human glutathione transferases and epoxide hydrolases in the metabolism of xenobiotics. Environ Health Perspect 1997; 105:791–799.
16. Townsend D, Tew K. Cancer drugs, genetic variation and the glutathione-*S*-transferase gene family. Am J Pharmacogen 2003; 3:157–172.
17. McLellan RA, Oscarson M, Alexandrie AK, et al. Characterization of a human glutathione S-transferase mu cluster containing a duplicated GSTM1 gene that causes ultrarapid enzyme activity. Mol Pharmacol 1997; 52:958–965.
18. Board PG, Webb GC, Coggan M. Isolation of a cDNA clone and localization of the human glutathione S-transferase 3 genes to chromosome bands 11q13 and 12q13–14. Ann Hum Genet 1989; 53(Pt 3):205–213.
19. Stucker I, Hirvonen A, de Waziers I, et al. Genetic polymorphisms of glutathione S-transferases as modulators of lung cancer susceptibility. Carcinogenesis 2002; 23:1475–1481.
20. Thier R, Pemble SE, Kramer H, Taylor JB, Guengerich FP, Ketterer B. Human glutathione S-transferase T1-1 enhances mutagenicity of 1,2-dibromoethane, dibromomethane and 1,2,3,4-diepoxybutane in Salmonella typhimurium. Carcinogenesis 1996; 17:163–166.
21. http://www.louisville.edu/medschool/pharmacology/NAT.html.
22. Meyer UA, Zanger UM. Molecular mechanisms of genetic polymorphisms of drug metabolism. Annu Rev Pharmacol Toxicol 1997; 37:269–296.
23. Nowell SA, Massengill JS, Williams S, et al. Glucuronidation of 2-hydroxyamino-1-methyl-6-phenylimidazo[4, 5-b]pyridine by human microsomal

UDP-glucuronosyltransferases: identification of specific UGT1A family iso-forms involved. Carcinogenesis 1999; 20:1107–1114.

24. Rothman N, Smith MT, Hayes RB, et al. Benzene poisoning, a risk factor for hematological malignancy, is associated with the NQO1 609C– > T mutation and rapid fractional excretion of chlorzoxazone. Cancer Res 1997; 57:2839–2842.

25. Moran JL, Siegel D, Ross D. A potential mechanism underlying the increased susceptibility of individuals with a polymorphism in NAD(P)H:quinone oxidor-eductase 1 (NQO1) to benzene toxicity. Proc Natl Acad Sci USA 1999; 96:8150–8155.

26. Costa LG, Cole TB, Jarvik GP, Furlong CE. Functional genomic of the para-oxonase (PON1) polymorphisms: effects on pesticide sensitivity, cardiovascular disease, and drug metabolism. Annu Rev Med 2003; 54:371–392.

27. De Boer J, Hoeijmakers JH. Nucleotide excision repair and human syndromes. Carcinogenesis 2000; 21:453–460.

28. Balajee AS, Bohr VA. Genomic heterogeneity of nucleotide excision repair. Gene 2000; 250:15–30.

29. Friedberg EC. DNA damage and repair. Nature 2003; 421:436–440.

30. Shen MR, Jones IM, Mohrenweiser H. Nonconservative amino acid substitu-tion variants exist at polymorphic frequency in DNA repair genes in healthy humans. Cancer Res 1998; 58:604–608.

31. Boiteux S, Radicella JP. The human OGG1 gene: structure, functions, and its implication in the process of carcinogenesis. Arch Biochem Biophys 2000; 377:1–8.

32. Kohno T, Shinmura K, Tosaka M, et al. Genetic polymorphisms and alterna-tive splicing of the hOGG1 gene, that is involved in the repair of 8-hydroxygua-nine in damaged DNA. Oncogene 1998; 16:3219–3225.

33. Jaiswal M, LaRusso NF, Nishioka N, Nakabeppu Y, Gores GJ. Human Ogg1, a protein involved in the repair of 8-oxoguanine, is inhibited by nitric oxide. Cancer Res 2001; 61:6388–6393.

34. Haufroid V, Jakubowski M, Janasik B, et al. Interest of genotyping and pheno-typing of drug-metabolizing enzymes for the interpretation of biological mon-itoring of exposure to styrene. Pharmacogenetics 2002; 12:691–702.

35. Verdina A, Galati R, Falasca G, et al. Metabolic polymorphisms and urinary biomarkers in subjects with low benzene exposure. J Toxicol Env Heal A 2001; 64:607–618.

36. Yang M, Kunugita N, Kitagawa K, et al. Individual: differences in urinary cotinine levels in japanese smokers: relation to genetic polymorphism of drug-metabolizing enzymes. Cancer Epidemiol Biomarkers Prev 2001; 10:589–593.

37. Pavanello S, Gabbani G, Brugnone F, Maccacaro G, Clonfero E. Influence of GSTM1 genotypes on ANTI-BPDE-DNA adduct levels in mononuclear white blood cells of humans exposed to PAH. Int Arch Occup Environ Health 1999; 72:238–246.

38. Rojas M, Alexandrov K, Cascorbi I, et al. High benzo(a)pyrene diol-epoxide DNA adduct levels in lung and blood cells from individuals with combined CYP1A1 MspI/MspI-GSTM1*0*0 genotypes. Pharmacogenetics 1998; 8: 109–118.

39. Palli D, Vineis P, Russo A, et al. Diet, metabolic polymorphisms and DNA adducts: the EPIC-Italy cross-sectional study. Int J Cancer 2000; 87:444–451.
40. Matullo G, Palli D, Peluso M, et al. XRCC1, XRCC3, XPD gene polymorphisms, smoking and 32P-DNA adducts in a sample of healthy subjects. Carcinogenesis 2001; 22:1437–1445.
41. Hou SM, Falt S, Angelini S, et al. The XPD variant alleles are associated with increased aromatic DNA adduct level and lung cancer risk. Carcinogenesis 2002; 23:599–603.
42. Lunn RM, Langlois RG, Hsieh LL, Thompson CL, Bell DA. XRCC1 polymorphisms: effects on aflatoxin B-1-DNA adducts and glycophorin A variant frequency. Cancer Res 1999; 59:2557–2561.
43. Wong RH, Du CL, Wang JD, Chan CC, Luo JCJ, Cheng TJ. XRCC1 and CYP2E1 polymorphisms as susceptibility factors of plasma mutant p53 protein and anti-p53 antibody expression in vinyl chloride monomer-exposed polyvinyl chloride workers. Cancer Epidemiol Biomarkers Prev 2002; 11:475–482.
44. Somorovska M, Jahnova E, Tulinska J, et al. Biomonitoring of occupational exposure to styrene in a plastics lamination plant. Mutat Res Fundament Molec Mech Mutagen 1999; 428:255–269.
45. Vodicka P, Soucek P, Tates AD, et al. Association between genetic polymorphisms and biomarkers in styrene-exposed workers. Mutat Res 2001; 482:89–103.
46. Abdel-Rahman SZ, Ammenheuser MM, Ward B. Human sensitivity to 1,3-butadiene: role of microsomal epoxide hydrolase polymorphisms. Carcinogenesis 2001; 22:415–423.
47. McGuire MC, Nogueira CP, Bartels CF, et al. Identification of the structural mutation responsible for the dibucaine-resistant (atypical) variant form of human serum cholinesterase. Proc Natl Acad Sci USA 1989; 86:953–957.
48. Goodall R. Association of clinical biochemists analytical investigations standing committee. Cholinesterase: phenotyping and genotyping. Ann Clin Biochem 2004; 41(Pt 2):98–110.
49. Clark DW. Genetically determined variability in acetylation and oxidation. Therapeutic implications. Drugs 1985; 29:342–375.
50. Sharma SK. Antituberculosis drugs and hepatotoxicity. Infect Genet Evol 2004; 4:167–170.
51. Weber WW, Hein DW. Clinical pharmacokinetics of isoniazid. Clin Pharmacokinet 1979; 4:401–422.
52. Mackness B, Durrington PN, Mackness MI. Low paraoxonase in Persian Gulf War Veterans self-reporting Gulf War Syndrome. Biochem Biophys Res Commun 2000; 276:729–733.

7

Identification and Use of Biomarkers in Preclinical Toxicologic Safety Assessment

Donna M. Dambach

Discovery Toxicology, Pharmaceutical Research Institute, Bristol-Myers Squibb, Princeton, New Jersey, U.S.A.

Jean-Charles Gautier

Molecular and Cellular Toxicology, Sanofi-Aventis, Vitry-sur-Seine, France

INTRODUCTION

The aim of this chapter is to offer conceptual and practical consideration on the process of identification of biomarker needs and on the development and application of biomarker platforms for the preclinical assessment of potential safety issues. The chapter will focus on pharmaceutical drug discovery and early development phases, which encompass target identification and validation, compound lead optimization, and preclinical development studies. The use and integration of biomarker data with traditional toxicology endpoints in the development of a risk assessment recommendation are also considered.

In agreement with the NIH Biomarkers Definitions Working Group (1), biomarkers are defined here as measurable and quantifiable characteristics that serve as indicators of pathologic or pharmacologically related events. As such, endpoints that fall under the definition of biomarker would include any semiquantitative or quantitative measurement that will define potential biological outcomes. This would include not only the traditional physiological and biofluid endpoint measurements from blood or urine but also measurable endpoints developed from in vivo or in vitro methods that serve as surrogate indicators of possible adverse events in preclinical species and/or humans. Likewise, the concept of "bridging" biomarkers of toxicity would therefore include not only those biomarkers that span use during in-life studies in preclinical species and also in humans, but also in vitro or ex vivo study results used as surrogate biomarkers that accurately "predict" a toxic outcome in preclinical species and/or humans or to establish in vitro–in vivo correlations.

One of the most important first steps of toxicity biomarker identification is a clear understanding and determination of the particular purpose the biomarker will serve. In particular, toxicity biomarkers that pertain to the assessment of an undesired pharmacologically-mediated effect for a particular molecular target may be identified, in which case, useful application may require the development of single or multiple bridging-type biomarkers for use as counter-screens during early discovery for safety optimization and for continued assessment during both preclinical in-life studies and in clinical trials. The biomarkers would be used during lead optimization to determine if the undesired toxic effect can be dissociated from the desired pharmacology, and during in-life studies or clinical trials to serve as indicators of the adverse effect and to help in determining therapeutic ranges. Other considerations for the application of a particular toxicity biomarker may include whether, as in the case of potential drug-related target organ toxicity, the goal is to identify a biomarker that can be used as a general screen for particular organ-related toxicity in a high-throughput manner or the goal is to identify biomarkers specifically related to a mechanistic pathway. These very different objectives dramatically define the type of studies necessary to identify a potential toxicity biomarker, the degree of validation necessary to apply such a biomarker in a meaningful manner, and, finally, how the data will impact the risk assessment process.

In general, the predominant preclinical applications of toxicity biomarker data include compound lead optimization, the development of a therapeutic index using pharmacodynamic markers and toxicity biomarkers, risk assessment interpretation and recommendations using biomarker data, and the identification of the relevant toxicity biomarkers and assay platforms that will be useful during in-life toxicity studies as well as clinically.

TARGET IDENTIFICATION AND VALIDATION: IDENTIFICATION OF POTENTIAL PHARMACOLOGY-RELATED TOXICITY BIOMARKERS

The initial assessment of toxicity biomarker needs begins with the identification of a potential molecular target. The target may be novel or, more typically, is one that has been identified in the literature. Thus an initial biological understanding of the target and the potential for toxicity when its activity is altered is acquired by discussion with the discovery therapeutic area scientists to understand the proposed pharmacological application to the target. Further, a review of the current literature is necessary in the context of the proposed pharmacological application to achieve an understanding of the potential toxicity issues. Such a review may lead to an immediate identification of potential target organ toxicity or undesired pharmacological effects for which biomarkers are known or for which new biomarkers may need to be generated to assess potential toxicity. At this stage, the biomarker assessment is strictly based on potential effects caused by alteration of the molecular target, and not on the potential for chemical structure-based toxicity, as compound series are often not yet identified.

The experimental paradigms used during target discovery also lend themselves to the identification of potential toxicity issues (2,3). This would include an understanding of related targets, e.g., isoforms, and the selectivity of the target versus these related forms. This generally requires the generation of in vitro binding or functional assays to assess selectivity, and the examination of tissue distribution of the target or related targets in both human and preclinical species tissues by methods such as tissue microarrays, northern analysis, RT–PCR, in situ hybridization, western analysis, enzyme linked immunosorbent assay (ELISA), and/or immunohistochemistry. The discovery biologist will use these approaches to verify the presence of the target, whereas the toxicologist will use these approaches to identify organs that may be affected by potential off-target or exaggerated activity. Understanding the cross-species conservation of the target also assists in determining the appropriate use of preclinical species as models during the assessment of potential mechanism-based toxicity. In addition to tissue distribution, this would include evaluation of the gene and protein homology and the differences in target binding affinities across species. In the instance in which a target is highly specific for humans, e.g., therapeutic monoclonal antibody, human-specific assays of potential target-related toxicity have to be developed, and the preclinical species can only be used to evaluate potential off-target toxicity.

Genetically modified (GM) animals, in particular mice, have been extensively utilized during the target identification and validation phases (4,5). Likewise, GM animals have utility in safety assessment. In particular, phenotypic assessment of GM mice can give an idea of a "worst-case scenario" related to the complete loss or exaggeration of function of a molecular target, which may be the only practical means available for a physiologically integrated evaluation of novel targets. This type of assessment has been used with success for target validation. In particular, Zambrowicz et al. (2003) found a good correlation between the phenotypes of knockout mice and realized the clinical efficacy of the intended targets for the 100 best-selling drugs (6). Thus, this initial phenotypic assessment can be used to identify biomarker needs to monitor toxicity in the organ(s) identified.

However, there are two major issues limiting the interpretive use of GM mice. First, the phenotypic changes seen may more closely mimic developmental defects from complete loss of target and not be representative of the more likely partial inhibition in an adult population administered a drug. In addition, the gene deletion may result in embryonic lethality and assessment of an adult phenotype would not be possible. Additional biomarkers, assays, or investigative studies may be necessary at some point to provide insight into the relevance and mechanism of the potential toxicity in an adult population for a toxicity identified using GM mice. Second, in many cases the embryonic or developmental loss of a target does not affect the development of an animal, which appears phenotypically normal. This is widely acknowledged to be due to some level of functional redundancy or compensatory mechanism allowing for maintenance of normal function (5,7). This outcome may, in fact, predict the outcome in the adult population; alternatively, the compensatory mechanisms may mask a potential effect.

Nonetheless, the development of biomarkers based on examination of a GM animal phenotype is useful especially as it may relate to truly novel targets, potential reproductive or developmental toxicity, and as indicators of potential pharmacologically-mediated organ toxicity. There is also the opportunity to use more refined GM animals for safety assessment, mechanistic investigation, and biomarker identification that may be more applicable to an adult population. These include the use of conditional knock-out mice, dominant negative transgenic mice, "humanized" transgenic mice, and heterozygous mice. These GM models are often applied in a more directed manner as tools for investigative studies, which are discussed later in the chapter.

In summary, during the target validation phase, biomarker assessment of potential target organ toxicity due to pharmacological activity is identified by literature assessment, tissue distribution studies, and evaluation of GM animals, if they exist. These data can be used to generate an initial toxicity risk assessment strategy that includes biomarkers, which can be applied to monitor potential toxicity during the lead optimization and development phases.

DISCOVERY LEAD OPTIMIZATION: BIOMARKER ASSESSMENT OF PHARMACOLOGY-RELATED AND CHEMICAL-RELATED TOXICITY

At this stage in the drug discovery process, added to assessment of pharmacology-related toxicity is the evaluation of chemical-based toxicity. As such, the toxicity assessment strategy includes utilization of biomarkers related to the particular molecular target, as well as indicators of issues associated with compound chemistry. During lead optimization, applications of toxicity biomarker data include compound ranking and/or structure–activity relationship (SAR) investigation for identification of an efficacious compound with an optimal safety profile, the initial development of a thera-peutic index using pharmacodynamic markers from in vitro assays or in vivo disease models compared to the toxicity biomarkers, a risk assessment inter-pretation of biomarker data, and with respect to any identified safety issues, the identification of the suite of relevant toxicity biomarkers and assay plat-forms that will be useful during in-life toxicity studies and in clinical trials.

Fundamental to the process of target proof-of-concept is the use of in vitro models and animal models. These approaches are utilized in a similar manner as surrogate models for the assessment of potential off-target or chemical-based toxicity, and the same criteria are also applied to these toxi-city models, i.e., the molecular target of interest is expressed and/or the model system has some relevance to in vivo application (8). With respect to both pharmacology-based and chemical-based toxicity, a major concern is off-target activity due to binding of related molecular targets or due to a compound substructure interacting with nontarget sites. An additional area of concern is toxicity related to the metabolic fate of a compound. As such, a significant aspect of risk assessment during the preclinical discovery period is oriented toward these types of assessment. Many surrogate biomarker platforms already exist in later development to assess these issues, e.g., geno-toxicity assays and in-life safety assessments; however, these assessments are now often initiated during the discovery period through the use of additional biomarker platforms that take advantage of in vitro systems and the applica-tion of molecular-based technologies. The goals of these earlier assays are to: (i) serve as higher throughput screens to "flag" potential liabilities or as predictors of an outcome, i.e., those that have good concordance or high sensitivity and specificity, and (ii) have minimal compound requirements.

During lead optimization, the use of indicator assays for safety assess-ment of compounds or compound series in parallel, with refinement of target efficacy, leads to a more efficient use of resources and time. Early in this process, based on the sheer number of different compounds (tens to hundreds), there is a need to effectively select a manageable number of the most promising candidates. One practical approach is to incorporate a multi-tiered safety evaluation scheme that uses both in vitro and in vivo platforms to sequentially remove the most undesirable compounds, while building a relevant data set for canditate compounds, thereby resulting in a more complete risk assessment. Specifically, the sequential assessment is part of a decision-tree algorithm that begins with higher throughput screens that may have a high false-positive rate, but will also have a low false-negative rate. The results of these sentinel screens are then verified by a second-tier assay that has better sensitivity, specificity or relevance for the outcome. As such, in vitro assay suites and in vivo studies can be used to progressively verify the previous assay results, as well as add to the assessment of the relevance to humans and an understanding of specific mechanisms of toxicity. Utilizing multiple endpoints for risk analysis will also help to overcome the limitations of a single endpoint, e.g., using preclinical species alone to predict outcomes in humans. Examples of biomarker platform applications used during the discovery phase are described in the following sections. The basic concepts described can be applied to any area of biomarker development for safety assessment.

In Vitro System Applications

Safety Pharmacology Biomarkers

In vivo assessment of safety pharmacology using physiological and clinical pathology biomarkers is an established standard of preclinical safety assessment that is a part of International Conference for Harmonization (ICH) guidelines (9). Addition of in vitro biomarker platforms for particular safety pharmacology organ assessment during the lead optimization phase provides an earlier indication of potential safety issues (10,11). This type of strategy not only provides a mechanism to evaluate structurally distinct chemical series for concurrent efficacy and safety optimization, but also buys time for follow-up studies to verify any suspect findings and determine their relevance (11–13).

One of the most mature examples of this strategy is the evaluation of cardiac QT prolongation. Drug-related prolongation of the electrocardiographic QT interval has a high associated risk for the development of the potentially fatal "torsades de pointes" arrhythmia, which in turn has been strongly associated with blockage of the cardiac potassium channel containing subunits encoded by the *hERG* gene (human ether-a-go-go) (14). The elucidation of this mechanistic relationship has led to the development of high-throughput hERG binding assays and medium throughput heterologous cellular hERG expression systems that utilize electrophysiological patch clamp analysis to measure functional changes in the ion channel that are predictive of clinical outcome (14,15).

An obvious strategy for the application of these assays in a discovery setting would be to utilize them in a sequential manner to initially screen larger numbers of structurally diverse compounds with the higher-throughput assay and use the cell-based system as a next step to assess the functional relevance of the screening assay for the chemical candidate or series. This would be followed by further assessment in an integrated functional system using ex vivo tissue models, e.g., Purkinje fiber action potential assessment, and/or in vivo evaluation in telemeterized animals (15). In these higher tier, integrated models, drug-related effects on the hERG channel are placed in the context potential drug-related effects on other ion channels involved in cardiac depolarization and repolarization, e.g., calcium and sodium channels, which may have either mitigating or exacerbating effects. Together, this type of assessment may not only predict the potential outcome but also the underlying mechanism when an effect is present.

In addition, exposure relationships acquired during in vivo studies can be used to generate therapeutic indices and to generate bridging in vitro–in vivo exposure correlations to assess potential clinical risk. This is a classic example of the integrated use of these tiered assays for decision-making regarding the lead optimization and advancement of a compound (16). To this end, a therapeutic index recommendation of $\geq$30-fold has been suggested as an indicator of reduced clinical cardiac QT prolongation liability. This particular index is based on in vitro–in vivo correlations between hERG assay IC_{50} values and the highest anticipated clinical exposures (unbound drug) for a set of pro- and non-proarrhythmic drugs (14). These types of surrogate systems are also immediately useful in defining offending SAR during this lead optimization process.

Similar sequential assessment strategies can be put in place for a more generalized assessment of other off-target binding (11,17). First-tier screening for a large number (>10) of predominantly human physiological targets, encompassing receptors, ion channels, transporters, and enzymes, can be accomplished by the use of binding assays that are available commercially or which can be developed in-house. In this paradigm, binding of a candidate drug is typically assessed at a single concentration. Interpretation of significant binding or inhibition of function are based on the pharmacological target, the physiological relevance of the off-target interaction, and assessment of the safety window with respect to either in vitro pharmacodynamic parameters or in vivo efficacy exposures. Further guidance can be obtained by comparing the binding data to known positive controls included in the screen. Off-target interactions deemed to be potentially significant can be further characterized by follow-up IC_{50} and selectivity (K_i) determination to allow for more precise safety window assessment.

Equally important are follow-up functional assessments to determine the significance of the binding and the type of activity, i.e., agonist or antagonist. Functional assessments can be accomplished either by in vitro, ex vivo, or in vivo methods. In vitro and ex vivo platforms often involve the use of primary cell cultures or cell lines, co-cultures or isolated organs, such as aortic rings, and the measurement of the relevant biomarker or physiologic parameter associated with the particular off-target binding in question. Physiological endpoints are often the typical biomarkers of activity in vivo, such as changes in blood pressure or heart rate. In many instances, the binding targets and their physiological effects are conserved across species; therefore, functional assays serve as a reasonable bridging biomarker to assess the relevance of off-target binding and to further refine safety intervals. However, species differences do exist and, if known, the relevance of a finding in a species with a particularly heightened sensitivity should be a component of the overall interpretation of the relevance to humans. Additional investigative work may be necessary to clarify or define the surrogate species-to-human relationship. Data generated from these surrogate safety pharmacology assays can be used to formulate a biomarker strategy to monitor for these effects during in-life studies.

Hepatotoxicity Biomarkers

With respect to target organ toxicity, more successful prediction of idiosyncratic hepatotoxicity has been a recognized need in the pharmaceutical industry for some time, as indicated by the number of drug withdrawals and the severity of the outcome, i.e., liver failure and death (18). Data suggest that idiosyncratic reactions are likely the result of multiple factors including individual-specific responses (18). Further, this type of toxicity occurs with very low frequency in humans (1 in 10,000 to 1 in 100,000) and therefore it is impractical to appropriately power preclinical animal studies. Finally, due to the lack of sufficient data, it is difficult to assess the value of preclinical animal studies to predict hepatotoxicity in humans (19,20). As such, there is extensive literature related to hepatoxicity prediction. Commonly described paradigms for the predictive assessment of liver toxicity include both in vitro and in vivo assessments (12,21–26). In particular, strategies to evaluate the potential for hepatototoxicity have taken on the use of immortalized cell lines as well as the use of primary human cell cultures to better approximate the metabolizing enzyme content of the human liver (21,24,27,28). Comparison of results from in vitro primary cultures from preclinical species to results from in vivo toxicity studies in preclinical species allows determination of in vitro–in vivo correlations. Further comparisons can then be made between human and preclinical species primary cultures to help assess relevance to humans. Co-culture systems, liver slices and whole, perfused liver systems may also be used in a similar manner. However, these systems are not conducive to high- or medium-throughput screening and therefore are often utilized during investigative toxicology studies (21–23,29,30).

Although general cytotoxicity is the most common endpoint used to screen for hepatotoxicity, the measurement of specific endpoints to assess underlying mechanisms of cytotoxicity, e.g., apoptosis or mitochondrial dysfunction, provides further insight for investigative purposes, as well as refinement of relevant biomarker information (24). These in vitro surrogate systems may also be used as part of a larger profiling paradigm to characterize the metabolic fate of compounds and whether metabolism contributes to toxicity. For example, primary hepatocyte cultures can be used to assess the potential for drug–drug interactions, such as CYP450 induction by a compound, and to identify metabolites (31,32). Additional in vitro metabolic assessments include determination of whether a compound is a significant substrate for specific phase I enzymes using isolated microsomal or supersomal preparations (metabolic stability) or phase II enzymes using primary human hepatocytes, whether a compound acts as an inhibitor of a particular CYP450 enzyme, and whether a formed metabolite is reactive, leading to macromolecular adduct formation or to enzymatic inactivation (32–34). Immortalized cell lines that overexpress individual human CYP450 isoenzymes in the absence of phase II enzymatic activity and that can be used to predict the potential for direct or metabolism-mediated acute hepatotoxicity have also been developed (26,35).

Analyzing the results of each of these composite surrogate assays in the total context of all assay data yields a much more informed risk assessment of the compound. Identification of a potential liability using these methods may then initiate a decision-analysis algorithm, such as whether to identify compounds with better metabolic and safety profiles, or whether other favorable characteristics of the compound warrant further metabolic and safety characterization. For example, drug metabolism data can be used to select the most relevant preclinical species for further in vivo toxicokinetic and safety studies to assess the fate of a compound in an integrated system. If drug metabolism data suggests that a potential toxicity may be mediated by alteration of a particular enzyme, e.g., polymorphism, the susceptibility of compound-related hepatotoxicity can potentially be modeled in hepatocytes from animal species that have specific enzyme defects or in transgenic mice that have gene deletions for specific enzymes (25).

In vitro hepatocyte culture systems, as well as liver samples from in-life studies, are one of the most frequently used cell types for biomarker discovery, especially with regard to the use of molecular profiling technologies, i.e., transcriptomics, proteomics, and metabonomics, as evidenced by the vast literature. These technologies have been most commonly utilized in the following ways: (i) as a component of traditional investigative toxicology studies that contribute to hypothesis-driven research through which potentially useful organ-specific or mechanism-based toxicity biomarkers have been identified, (ii) to identify characteristic or signature patterns that allow assessment of similarity to known toxicants, and (iii) for the refinement or enhancement of current biomarker platforms (36–38). Although hepatocytes are used here as a relevant example, these approaches can be applied to any cell culture or organ system platform.

Genotoxicity Biomarkers

Compound-induced mutagenicity and clastogenicity are significant barriers to compound development. This has also become an issue for the newer generation cytostatic oncology drug classes, for which treatment regimes are more representative of chronic disease management. The Ames bacterial reverse mutation assay and both the in vitro chromosomal aberration and in vivo erythrocyte micronucleus assays serve as standard indicator assays for mutagenicity and clastogenicity, respectively, and are necessary for investigational new drug applications (39). Typically these assays are performed during later stages of preclinical development and require substantial amounts of compound, i.e., gram amounts. A number of medium-through-put in vitro assays that require small amounts of compound, e.g., 2 to 30 mg, have been developed to examine the mutagenic and clastogenic potential of compounds. The small compound requirements and faster throughput have made these assays very amenable to application during early drug discovery, with the goals being to identify potential issues and develop an understanding of SAR in order to design these characteristics out of the compound.

There are several non-GLP (good laboratory practice) mutagenicity assays that have been used in this capacity, such as three assays that are derived from the standard GLP Ames the plate-based miniaturized and abbreviated Ames assay; the non-plate-based Ames II assay; and an assay that is based on inducing the DNA repair apparatus, the SOS chromotest (40–43). Each of these assays have been reported to have greater than 85% concordance with the standard GLP Ames, thus these assays can be utilized as surrogates for Ames testing to identify potential mutagenicity issues during lead optimization. Furthermore, data generated from these assays can be coupled with in silico computational mutagenicity SAR databases, such as DEREK for Windows (Lhasa Limited, Leeds, U.K.), so that SAR testing can be performed to identify the offending chemophore with the goal of removing the mutagenic potential while maintaining efficacy (44–46). A similar approach has been adopted to examine the clastogenic potential of compounds via utilization of either the in vitro chromosome aberration or in vitro micronucleus assays (47), the latter of which has been reported to have 80% or more concordance with the in vivo erythrocyte micronucleus assay (48,49). In addition to detection of potential clastogens, the in vitro micronucleus assay will also detect mutagens and aneugens (50). Thus, these assays for genotoxicity that exhibit good concordance to regulatory standard assays are examples of bridging biomarkers for these endpoints. As a result, these assays can be applied much earlier in the discovery process so that compounds can be optimized away from the potential issue of genotoxicity, resulting in greater compound success and far greater cost savings.

There has also been extensive work to develop assays for nongenotoxic carcinogenicity through the use of mammalian cell transformation assays, which can actually identify both nongenotoxic and genotoxic compounds (50). However, these assays are labor-intensive and because of the uncertainties of extrapolating data obtained in these systems to predict complex tumorogenesis biology in vivo, these assays have been used predominantly as tools to investigate compound-related mechanisms of carcinogenicity (51).

In Vivo System Applications

During the discovery phase, there are several opportunities for in vivo toxicity assessment. Examples include evaluation of animals during efficacy studies with additional disease-free satellite animal groups administered higher doses of compound (e.g., $\leq$10-fold margin), single ascending-dose toxicokinetic/tolerability studies, and short-term (<4-week) exploratory toxicology studies. During such studies, traditional biomarkers utilized for toxicity assessment, e.g., physiology measurements, clinical hematology and biochemical parameters, macroscopic and microscopic tissue evaluation, as well as specific biomarkers of potential issues identified during target validation and through in vitro indicator assays, can be assessed in the context of in vivo exposures. Additionally, there is an opportunity to assess the potential for unexpected compound-related toxicity in animal disease models, for which the systemic effects of a disease process may lead to exacerbation of toxicity (52).

The identification or confirmation of a potential toxicity during in-life studies provides an early safety window estimate that can then be applied to human dose projections. This also allows for more focused development of clinically appropriate bridging biomarkers. Investigative toxicology studies can be initiated to examine potential mode or mechanism of toxicity, i.e., whether pharmacology- or chemically-based, and relevance to humans, e.g., species-specific issues. Information gained during these investigations will contribute to compound advancement decisions, refinement of useful biomarkers, and new strategies for back-up programs including the development of counterscreens.

Any biomarker platform can be utilized during these early in-life studies, and often the most commonly utilized biomarkers are those that are well established and validated, i.e., physiological measurements and clinical hematology and biochemistry parameters derived from blood and urine. In recent years, technological advancements have allowed a greater use of other molecular endpoints, e.g., mRNA levels and imaging modalities (53,54), many of which can be transferred directly to clinical use. Historically, investigative studies have been and will continue as the principal source of biomarker discovery. This is inherent in the methodology by which the delineation of the mechanism of toxicity results in the discovery of its components, and these in turn may have predictive value. This topic will be discussed in greater detail in the next section.

PRECLINICAL DEVELOPMENT: APPLICATION AND REFINEMENT OF BIOMARKERS

Biomarker Applications

In vivo models of disease are often not available and the first in vivo safety assessment is made during studies in support of the development of a drug. Testing requirements to support a new drug application have been specified under the ICH guidelines and consist of escalating single and repeated administrations in at least two animal species (one rodent and one non-rodent species) in order to find the target organs for toxicity and to evaluate the possibility for safety margin. There are also guidelines to assess neurologic, ophthalmologic, cardiovascular, respiratory, and renal functions (safety pharmacology), genotoxicity and carcinogenicity, reproductive and developmental toxicity, immunotoxicity, and toxicokinetics (55). The assays outlined in the ICH guidelines are, in effect, surrogate assays used to predict potential toxicity and include both in vitro assays and in vivo studies. Results obtained from these studies are used to determine the starting dose in phase I clinical trials, to guide the monitoring of potential side effects in healthy volunteers and during proof-of-concept studies, and to define potential adverse effects for labeling. It is during these toxicity studies that the synthesis of all of the biomarker data gained during discovery may be applied. At the transition from discovery to early development, the biomarker data generated can be used to develop a risk assessment summary and biomarker monitoring strategy, and to detail issues that need further investigation.

Identification of toxicity during an in-life study, whether predicted or unexpected, will necessitate some degree of investigation of that toxicity to characterize the underlying mechanism, e.g., pharmacology- or chemical-based, and the relevance to humans. Data previously obtained during discovery can be used to support any additional investigative work and conclusions. This investigation will include the identification of potential biomarkers of toxicity that may be useful clinically to assess toxicity and to drive development with quantitative safety margins. Identified biomarkers of toxicity are also used to develop in vitro-based or in vivo-based counter-screens to assist in the selection of back-up compounds.

Biomarker Considerations

Ideally, to be of practical use in the development phase of drug candidates, a biomarker of toxicity should be sensitive, specific for the toxicological change, and detectable in easily accessible tissues samples. Traditional indicators of target organ toxicity used in preclinical safety studies consist of a battery of clinical pathology parameters in blood and urine coupled with histopathologic examination of altered tissues. Several analytes and enzymes are used to assess the integrity and the function of organs. For example, serum transferases (both ALT; aspartate aminotransferase and AST; alanine aminotransferase) and alkaline phosphatase are common indicators of hepatocellular and hepatobiliary injury, respectively. Serum creatinine and urea are markers of the renal clearance of nitrogenous waste and thus of the kidney function. However, it is noteworthy to say that changes in clinical pathology parameters must be interpreted in the context of knowledge of pathophysiology and the known effects of the compounds tested. For example, the transferase AST is not only found in the liver but also in the muscle. So, in case of a compound suspected to create lesions of the muscle, other enzymes like sorbitol dehydrogenase (SDH) (liver-specific) and creatine kinase (CK) (muscle and brain) could be used to differentiate source(s) of AST. Likewise, anticonvulsant drugs have been shown to elevate serum transferase, gamma-glutamyltransferase (GGT), and alkaline phosphatase activities in preclinical species and humans in the absence of histological evidence of hepatic injury (56–59). Further, serum creatinine and urea levels are influenced by nonrenal sources and other adverse effects, including changes in protein synthesis and degradation resulting from lesions of the muscle.

The conventional clinical pathology indicators of toxicity also have well-known limitations. For example, a significant rise of serum creatinine and urea occur only once there has been extensive nephron damage, i.e., greater than 50%, and therefore these biomarkers are rather insensitive indicators of renal injury. Further, serum transferases in rodents may not be optimal predictors for human liver toxicity. Thus, not only is there a continual drive to identify more sensitive and more predictive biomarkers of toxicity in preclinical studies, but also a continual re-evaluation of potentially new uses of established biomarkers. Enhanced biomarker sensitivity and predictivity may come not only from newly identified biomarkers but also from a better understanding of the limitations of current biomarkers, which may lead to the use of different suites of biomarkers together or to novel uses for known biomarkers.

The most commonly utilized, clinically-relevant bridging biomarkers fall into two major categories: (i) those that are validated in both preclinical species and humans, i.e., clinical pathology parameters; and (ii) those validated or well-established in humans that are applied "back" to preclinical species. These strategies are more amenable to the resource and time restrictions that are placed on drug discovery and development. In the first case, there is a vast data and knowledge base related to the validation and limitations of these established biomarkers, while in the latter case, the biomarker for the definitive species, humans, already exists. To illustrate this point, the troponin biomarkers, which are currently used clinically to detect myocardiac infarction (60,61), are currently being evaluated to better understand their usefulness in preclinical studies by the International Life Sciences Institute/Health and Environmental Sciences Institute (ILSI/HESI) Initiative on biomarkers of toxicity (62). The focus of the on-going studies is to validate a set of commercial troponin assays by establishing the degree of immunoreactivity and imprecision across species. These studies are needed to define practical utility in preclinical species, i.e., establish thresholds of troponin response and diagnostic windows in rat, dog, and monkey, and to correlate troponin response with cardiac histopathology.

Another example of biomarkers which are used clinically and which could potentially be applied in preclinical studies are urinary GSTα and GSTπ for proximal and distal tubular lesions of the kidney, respectively. Studies performed in human volunteers showed that urinary GSTα and GSTπ were more sensitive than plasma creatinine to detect drug-induced nephrotoxicity (63,64). A validation study is also under way with ILSI/HESI to establish scientific and regulatory acceptance of these two biomarkers for preclinical studies (62). These ILSI/HESI activities will hopefully also result in a more defined and efficient process of biomarker validation and regulatory submission.

There are two practical issues that often occur during the identification and application of bridging biomarkers. First, in some cases, reagents that may be used to measure biomarkers in humans may not be available for preclinical species, and secondly, a biomarker used preclinically may not be acceptable clinically. In both cases, related or surrogate biomarker(s) must be identified. For example, the measurement of interleukin-2 (IL-2) as an indictor of T-lymphocyte function can be performed by ELISA or western blot techniques using isolated peripheral blood mononuclear cells (PBMC) in humans. However, IL-2-specific antibodies do not exist for all preclinical species. Measurement of changes in IL-2 expression in PBMC in these species can be accomplished using RNA-based methods, as the sequences for IL-2 for different species are available in GenBank. Therefore, during the development of an IL-2 biomarker for PBMC, the strategy may entail utilization of an RT–PCR-based IL-2 endpoint preclinically, followed by a characterization of the temporal relationship of IL-2 mRNA expression and IL-2 protein expression in human PBMC as a study to bridge the relationship of the two different molecular endpoints for IL-2. With this knowledge, the effects causing alteration of IL-2 mRNA expression in preclinical models can be directly related to IL-2 protein changes in humans.

With respect to the concept of a clinically acceptable biomarker, the most important consideration is the ability to collect samples in a relatively noninvasive manner. Thus, whereas it is feasible to collect any tissue during preclinical studies, this is an obvious limitation clinically. Therefore, during preclinical biomarker development, consideration must be given to identifying the most appropriate biomarker measurement and then determining the most applicable platform for measurement clinically. This may require studies to identify surrogate bridging markers.

Contribution of Molecular Profiling Technologies to Biomarker Development

Recent scientific and technological advances have provided new opportunities to find new or novel biomarkers of toxicity for preclinical studies. These advances include improved mechanistic knowledge on cell signaling, gene structure and function, and cell death, as well as the development of high-throughput molecular profiling, a.k.a "-omics" technologies. The contribution of molecular biology to biomarker discovery has been to provide a more detailed understanding of the molecular regulation of potentially useful biomarkers, which has resulted in re-assessment of their use and limitations and, in some instances, has resulted in refinement in their application. Molecular profiling, i.e., transcriptomics, proteomics, and metabonomics, has often provided a broader view of molecular events taking place along affected cellular pathways. This has contributed to a relational understanding of how the molecular changes relate to the eventual toxic outcome as determined by traditional endpoints, such as histology, and the identification of biomarkers that predict a potential specific toxicity, e.g., testicular or liver toxicity, or a particular mechanistic pathway (65,66). This allows for selection of sets of genes, proteins, or small molecular weight molecules that can be used as biomarker suites.

The toxicogenomics approach has proven to be a particularly useful tool used to gather information on the mechanism(s) of pharmaceutical agents or classical toxins (67,68). In some cases, microarray experiments allow identification of new gene expression changes that correlate highly with toxicity. This approach has been successfully used to identify Kidney Injury Molecule-1 (KIM-1) and clusterin as potential, noninvasive biomarkers of nephrotoxicity in rodents (69). Indeed, these genes are expressed at low levels in normal rodent kidney, but their expression is increased with kidney damage. Increased protein expression correlated well with changes in gene expression for these targets in many species, including rodents and humans. Importantly, KIM-1 protein expression has been measured in the urine of humans after renal ischemic injury (70). KIM-1 is an example of a newly identified bridging biomarker that can monitor renal damage in both rodents and humans in a way that is potentially more sensitive than the current measurements.

Gene expression profiling may also be potentially useful to predict long-term toxic events from short-term studies. For example, the identification of molecular biomarkers capable of predicting a positive result in a two-year carcinogenicity study after only a short repeat dose in vivo toxicology study would be of significant value for preclinical safety assessment. By correlating the resulting data with an estimated carcinogenic potential of several compounds and dose levels, Kramer et al. identified several candidate molecular markers of rodent nongenotoxic carcinogenicity, including transforming growth factor beta stimulated clone 22 (TSC-22) and NAD(P) H cytochrome P450 oxidoreductase (CYP-R) (71). Other researchers were able to derive a combination of genes that may be distinctive for genotoxic carcinogens in short-term in vivo studies and may represent the main pathways affected early after exposure to this compound class (72). Although these findings seem promising, much work remains to be done to evaluate and validate these potential biomarkers of carcinogenesis in longer-term studies and to assess their biological significance.

Given the potential of gene expression profiling to improve the safety assessment of new drug candidates, the FDA has recently issued the final guidance on "Pharmacogenomic Data Submissions" (see website http:// www.fda.gov/cder/genomics) (73), which provides recommendations to sponsors on pharmacogenomic data submission requirements, with an interest in genomic data related to safety assessment. According to the guidance, no submission is needed for exploratory or research biomarkers, but voluntary genomic data submission (VGDS) is encouraged in an attempt to enhance understanding of relevant scientific issues related to genomics data among FDA scientists and to prepare them to appropriately evaluate future submissions. The purpose is to create a generalized pathway for accelerating development of new technologies. The guidance recognizes that gene expression data sets could ultimately be viewed as biomarkers. A distinction is made between "known valid biomarker" (for which validity is accepted by the broad scientific community) and "probable valid biomarker" (for which the sponsor owns data to establish biomarker as valid but not yet widely accepted). Discussions are on-going on issues such as the standardization of genomics platforms, interpretation of large data sets, and the process for validation of biomarkers in order to make gene expression data suitable for regulatory decision-making. A similar process would likely apply in the future for data derived from proteomics and metabonomics platforms.

CONCLUSIONS: USE OF BIOMARKER DATA FOR HAZARD AND SAFETY RISK ASSESSMENT

Goals and Integration of Biomarker Data for Compound Selection

As stated earlier, the overall goals of utilizing toxicity biomarkers during drug development are to identify potential toxicity issues and to assess their relevance to humans with respect to a particular drug target, so that an efficacious drug with the best safety profile is advanced. Practically, what this entails is the identification of biomarker needs, the establishment of biomarker platforms that will reliably measure desired endpoints, and the development of testing strategies to verify and determine the relevance of the data for rational decision-making related to safety issues. Furthermore, by "flagging" the potential liabilities early on in discovery and attempting to understand their relevance, more useful recommendations and guidance with regard to follow-up studies or monitoring during the development process may be possible.

The application of the biomarker should be rigorously defined and the endpoints evaluated based on real clinical outcomes for predictive assays or outcomes that have a mechanistic basis. Data obtained from these systems should not stand alone, but should be used as part of a multi-tiered approach and assessed in combination with other toxicology, efficacy, and toxicokinetic parameters including traditional in vivo studies. Finally, care must be taken to relate biomarker measurements to in-life or projected human exposures for efficacy and toxicity so that they can be used to generate rational therapeutic index measurements. There is a continual need for more sensitive, more specific, and predictive biomarkers of toxicity. The compilation of data from well-validated in vitro systems, new technology platforms, and more traditional toxicity studies will also likely result in the continual re-examination, re-definition, and refinement of current bio-markers. When deriving a toxicity biomarker strategy, a balance must be struck between the overall goal of identifying the drug with the best safety profile and fulfilling a medical need that makes sense both scientifically and economically. The identification of a liability may not necessarily result in a no-go decision for a particular compound, but it will initiate an evalua-tion of all other profiling data for that compound and a comparison to other compounds from the same or a different chemical series, as well as decisions about the types of post hoc analyses necessary to verify the result. However, identification of a diversity of potential liabilities for a compound by surro-gate assays may, in fact, lead to a decision to identify a compound or chemical series with fewer issues.

Limitations

The limitations of the toxicity biomarkers identified must be realistically acknowledged so as not to overestimate or underestimate their utility. For example, a toxicity biomarker measured in an in vitro cell culture model system that is used to evaluate potential in vivo toxicity has two immediately apparent limitations. First are the differences inherent to immortalized, transformed cell lines, and second is the inability to account for diverse cell population interactions leading to toxicity when using a single cell type culture system. Cell lines are, by definition, genotypically and phenotypi-cally altered and therefore may not possess the same complement of surface receptors or signal transduction pathways as intact cells (28), in which case the use of primary cell cultures that more closely approach the adult cell type differentiated state may be more relevant. Assay conditions are also highly unnatural when compared with in vivo conditions. Also, many toxic events are related to multiple cell interactions and therefore may not be appropriately modeled even with primary cultures of single cell types. Con-sequently, in vitro co-culture cell cultures or organ slice systems may be more relevant when different cell types are implicated in the mechanism of toxicity (22,30). In vitro systems are used for reasons of practicality and reproducibility, and when the limitations of these systems are taken into consideration with regard to interpretation, and post hoc analyses are used to verify the results, such systems can be utilized. However, consideration must be given to the utility of the data generated and the nature of follow-up investigative strategies to allow an assessment of relevance in humans.

Validation

The Biomarkers Validation Working Group has proposed that the process of linking the predictive value of surrogate biomarkers to clinical endpoints be termed evaluation, whereas the term validation be reserved for characterizing performance characteristics of a biomarker or assay (1). In either case, depending on the intended use of the biomarker platform, there are variable levels of evaluation and validation. For example, for counter-screen assays or biomarkers that are being used during the discovery phase in a limited manner, e.g., for use with a single therapeutic target, often the number of compounds tested to evaluate the utility of the screen is small ($\leq$30 compounds), whereas in the case of a high-throughput screen to be used for general optimization purposes, hundreds of compounds are tested as the validation set and additional compounds with known clinical outcomes that pertain to that screen are applied as test sets. In most cases, the assay platforms that are employed have been previously described in the literature so that there is some understanding of their limitations. Biomarkers utilized during in-life studies and proposed for clinical use that are novel require evaluation in thousands of individuals and therefore, although these biomarkers may be initially evaluated during phase I and phase II studies, they are by no means fully validated. Therefore, as mentioned previously, the identification and successful validation of a novel biomarker or biomarker suite is rather rare, but more commonly, because of time and resource constraints, established biomarkers are utilized either in traditional applications or in new applications. The newly evaluated use of C-reactive protein as an indicator of cardiovascular disease risk is a recent example of this scenario (74,75).

REFERENCES

1. Biomarkers Definitions Working Group. 2001. Biomarkers and surrogate endpoints: preferred definitions and conceptual framework. Clin Pharm Ther 2001; 69:89–95.
2. Schneider M. A rational approach to maximize success rate in target discovery. Arch Pharmacol Med Chem 2004; 337:625–633.
3. Sams-Dodd F. Target-based drug discovery: is something wrong? Drug Disc Today 2005; 10:139–147.
4. Harris S, Foord SM. Transgenic gene knock-outs: functional genomics and therapeutic target selection. Pharmacogen 2000; 1:433–443.

5. Toernell J, Snaith M. Transgenic systems in drug discovery: from target identification to humanized mice. Drug Disc Today 2002; 7:461–470.
6. Zambrowicz BP, Sands AT. Knockouts model the 100 best-selling drugs-will they model the next 100? Nature Rev Drug Disc 2003; 2:38–51.
7. Rudman DG, Durham SK. Utilization of genetically altered animals in the pharmaceutical industry. Toxicol Pathol 1999; 27:111–114.
8. Williams PD. The role of pharmacological profiling in safety assessment. Regul Toxicol Pharmacol 1990; 12:238–252.
9. International Conference on Harmonization (ICH), Safety Pharmacology Studies for Human Pharmaceuticals, 2000.
10. Harry GJ, Billingsley M, Bruinink A, et al. In vitro techniques for the assessment of neurotoxicity. Environ Health Perspect 1998; 106(suppl 1):131–158.
11. Wakefield ID, Pollard C, Redfern WS, Hammond TG, Valentin J-P. The application of in vitro methods to safety pharmacology. Fundament Clin Pharmacol 2002; 16:209–218.
12. Sasseville VG, Lane JH, Kadambi VJ, et al. Testing paradigm for prediction of development-limiting barriers and human drug toxicity. Chem Biol Interact 2004; 150:9–25.
13. Li AP. A comprehensive approach for drug safety assessment. Chem Biol Interact 2004; 150:27–33.
14. Redfern WS, Carlsson L, Davis AS, et al. Relationships between preclinical cardiac electrophysiology, clinical QT interval prolongation and torsade de pointes for a broad range of drugs: evidence for a provisional safety margin in drug development. Cardiovasc Res 2003; 58:32–45.
15. Guth BD, Germeyer S, Kolb W, Markert M. Developing a strategy for the nonclinical assessment of proarrhythmic risk of pharmaceuticals due to prolonged ventricular depolarization. J Pharmacol Toxicol Method 2004; 49:159–169.
16. Roden DM. Drug-induced prolongation of the QT interval. N Engl J Med 2004; 350:1013–1022.
17. Mattheakis LC, Savchenko A. Assay technologies for screening ion channel targets. Curr Opin Drug Disc Develop 2001; 4:124–134.
18. Lee WM. Drug-induced hepatotoxicity. New Engl J Med 2003; 349:474–485.
19. Ballet F. Hepatotoxicity in drug development: detection, significance, and solutions. J Hepatol 1997; 26:26–36.
20. Olsen H, Betton G, Robinson D, et al. Concordance of the toxicology of pharmaceuticals in humans and in animals. Reg Tox Pharm 2000; 32:56–67.
21. Guillouzo A, Morel FA, Fardel O, Meunier B. Use of human hepatocyte cultures for drug metabolism studies. Toxicology 1993; 82:209–219.
22. Guillouzo A, Morel FA, Langouet S, Maheo K, Rissel M. Use of hepatocyte cultures for the study of hepatotoxic compounds. J Hepatol 1997; 26(suppl 2):73–80.
23. Groneberg DA, Grosse-Siestrup C, Fischer A. In vitro models to study hepatotoxicity. Toxicol Pathol 2002; 30:394–399.
24. Xu JJ, Diaz D, O'Brien PJ. Applications of cytotoxicity assays and pre-lethal mechanistic assays for assessment of human hepatotoxicity potential. Chem Biol Interact 2004; 150:115–128.

25. O'Brien PJ, Chan K, Silber PM. Human and animal hepatocytes in vitro with extrapolation in vivo. Chem Biol Interact 2004; 150:97–114.
26. Dambach DM, Andrews BA, Moulin F. New technologies and screening strategies for hepatotoxicity: use of in vitro models. Toxicol Pathol 2005; 33:17–26.
27. Li AP, Maurel P, Gomez-Lechon MJ, Cheng LC, Jurima-Romet M. Preclinical evaluation of drug–drug interaction potential: present status of the application of primary human hepatocytes in the evaluation of cytochrome P450 induction. Chem Biol Interact 1997; 107:5–16.
28. Riley RJ, Kenna JG. Cellular models for ADMET predictions and evaluation of drug–drug interactions. Curr Opin Drug Disc Develop 2004; 7:86–99.
29. Ulrich RG, Bacon JA, Cramer CT, et al. Cultured hepatocytes as investigational models for hepatic toxicity: practical applications in drug discovery and development. Toxicol Lett 1995; 82/83:107–115.
30. Vickers AEM, Fisher RL. Organ slices for the evaluation of human drug toxicity. Chem Biol Interact 2004; 150:87–96.
31. Fuhr U. Induction of drug metabolizing enzymes. Clin Pharmacokinetic 2000; 38:493–504.
32. Rodrigues AD, Lin JH. Screening of drug candidates for their drug–drug interaction potential. Curr Opin Chem Biol 2001; 5:396–401.
33. MacGregor JT, Collins JM, Sugiyama Y, et al. In vitro human tissue models in risk assessment: report of consensus-building workshop. Toxicol Sci 2001; 59:17–36.
34. Li AP. Screening for human ADME/tox drug properties in drug discovery. Drug Disc Today 2002; 6:357–366.
35. Andrews B, Chen S, Zhu M, Moulin F, Flint O. Evaluation of cytochrome P450-mediated hepatotoxicity using a high throughput robotic system [abstract]. Drug Metabol Rev 2003; 35:413.
36. Lindon JC, Nicholson JK, Holmes E, et al. Metabonomics in toxicology: the COMET project. Toxicol Appl Pharmacol 2003; 187:137–146.
37. Yang Y, Blomme EAG, Waring JF. Toxicogenomics in drug discovery: from preclinical studies to clinical trials. Chem Biol Interact 2004; 150:71–85.
38. Petricoin EF, Rajapaske V, Herman EH, et al. Toxicoproteomics: serum proteomic pattern diagnostics for early detection of drug induced cardiac toxicities and cardioprotection. Toxicol Pathol 2004; 32:122–130.
39. International Conference on Harmonization (ICH). Genotoxicity: Specific Aspects of Regulatory Genotoxicity Tests for Pharmaceuticals S2A. Guidance for Industry. 1996.
40. Quillardet P, Hofnung M. The SOS chromotest: a review. Mutat Res 1993; 297:235–279.
41. Reifferscheid G, Heil J. Validation of the SOS/umu test using test results of 486 chemicals and comparison with the Ames test and carcinogenicity data. Mutat Res 1996; 369:129–145.
42. Gee P, Sommers CH, Melick AS, et al. Comparison of responses of base-specific *Salmonella* tester strains with the traditional strains for identifying mutagens: the results of a validation study. Mutat Res 1998; 30:115–130.
43. Fluckiger-Isler S, Baumeister M, Braun K, et al. Assessment of the performance of the Ames II assay: a collaborative study with 19 coded compounds. Mutat Res 2004; 558:181–197.

44. Pearl G, Livingston-Carr S, Durham S. Integration of computational analysis as a sentinel tool in toxicological assessments. Curr Top Med Chem 2001; 1:247–255.
45. He L, Jurs PC, Custer LL, Durham SK, Pearl GM. Predicting the genotoxicity of polycyclic aromatic compounds from molecular structure with different classifiers. Chem Res Toxicol 2003; 16:1567–1580.
46. Mattioni BE, Kauffman GW, Jurs PC, Custer LL, Durham SK, Pearl GM. Predicting genotoxicity of secondary and aromatic amines using data subsetting to generate a model ensemble. J Chem Inf Comput Sci 2003; 43:949–963.
47. Fenech M. The in vitro micronucleus technique. Mutat Res 2000; 455:81–95.
48. Miller B, Poetter-Locher F, Seelbach A, Stopper H, Utesch D, Madle S. Evaluation of the in vitro micronucleus test as an alternative to the in vitro chromosomal aberration assay: position of the GUM working group on the in vitro micronucleus test. Mutat Res 1998; 410:81–116.
49. Matsushima T, Hayashi M, Matsuoka A, et al. Validation study of the in vitro micronucleus test in a Chinese hamster lung cell line (CHL/IU). Mutagenesis 1999; 14:569–580.
50. Kowalski LA. In vitro carcinogenicity testing: present and future perspectives in pharmaceutical development. Curr Opin Drug Disc Develop 2001; 4:29–35.
51. MacGregor JT, Casciano D, Mueller L. Strategies and testing methods for identifying mutagenic risks. Mutat Res 2000; 455:3–20.
52. Boelsterli UA. Animal models of human disease in drug safety assessment. J Toxicol Sci 2003; 28:109–121.
53. Campbell DB. The role of radiopharmacological imaging in streamlining the drug development process. Q J Nucl Med 1997; 41:163–169.
54. Floyd E, McShane TM. Development and use of biomarkers in oncology drug development. Toxicol Pathol 2004; 32(suppl 1):106–115.
55. http://www.ich.org/UrlGrpServer.jser?@ID=276&@_TEMPLATE=254 (accessed March 2005).
56. Muller PB, Taboada J, Hosgood G, et al. Effects of long-term phenobarbital treatment on the liver in dogs. J Vet Intern Med 2000; 14:165–171.
57. Wall M, Baird-Lambert J, Buchanan N, Farrell G. Liver function tests in persons receiving anticonvulsant medications. Seizure 1992; 1:187–190.
58. Mendis GP, Gibberd FB, Hunt HA. Plasma activities of hepatic enzymes in patients on anticonvulsant therapy. Seizure 1993; 2:319–323.
59. Hoshino M, Heise CO, Puglia P, Almeida AB, Cukiert A. Hepatic enzyme levels during chronic use of anticonvulsant drugs. Arq Neuropsiquiart 1995; 53:719–723.
60. Wallace KB, Hausner E, Herman E, et al. Serum troponins as biomarkers of drug-induced cardiac toxicity. Toxicol Pathol 2004; 32:106–121.
61. McDonough JL, Van Eyk JE. Developing the next generation of cardiac markers: disease-induced modifications of troponin I. Prog Cardiovasc Disc 2004; 47:207–216.
62. http://hesi.ilsi.org/index.cfm?pubentityid=82 (accessed March 2005).
63. Goldberg ME, Cantillo J, Gratz I, et al. Dose of compound A, not sevoflurane, determines changes in the biochemical markers of renal injury in healthy volunteers. Anesth Analg 1999; 88:437–445.

64. Eger EI, Koblin DD, Bowland T, et al. Nephrotoxicity of sevoflurane versus desflurane anesthesia in volunteers. Anesth Analg 1997; 84:160–168.
65. Richburg JH, Johnson KJ, Schoenfeld HA, Meistrich ML, Dix DJ. Defining the cellular and molecular mechanisms of toxicant action in the testis. Toxicol Lett 2002; 135:167–183.
66. Waring JF, Jolly RA, Ciurlionis R, et al. Clustering of hepatotoxins based on mechanisms of toxicity using gene expression profiles. Toxicol Appl Pharmacol 2001; 175:28–42.
67. Reilly TP, Bourdi M, Brady JN, et al. Expression profiling of acetaminophen liver toxicity in mice using microarray technology. Biochem Biophys Res Commun 2001; 282:321–328.
68. Wang Y, Rea T, Bian J, Gray S, Sun Y. Identification of the genes responsive to etoposide-induced apoptosis: application of DNA chip technology. FEBS Lett 1999; 445:269–273.
69. Amin RP, Vickers AE, Sistare F, et al. Identification of putative gene based markers of renal toxicity. Environ Health Perspect 2004; 112: 465–479.
70. Han WK, Bailly V, Abichandani R, Thadhani R, Bonventre JV. Kidney Injury Molecule-1 (KIM-1): a novel biomarker for human renal proximal tubule injury. Kidney Int 2002; 62:237–244.
71. Kramer JA, Curtiss SW, Kolaja KL, et al. Acute molecular markers of rodent hepatic carcinogenesis identified by transcription profiling. Chem Res Toxicol 2004; 17:463–470.
72. Ellinger-Ziegelbauer H, Stuart B, Wahle B, Bomann W, Ahr HJ. Characteristic expression profiles induced by genotoxic carcinogens in rat liver. Toxicol Sci 2004; 77:19–34.
73. http://www.fda.gov/cder/genomics (accessed March 2005).
74. Rohde PM, Buring JE, Shih J, Matias M, Hennekens CH. Survey of C-reactive protein and cardiovascular risk factors in apparently healthy men. Am J Cardiol 1999; 84:1018–1022.
75. Ridker PM, Hennekens CH, Buring JE, Rifai N. C-reactive protein and other markers of inflammation in the prediction of cardiovascular disease in women. N Engl J Med 2000; 342:836–843.

8

Use of Biomarkers in Clinical Toxicology and Clinical Trials: A Critical Assessment of QTc Interval Prolongation as a Biomarker

Daniel Bloomfield

*Department of Clinical Pharmacology, Merck Research Laboratories,
Merck & Co., Inc., Rahway, New Jersey, and Columbia University College of
Physicians and Surgeons, New York, New York, U.S.A.*

John A. Wagner

*Department of Clinical Pharmacology, Merck Research Laboratories,
Merck & Co., Inc., Rahway, New Jersey, and Thomas Jefferson University,
Philadelphia, Pennsylvania, U.S.A.*

INTRODUCTION

In this chapter, key terms—biomarker, surrogate endpoint, validation, and qualification—are carefully defined to clarify the various meanings with which these terms are often used. With these terms defined, a conceptual framework is provided for the development and utilization of biomarkers in drug development and in clinical practice.

A detailed discussion of prolongation of the QT interval provides a useful example of issues related to the clinical use of toxicologic biomarkers. Over the past 10 years, there has been considerable interest and concern regarding the ability of some non-antiarrhythmic drugs to delay cardiac ventricular repolarization as measured by prolongation of the QT interval on the surface electrocardiogram (ECG) and cause torsade de pointes (TdP) (1). Based on this paradigm, the QT/QTc interval from the 12-lead ECG has been used as a biomarker predictive of this undesirable clinical outcome. A brief review of the biology of ventricular repolarization and its imperfect association with TdP will follow providing the necessary background for a critical assessment of QTc prolongation as a biomarker within the context of the conceptual framework outlined for the development and utilization of biomarkers. This chapter will review a number of experimental paradigms, clinical and nonclinical, that have been utilized to evaluate the propensity of a drug to prolong the QTc interval (as a biomarker for an increased risk of developing TdP). Finally, the regulatory implications of the use of QTc as a biomarker are discussed including the recent efforts by International Conference on Harmonization (ICH) to achieve consensus in generating guidelines for the evaluation and use of drugs associated with prolongation of the QTc interval.

CONCEPTUAL FRAMEWORK FOR THE USE AND DEVELOPMENT OF BIOMARKERS

Definitions of biomarkers and related terms have recently been refined by a Biomarkers Definitions Working Group with members from the U.S. Food and Drug Administration (FDA), National Institutes of Health (NIH), academics, and industry (2). The term biomarker is the most general case; it refers to any useful characteristic that can be measured and used as an indicator of a normal biologic process, a pathogenic process, or a pharmacologic response to a therapeutic agent (2). A clinical endpoint actually quantifies a characteristic related to how a patient feels, functions, or survives, and a surrogate endpoint is a biomarker that is meant to substitute for a clinical endpoint. Surrogate endpoints are really a subset of biomarkers and there are relatively few biomarkers that qualify for the evidentiary status of surrogate endpoints. Surrogate endpoints are also referred to as surrogate markers in the biomarker literature. The Biomarkers Definitions Working Group has pointed out that the term surrogate endpoint is preferred because the use of this term properly connotes that the biomarker is being used to substitute for a clinical endpoint (2).

Validation and qualification are other key terms used for discussion of biomarkers. Validation (method or assay validation) is the assessment of the assay or measurement performance characteristics including sensitivity, specificity, and reproducibility. Qualification (also known as clinical validation or evaluation) is the evidentiary process of linking a biomarker with biology and a clinical endpoint (3). The biomarker literature occasionally uses validation and qualification synonymously; however, this should be avoided because the validation and qualification processes must be distinguished, and the term validation does not adequately describe the qualification process (2,3).

Biomarkers require validation in most circumstances. Validation of biomarker assays is a necessary component to delivery of high-quality research data necessary for effective use of biomarkers. Qualification is necessary for use of a biomarker as a surrogate endpoint. Qualification is a graded process by which evidence is acquired linking a biomarker with a clinical endpoint such that it can be used as a surrogate endpoint; it is not necessarily an all or none characterization.

Typically, an understanding of pathophysiology governs development of biomarkers. Pathophysiology leading to a specific disease outcome is typically a multistep process. A putative biomarker may be (i) involved in the pathophysiology of a disease outcome, (ii) related, but not directly involved in the pathophysiology of a disease outcome, or (iii) not involved in the pathophysiology of a disease outcome. Thus, one putative biomarker may be identical to a pathophysiologic step leading to the disease outcome. Another putative biomarker may not be directly involved in the pathophysiology of the disease outcome, but directly correlated with one of the steps leading to the disease outcome, and is, in turn, correlated with the disease outcome. A third putative biomarker may not be involved in the pathophysiology of the disease outcome and also not correlated with the disease outcome. The first two theoretical examples of biomarkers rationally fit into the pathophysiologic cascade of a disease outcome; confirmatory studies may demonstrate these measures as appropriate biomarkers. However, a rational basis for the third putative biomarker is relatively lacking. Despite a rational basis for biomarker selection, a biomarker must be qualified as a surrogate endpoint through well-controlled clinical studies. High serum total cholesterol and LDL-cholesterol are regarded as key pathophysiologic steps leading to coronary atherosclerosis. High serum lipids are thought to lead to an excessive lipid burden in the coronary vessel wall, ultimately resulting in atherosclerosis and associated sequelae. Thus, a rational basis exists for recommending total cholesterol as a biomarker of coronary atherosclerosis. Furthermore, a rational basis exists for use of total cholesterol measurements as a biomarker for the efficacy of lipid lowering therapeutics such as hydroxy-methylglutaryl coenzyme A (HMG-CoA) reductase inhibitors. However, it was critical to acquire experience in well-controlled clinical trials to qualify the use of total cholesterol as a surrogate endpoint for atherosclerosis. The 4444 patient Scandinavian Simvastatin Survival Study (4S) provided the critical evidence to qualify total cholesterol as a surrogate endpoint for atherosclerosis events and overall mortality (4). Previous to this study, there were suggestions that reduction in total cholesterol may be associated with increased noncardiac mortality, including cancer and violent deaths, despite a correlation between total cholesterol and deaths due to atherosclerosis. 4S established that simvastatin decreased overall mortality in association with decreased serum total cholesterol and LDL-cholesterol. This study not only qualified total cholesterol as a surrogate endpoint for atherosclerosis events and overall mortality, but also laid the groundwork for use of total cholesterol in general medical practice. Biomarkers are also clearly useful prior to qualification as surrogate endpoints. Thus, total cholesterol was useful in the development of HMG-CoA reductase inhibitors prior to its qualification as a surrogate endpoint. For example, total cholesterol measurements were successfully used as a pharmacodynamic marker in a phase II dose-ranging study of simvastatin to aid in dose selection (5).

Commonly, biomarkers and surrogate endpoints are often conceptualized with reference to measurement of efficacy, but biomarkers of safety and tolerability or toxicologic biomarkers are equally important. Routine toxicologic biomarkers are in widespread use in general clinical practice and are also used in the clinical trial setting. Examples of commonly used toxicologic biomarkers include creatinine as a biomarker of renal dysfunction and transaminase determinations as a biomarker for hepatic dysfunction. This chapter will explore in greater depth issues surrounding the use of the electrocardiographic QT interval as an emerging biomarker predicting risk for cardiac arrhythmias including TdP.

QT/QTc INTERVAL AS A TOXICOLOGIC BIOMARKER

The QT interval represents the total duration of ventricular depolarization and subsequent repolarization, and is measured from the beginning of the QRS complex to the end of the T wave (Fig. 1). Prolonged ventricular repolarization creates an electrophysiological environment in which there is a greater risk of developing life-threatening cardiac arrhythmias such as TdP in certain circumstances and in response to a number of different stimuli. The potential for drugs to cause TdP has been elucidated over the past 50 years (Fig. 2). During this time, a link between TdP and a prolonged QT interval was identified although the epidemiology of this relationship has

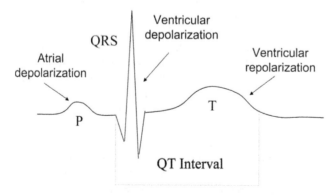

Figure 1 Illustration of the surface electrocardiogram.

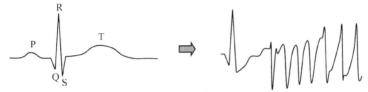

·1918: Quinidine introduced as an anti-arrhythmic

·1920s: Episodes of syncope and 'pseudofibrillation' observed in quinidine patients

·1963: First reports of sudden arrhythmic deaths with phenothiazine antipsychotics

·1966: Dessertenne coins the term 'torsade de pointes' (TdP)

·1970s: Various other drugs found to cause TdP

·1988: Prenylamine (anti-anginal) - first drug withdrawn from sale due to TdP

·1990s: Growing concern about deaths from drug-induced TdP

·1997: CPMP publish a 'Points to Consider' document (CPMP/986/96) on detection of torsadogenic propensity in non-cardiovascular drugs

·1997- Terfenadine, sertindole, astemizole, grepafloxacin, cisapride, droperidol and levomethadyl withdrawn from major markets due to TdP

Figure 2 Example of TdP and history of the relationship between QT and TdP.

not been well quantified. While there is a qualitative relationship between QT prolongation and the risk of TdP (especially for drugs that cause substantial prolongation of the QT/QTc interval), the risk of TdP is not a simple linear function of the QT/QTc interval, nor of the extent of prolongation of the QT/QTc interval during drug therapy (6). Antiarrhythmic agents whose mechanism of action is prolongation of ventricular repolarization, such as sotalol, dofetilide, and ibutilide, can prolong the QT interval by more than 50 milliseconds at clinically prescribed doses which may be therapeutic or which may cause TdP. Because the risk of TdP with these drugs is more than 1% (7–9), in-hospital cardiac monitoring is recommended for the initiation of treatment with these agents. On the other hand, there are drugs that block IKr and prolong the QT interval but have not been associated with TdP (e.g., verapamil and amiodarone) (10,11). However, the risk to the general public from antiarrhythmic drugs that prolong QT interval is relatively small because these drugs include a clear warning in their label, are used relatively infrequently, and tend to be prescribed only by highly trained specialists after a careful assessment of the potential risks and benefit in a given patient.

Of greater concern to public health is the potential risk of noncardiac drugs known to prolong the QT/QTc interval, especially given the large number of patients who may take these drugs often for non–life threatening illnesses. In most cases, the effect of these drugs on ventricular repolarization represents an off-target mechanism and these drugs have only a modest effect on the QT/QTc interval (12–16). However, prolongation of the QT interval when associated with the occurence of polymorphic ventricular tachycardia or TdP, has been the most common cause of the withdrawal or restriction of the use of drugs. Nine structurally unrelated drugs marketed for a range of noncardiovascular indications have been removed from the market or had their availability severely restricted because of this rare form of toxicity (terfenadine, astemizole, grepafloxicin, terodiline, droperidol, lidoflazine, sertindole, levomethadyl, and cisapride) (17). Cases of TdP have been reported with these noncardiovascular drugs despite mean increases in the QT interval as small as 5 to 10 milliseconds in populations of patients (12,18).

Recent efforts have strived to achieve consensus in generating guidelines for the evaluation of the pro-arrhythmic potential of new chemical entities using prolongation of QTc interval as a biomarker for an increased risk of TdP. The ICH S7B nonclinical guidance document ["Nonclinical Evaluation of the Potential for Delayed Ventricular Repolarization (QT Interval Prolongation) by Human Pharmaceuticals"] and the ICH E14 clinical guidance document ("The Clinical Evaluation of QT/QTc Interval Prolongation and Proarrythmic Potential for Non-Antiarrythmic Drugs") are being prepared as part of the ICH process and the step 3 draft was just released in June 2004 (19). These guidances call for a rigorous nonclinical and clinical assessment of the propensity of a drug to cause QT/QTc prolongation. These guidances are discussed in detail later in this chapter.

BIOLOGICAL ISSUES WITH QTc AS A BIOMARKER

Link Between Prolonged QTc and TdP

The evidentiary link between a prolonged QT interval and TdP has been elegantly demonstrated in both animal and human models. When ventricular repolarization is delayed and the QT interval is prolonged, there is an increased risk of ventricular tachyarrhythmia, including TdP. Prolongation of the QT interval on the surface ECG is a reflection of prolongation of ventricular repolarization, as determined by the duration of the cardiac action potential in individual myocytes. This is a complex physiological process integrating the activities of many membrane ion channels and transporters and is affected by multiple factors including, but not limited to, intracellular and extracellular ion concentrations, membrane potential, cell-to-cell electrical coupling, heart rate, and autonomic nervous system activity. The metabolic state (e.g., acid–base balance) and location and type of cardiac cell are also important. Repolarization of the action potential is the result of the efflux of potassium via the rapidly and slowly activating components of the delayed rectifier potassium current, IKr, and IKs. The human ether-a-go-go-related gene (*hERG*) and *KvLQT1* gene encode pore-forming proteins that are thought to represent the α-subunits of the human potassium channels responsible for IKr and IKs, respectively. The most common mechanism of QT interval prolongation by pharmaceuticals is inhibition of the delayed rectifier potassium channel that is responsible for IKr.

With this in mind, the use of QT prolongation appears to be an attractive biomarker for the risk of TdP not only because it represents part of the pathogenic process for TdP but also because the measurement of the QT interval on the surface seems simple and is so readily available. However, QT interval prolongation is an imperfect biomarker for a number of reasons.

First, the link between a prolonged QT interval and the pathogenesis of TdP is extraordinarily complex. While there is a qualitative relationship between QT prolongation and the risk of TdP, especially for drugs that cause substantial prolongation of the QT/QTc interval, the risk of TdP is not a simple linear function of the QT/QTc interval, nor of the extent of prolongation of the QT/QTc interval during drug therapy. In patients with either congenital or acquired (drug-induced) long QT syndrome, the occurrence of TdP is modulated by a number of other factors such as increases in sympathetic nervous system activity, hypokalemia, hypomagnesemia, transient or persistent bradycardia, or irregularities in cardiac rhythm due to sinus pauses, or atrial or ventricular ectopy. In congenital long QT syndrome, there is a relationship between the absolute length of the QT interval and the risk of TdP although this relationship is not strong. Further highlighting the complexity of this relationship are drugs that block IKr, prolong the QT interval, but have not been associated with TdP (e.g., verapamil and amiodarone) (10,11).

Recently, it has become increasingly clear that it is the heterogeneity of action potential prolongation throughout the heart that creates the vulnerability to TdP rather than just an absolute increase in repolarization. The QT interval as measured from the surface ECG represents the summation and spatial averaging of the action potential duration throughout the heart. While an increase in QTc interval is consistent with a prolongation of action potential duration within the heart, there is growing interest in developing measurements of the spatial and temporal heterogeneity of ventricular repolarization. This is an extremely active area of research seeking to define a repolarization biomarker with a more direct relationship to the pathogenesis of TdP.

Intrinsic Variability in the QT Interval

Second, the large variability in the QT/QTc interval is a major obstacle to obtain adequate validation of this biomarker. This variability is derived from the intrinsic physiological variability of ventricular repolarization as well as from methodological issues related to the measurement of ventricular repolarization using the QT/QTc interval. The large amount of intrinsic variability in cardiac repolarization stems from a number of sources including the dependence of QT interval on heart rate, the status of the autonomic nervous system, and gender.

QT Interval and Heart Rate

Because of its inverse relationship to heart rate, the QT interval is routinely transformed (normalized) by means of various formulas into a heart rate independent or "corrected" value known as the QTc interval. The QTc interval is intended to represent the QT interval at a standardized heart rate (60 bpm using Bazett's correction formula). However, it is not clear whether the risk of developing TdP is more closely related to an increase in the absolute QT interval or an increase in the relative (corrected) QT interval (QTc). Most drugs that have caused TdP clearly increase both the absolute QT and the QTc (hereafter called QT/QTc).

The goal of correcting the QT interval for heart rate is to obtain a corrected QT interval that is statistically independent of the heart rate (or RR interval, which equals the interval between two heart beats or 60,000/heart rate) (Fig. 3). Numerous correction formulas have been proposed in the ECG literature, reflecting the variety of statistical models which have been fit to the data. The most popular corrections are the Bazett (20) and Fridericia (21) formulas. Both are based on the simple power model $QT = aRR^b$, with $QTc = QT/RR^b$. Bazett (20) corroborated the previously

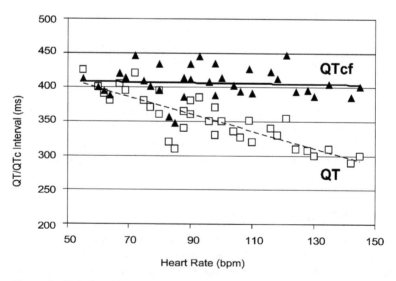

Figure 3   Relationship between QT and HR.

observed relationship between the "ventricular systole" (QT) and the square root of the "heart cycle" (RR) by using data from 40 normal healthy young male and female subjects. This relationship is known as "square root correction formula," $QTcB = QT/RR^{1/2}$. Fridericia (21) examined 50 normal healthy male and female subjects. In order to study high heart rates, he also included nine healthy children. In deriving his formula, Fridericia used the log–log transformation of the power model, $\log QT = a + b \log RR$, and fit the transformed model to the data to find least squares estimates. His estimate of b was 0.3558. He rounded his estimate of b to $1/3$ and thus his correction is $QTcF = QT/RR^{1/3}$.

The corrections of Bazetts' and Fridericias' can produce similar or different QTc intervals for the same QT interval, depending on the heart rate. For RR values less than one second (heart rates greater than 60 bpm), the square root function is smaller than the cube root function and the Bazett-corrected QT interval will be larger than the Fridericia-corrected QT interval. Thus at high heart rates, QTcB is much larger than QTcF and the Bazett formula is said to "overcorrect," whether or not there is a treatment effect. For example, with a fixed QT interval of 400 milliseconds and a heart rate of 80 bpm, $QTcB = 462$, and $QTcF = 440$. Thus, when a drug increases the heart rate substantially but does not truly prolong the QT interval, the use of Bazett's formula can inflate the chance of concluding a positive QT/QTc signal when such a signal does not exist. Similarly, Fridericia's correction can undercorrect at low heart rates.

An alternative approach to correcting QT interval for heart rate is to generate either study-specific or subject-specific correction formulas based on the observed relationship between QT interval and heart rate using either all ECGs from a given study, or all ECGs from a given subject at baseline. In any specific study, linear or log-linear models can be used to derive an empirical population- or subject-specific correction based on the observed QT/RR baseline (pre-drug) data including ECGs from all subjects in the study (22–24). The baseline correction is then applied to all pre- and post-drug data. Baseline corrections depend heavily on the clinical assumptions that the baseline data represent the subjects' physiological condition in the absence of any effects of the drug or unaffected by experimental conditions that may exist during the active treatment phase, and that the QT/RR relationship stays the same before and after drug administration, whether or not the heart rate changes. These assumptions need to be verified and their impact on the resulting inferences needs to be evaluated at the time of a specific analysis. Corrections derived from or including data from the active treatment period are not recommended.

Subject-specific corrections may be preferable to population-based correction formulas in studies with multiple ECG recordings per subject at baseline (23), but their effective use depends on an adequate range of heart rates (to accurately characterize the relationship between QT interval and heart rate) in the baseline data for each subject. This can present a problem in clinical trials because subjects are resting and their heart rates do not usually vary much. In such situations, an individually derived correction based on a narrow range of heart rate pretreatment may not be the most accurate correction available to correct for on-treatment QT measurements and can lead to false conclusions.

No single correction formula will work for every dataset, and therefore understanding the limitations of each correction is critical (25). The corrections of Bazett and Fridericia are based on simple models and are easy to understand. Both formulas produce similar results when the range of heart rates is not extreme. Bazett's correction is often used despite its shortcomings because the vast majority of studies have used this formula and it thus provides for a direct comparison with data generated with other compounds. It can also be used as a tool to check consistency of the data, i.e., we expect large values of QTcB at high heart rates, and QTcB tends to be more variable. For most populations, however, Fridericia's formula generally provides a more accurate correction. Although the Fridericia correction is often designated as the primary correction, it is prudent to present the results using several corrections. Population and individual empirical corrections derived from baseline data can also be included. When statistical results differ because various corrections were applied to the same dataset, discrepancies should be explained and can usually be traced to the range of heart rates prior to and after drug administration, a change in heart rate, a change in the QT/RR relationship, or differences between subjects in individual QT/RR relationships. It is recommended that pre- and postdose RR intervals (or heart rates) as well as uncorrected QT intervals also be examined and analyzed in order to understand the relationships between the variables.

Recently, techniques have been developed to understand and model the QT/RR relationship in the presence of potentially confounding variables such as drug-induced heart rate changes. Such techniques include linear and nonlinear mixed effects modeling and PK/PD analysis of QT/QTc vs. concentration. Furthermore, researchers have attempted to use analysis of covariance and repeated measures models to reduce the chance to erroneously conclude the presence or absence of a QT signal (24).

Effect of Autonomic Conditions on Ventricular Repolarization

Autonomic conditions affect the sinus node as well as the ventricular myocardium (26). Autonomic nervous system changes influence the QT in at least two ways: (i) directly, through effects of the intervention on the ventricular myocardium and (ii) indirectly, via the associated change in HR and the accompanying effects of HR on the QT. HR is a major determinant of the QT. The QT has been shown to shorten predictably as HR increases in response to atrial pacing (27), a state in which autonomic conditions remain relatively constant over a wide range of HRs. In several studies, however, direct effects of autonomically active agents on the QT have been demonstrated when atrial pacing was used to control HR (26,28). For example, atropine shortens the QT and ventricular effective refractory period during pacing at a fixed heart rate. Magnano et al. demonstrated that isoproterenol is associated with much less QT shortening as heart rate increases as compared to the QT shortening that occurs with exercise or with atropine (29). In addition, isoproterenol was associated with complex morphological changes of the U wave, which may contribute to prolongation of the QT at high heart rates.

Based on these findings, the evaluation of the effects of a drug on cardiac ventricular repolarization needs to be done in carefully controlled conditions to reduce the variability in the measurement from autonomic nervous system influences. All comparisons between QT intervals from different treatment periods need to be made with the subject in the same position (supine). In addition, subjects should be supine and should be resting quietly for a few minutes prior to recording an ECG.

Effects of Gender on Ventricular Repolarization

Electrocardiographic and electrophysiologic differences between men and women have long been noted. Women have a higher intrinsic heart rate than men along with a longer corrected QT interval. While in general, women have a lower incidence of sudden cardiac death than men, drug-induced TdP and symptomatic long QT syndrome have a clear female predominance (31–33). Two-thirds of the cases of drug-induced TdP occur in women.

Clinical and experimental studies show that female gender is associated with a longer corrected QT interval at baseline and a greater response to drugs that block IKr, both of which facilitate the emergence of arrhythmia. This results most likely from a specific regulation of ionic channel expression by sex steroids, even though nongenomic effects may play a role as well. Estrogens facilitate bradycardia-induced prolongation of the QT interval and the emergence of arrhythmia, whereas androgens shorten the QT interval and blunt the QT response to drugs. Hence, underlying genetic defects of potassium channels that may be asymptomatic in normal conditions may precipitate drug-induced arrhythmia in women more frequently than in men. Even in the presence of a drug that mildly blocks IKr and seldom prolongs the QT interval, women are still more prone to drug-induced TdP, due to their reduced cardiac "repolarization reserve."

While there are clear gender differences in cardiac repolarization and while it appears that the female gender is more sensitive to TdP, the E14 guidance document does not make mention of the need to enroll women in "thorough QT studies."

Methodologic Issues with the Measurement of the QT Interval

The QT interval is measured from the beginning of the QRS complex to the end of the T wave. Even if the biology linking prolongation of the QT interval and the occurrence of TdP were more straightforward, there are still a number of issues related to the actual measurement of the QT interval that contribute to the variability and uncertainty about the optimum measurement of cardiac ventricular repolarization from the 12-lead ECG.

Unlike the onset of the QRS complex, a high amplitude and high frequency signal that is relatively easy to detect, the end of the T wave is a low amplitude and low frequency signal, which is difficult to detect with precision. When the QT interval is measured by eye on a standard 12-lead ECG (at a paper speed of 25 mm/sec), the precision of the end of T wave measurement is no better than 20 to 40 milliseconds (roughly 10% of the QT interval). A number of different computerized automated methods for measuring the end of the T wave have been described although each has its own biases and limitations and no single method has received general acceptance.

There is no consensus about which lead should be used. Historically, limb lead II has been used to measure the QT interval although the T wave tends to be longer in the precordial leads, especially lead V2 and V3. Some investigators have used a specific lead which is then very sensitive to the morphology of the T wave in that lead. The measurement of a QT interval in a lead with relatively flat T waves is extremely difficult because the end of the T wave is often hard to discern. Others have used the longest QT interval on a tracing, which means that comparisons might be made between one lead predose and another lead postdose. In addition, some of the most commonly used 12-lead ECG machines use a composite lead (either a superimposition of all 12 leads or the median of all 12 leads) to measure the QT interval (which is biased by the longest QT interval of all the leads).

One of the most difficult issues in the measurement of the QT interval is how to handle the measurement in the presence of a U wave. Low amplitude U waves are ubiquitous but often do not affect the measurement of the T wave because there is a clear distinction between the high amplitude T wave and a very low amplitude U wave. However, in certain situations, the T and U waves may be partially merged giving a humped appearance and making it virtually impossible to specifically measure QT interval as distinct from the QTU interval. Because of the confusion created by how to measure the QT interval in the presence of the U wave, most investigators specifically state that the U wave should not be included in the measurement of the T wave, and methods are provided to exclude the U wave (tangent method). The decision to exclude the U wave, however, is not intellectually consistent with knowledge that the presence of large-amplitude U waves represent a significantly increased risk of TdP.

Morphologic changes in the QT interval, the T wave, and the U wave have been recognized as having clinical significance although the predictive value of these drug-induced changes in ECG morphology has not been established (34–36). Newer analytic methods for assessing QTU morphology are being developed but remain to be validated (37). As such, at the present time, morphological abnormalities associated with drug therapy can be described and summarized from the data presented, in terms of the number and percentage of subjects in each treatment group having changes from baseline that represent the appearance or worsening of the morphological abnormality. Typically these data will be obtained as a part of the "thorough QT/QTc study."

Validation of QTc Interval Prolongation as a Biomarker for TdP

Given these biological and methodological issues with the use of QTc prolongation as a biomarker for TdP, it should be no surprise that the validation of this marker faces enormous hurdles. Validation of the performance characteristics of this biomarker would involve demonstrating its reliability and reproducibility on multiple levels. Within a single ECG, the measurement of the QTc interval is not robust. Different computerized algorithms for measuring the QTc interval result in very different measurements and there is no general agreement about which, if any, of these algorithms is optimal. Even when one algorithm is selected for a given study, changes in the heart rate and/or morphology of the T wave over the course of the study within an individual subject can result in an unstable measurement. A great deal of effort has been directed at improving the reliability of manually (human) read QTc intervals using electronically acquired ECGs with software systems that provide computerized calipers and screen resolutions of up to 1 millisecond per pixel. However, little has been published on the estimation of intrareader and interreader variability of manually read QTc intervals. Manually reading a large number of ECGs adds enormous costs to a study and adding these two sources of variability to the intrinsic variability of the QTc interval significantly increases the size of any study that seeks to quantify the effect of a drug or a biologic process on the QTc interval.

Within a given subject, the precision and reproducibility of the QTc interval is poor. In one study of 20 healthy normal male subjects (mean age approximately 40 years), Morganroth et al. performed 800 QT measurements from lead V5 on a 24-hour Holter recording (30). QT was corrected for heart rate using Bazett's correction (QTcB). Even after adjusting for heart rate using QTcB, mean QTcB variability was 76 ± 19 milliseconds (maximum 108 milliseconds). In another study, Pratt et al. evaluated 28 healthy volunteers (24 men) and 28 patients with a history of cardiovascular disease (mean age approximately 57–60 years) and examined the variability in QTc intervals using 40 ECGs collected during treatment with placebo in each subject (8). Mean QTc variability was 56 milliseconds (with a maximum of 156 milliseconds). This large amount of diurnal variation in the QT interval, even after correcting for heart rate using Bazett's correction formula, represents an important consideration in the validation of QTc prolongation as a biomarker.

Qualification of QTc Interval Prolongation as a Biomarker for TdP

Qualification of the QTc interval requires an assessment of the strength of the relationship between the biomarker and the endpoint of clinical interest. Many questions remain unanswered when considering qualification of QTc interval prolongation as a biomarker for TdP. A comprehensive discussion of these questions is beyond the scope of this chapter. In general, the epidemiology of the relationship between this biomarker (QTc prolongation) and the event of clinical interest (TdP) has not been well quantified. There is no question that a prolonged QT interval would not qualify as a surrogate endpoint as defined earlier. Yet, there is clearly enough relationship between a prolonged QTc interval and TdP to warrant concern. The assessment of the strength of the relationship is extraordinarily difficult in part because the clinical endpoint of interest, TdP, is so exceedingly rare and difficult to document. Moreover, a number of other modulating factors play an important role in linking a prolongation of QTc interval to the initiation of an arrhythmia such as changes in electrolytes and autonomic nervous system function as described earlier.

The extremely limited number of clinical endpoints are a major obstacle in defining a formal, statistically valid qualification of this biomarker. As mentioned earlier, even if there are no cases of TdP after exposing 5000 patients to the drug, the upper limit of the 95% confidence interval (CI) around the estimate for the risk of TdP would still be 1 in 1600 (0.000625), reflecting the potential for a very high incidence after marketing.

There are a number of other important questions that have not been adequately addressed. As discussed earlier, the link between a prolonged QT interval and the pathogenesis of TdP is extraordinarily complex. The link between QT prolongation and the risk of TdP is not a simple linear function of the QT/QTc interval. This calls into question the value of categorical analysis of data, which often uses a 60 milliseconds increase in QTc as an important signal for an increased risk. It is clear that a 60 milliseconds increase in QTc does not represent the same increase in risk if the increase is from 340 to 400 milliseconds compared to an increase from 450 to 510 milliseconds. The interaction between the change in QTc interval and the absolute QTc interval with respect to the risk of TdP has not been adequately evaluated. Important biological and epidemiological issues underlie these questions.

REGULATORY GUIDANCE ON THE USE OF QTc INTERVAL PROLONGATION AS A BIOMARKER

Despite the problems with validation and qualification of QTc interval as a biomarker for TdP, various experimental paradigms, clinical and nonclinical, have been utilized to evaluate the propensity of a drug to prolong the QTc interval. Recent efforts have strived to achieve consensus in generating guidelines for the evaluation and use of drugs associated with prolongation of the QTc interval. Regulatory guidance documents for the evaluation of pro-arrhythmic potential of new chemical entities are in development at the present time. The ICH S7B nonclinical guidance document ["Nonclinical Evaluation of the Potential for Delayed Ventricular Repolarization (QT Interval Prolongation) by Human Pharmaceuticals" June 10, 2004] and the ICH E14 clinical guidance document ("The Clinical Evaluation of QT/QTc Interval Prolongation and Proarrythmic Potential for Non-Antiarrythmic Drugs" June 10, 2004) were just released (19). These guidances call for a rigorous assessment of the propensity of a drug to cause QT/QTc Prolongation.

Each of these guidances makes a seminal contribution to drug development. The S7B Guidance adds the necessary depth, breadth, and clarity to the previously established S7A Guidance by specifying the nonclinical evaluation of the potential for drugs to delay ventricular repolarization (QT interval prolongation). The S7B guidance requires an in vitro IKr assay and an in vivo QT assay for all new chemical entities prior to the administration of the drug to man. These data are then interpreted in the context of other clinical and nonclinical data to provide an integrated risk assessment for the compound (Fig. 4). The E14 Guidance provides the standards for a robust clinical evaluation of the potential for drugs to delay ventricular repolarization. Unfortunately, the S7B and E14 Guidances are not harmonized sufficiently at this time. The S7B guidance states clearly that nonclinical testing is not only valuable but critical to assess the potential risk for humans, to design appropriate clinical tests, and to interpret clinical data. However, the strength and clarity of S7B is lost in the context of E14 where the value of the nonclinical risk assessment as outlined in S7B is lost. The E14 guidance does not accept the preclinical assessment (as outlined in S7B) as being able to exclude the possibility that a drug may cause QT/QTc prolongation.

There are no published examples of any drug with a completely clean nonclinical S7B assessment (or an assessment with a large margin between the expected clinical exposure and the exposure at which there is a nonclinical cardiovascular safety signal) that has caused TdP in the clinic. Therefore, it may not be necessary to conduct a thorough QT/QTc clinical study for all drugs. For drug development candidates that lack a nonclinical signal, it should be sufficient to collect ECGs during phase I studies evaluating a range of doses and from a subset of patients during the clinical program.

Nonclinical Testing Strategy

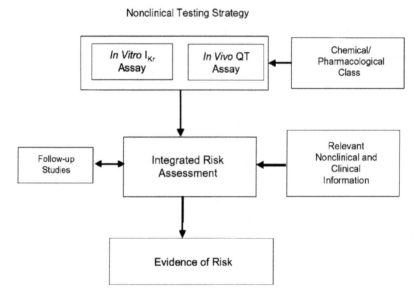

Figure 4   Nonclinical testing strategy in ICH S7B.

A thorough QT/QTc clinical study should be required for any development candidate with a nonclinical signal indicative of the potential for prolongation of ventricular repolarization in a range of exposures near projected clinical exposures.

Design and Conduct of a Thorough QT/QTc Study

The E14 guidance offers a number of very specific guidelines for conducting a "thorough QT/QTc study." The guidance states that "drugs should receive an electrocardiographic evaluation, beginning early in clinical development, typically including a single trial dedicated to evaluating their effect on cardiac repolarization ('thorough QT/QTc study')." For reasons that will be clear below, retrospective analyses of data from previously conducted clinical trials may not be acceptable to exclude the possibility of the effect of a drug on the QT/QTc interval. There are several key points made in the E14 guidance including (i) use of a positive control, (ii) parameters defining a negative study, (iii) characterization of a concentration–response relationship using exposures that are multiples above the expected therapeutic concentration, (iv) the need to reduce variability in the measurement of the QTc interval using replicate ECGs and a centralized core laboratory to measure QTc interval, (v) the complexity of correcting the QT interval for heart rate, and (vi) the need to provide continuous and categorical analyses of QTc interval.

Use of a Positive Control

The E14 guidance states clearly and unambiguously that studies need to include a positive control. The positive control is intended to serve as a method of ensuring assay sensitivity by providing a high degree of confidence that the study is able to detect differences of clinical significance. The confidence in the ability of the study to detect QT/QTc prolongation can be greatly enhanced by the use of a concurrent positive control group to establish assay sensitivity. On that basis, the positive control (whether pharmacological or nonpharmacological) should be well-characterized and consistently produce an effect corresponding to the largest change in the QT/QTc interval that is currently viewed as clinically not important to detect (a mean change of around 5 milliseconds or less).

Parameters Defining a Negative Study

The E14 guidance defines a negative "thorough QT/QTc study" as "one in which the upper bound of the 95% one-sided confidence interval for the largest time-matched mean effect of the drug on the QTc interval excludes 10 milliseconds. This upper bound was chosen to reflect the uncertainty related to the variability of repeated measurements."

The scientific basis for defining a negative "thorough QT/QTc study" as excluding an effect >10.0 milliseconds is not discussed or referenced in the guidance. There have been cases of TdP reported with noncardiovascular drugs in which mean increases in the QTc interval within the therapeutic concentration were as small as 5 to 10 milliseconds (14,15). However, it is unlikely that these drugs caused TdP with such modest increases in QTc interval; rather many if not all of the cases of TdP were reported when the concentration of the drug in question was likely extremely high because of coadministration of a metabolic inhibitor (14,38). Whether a drug could cause TdP at a concentration that only prolongs QTc by 10 milliseconds is unknown. In fact, there are a number of drugs that consistently prolong QTc by approximately 10 milliseconds at the therapeutic concentration in which TdP has not been reported (e.g., moxifloxacin).

Characterization of a Concentration–Response Relationship

The E14 guidance states that the duration of dosing or the dosing regimen should be sufficient to characterize the effects of the drug and its active metabolites at relevant concentrations including "exploration of concentrations that are higher than those achieved following the anticipated therapeutic doses" in order to characterize the relationship between the exposure and the QT/QTc interval response. A "thorough QT study" should include exposures that are three- to tenfold higher than the expected therapeutic concentration and which exceed the anticipated maximum exposures. In

addition, recognizing that the concentrations of a drug can be increased by
drug–drug or drug–food interactions involving metabolizing enzymes, the
draft guidance suggests that one way to achieve these high exposures is to
do the "thorough QT/QTc study" under conditions of maximum inhibition.
This approach calls for a detailed understanding of the absorption, distribution, metabolism, and excretion of the drug.

In order to properly characterize the exposure–response relationship,
the E14 guidance specifies that the timing of the collection of ECGs should
be guided by the available information about the pharmacokinetic profile of
the drug. This detailed characterization of the exposure–response relationship will require an analysis of the effect of a drug on the QT/QTc throughout the dosing interval with particular attention to ECG recordings made at
time points around the C_{max}.

Need to Reduce Variability in Measurement of QTc Interval

The E14 guidance recognizes that a critical problem in the measurement of
the QT/QTc interval is its intrinsic variability and states that it is "considered
essential to address intrinsic variability in the conduct of the 'thorough QT/
QTc study.' This can be accomplished in several ways, including the collection of multiple ECGs at baseline and during the study." The use of replicate
ECGs, multiple ECG time points, and time-matched baseline values has
important implications for the design of the "thorough QT/QTc study"
and the analysis of QT/QTc interval data within that study. This raises
important and complex problems with multiplicity in the "thorough QT/
QTc study" that are not addressed in the guidance.

In a discussion on the analysis and interpretation of QT/QTc interval
data, the E14 guidance specifically addresses the need for a centralized
interpretation of QT/QTc intervals: "The 'thorough QT/QTc study' would
warrant particularly careful attention to interval measurement. At present,
this would usually involve the measurement by a few skilled readers
(whether or not assisted by the computer) operating from a centralized
ECG laboratory. Readers of ECGs should be blinded to time, treatment,
and subject identifier, and one reader should read all the ECG recordings
from a given subject."

Complexity of Correcting QT Interval for Heart Rate

The E14 guidance also discusses the complexity of correcting QT interval
data with respect to heart rate. As the QT interval has an inverse relationship
to heart rate, the measured QT intervals are generally corrected for heart rate
in order to determine whether they are prolonged relative to baseline. Various correction formulas have been suggested, of which Bazett's and Fridericia's corrections are the most widely used. In early trials evaluating the

effects of a new drug on the QT/QTc interval in healthy volunteers, designed to detect relatively small effects (e.g., 5 milliseconds), it is important to apply the most accurate correction available (e.g., methods using individually derived relationships between RR and QT intervals). Because the best correction approach is a subject of controversy, uncorrected QT and RR interval data, heart rate data, as well as QT interval data corrected using the corrections of Bazett and Fridericia should be submitted in all applications, in addition to QT interval data corrected using any other formulas.

Continuous and Categorical Analyses of QTc Interval

With reference to the specific analyses of the QT/QTc interval data, the E14 guidance specifies that "the QT/QTc interval data should be presented both as analyses of central tendency (e.g., means, medians) and categorical analyses" as both can provide relevant information on clinical risk assessment. The effect of an investigational drug on the QT/QTc interval is most commonly analyzed using the largest time-matched mean difference between the drug and placebo (baseline-subtracted) over the collection period (e.g., hourly, weekly, monthly). Additional approaches to the assessment of central tendency could include analysis of time-averaged QT/QTc intervals or analysis of changes occurring at the C_{max} for each individual.

The guidance does not address any issues with reference to multiplicity generated by the use of the largest time-matched mean difference, which effectively requires all time points to meet the prespecified hypothesis and lie within the prespecified confidence limits (<10 milliseconds).

In addition, the guidance states that categorical analyses of QT/QTc interval data must also be presented. Categorical analyses of QT/QTc interval data are based on the number and percentage of patients meeting or exceeding some predefined upper limit value. Clinically, noteworthy QT/QTc interval signals might be defined in terms of absolute QT/QTc intervals (QTc >450, 480, and 500 milliseconds) or changes from baseline (QTc interval increases from baseline ≥ 30 and ≥ 60 milliseconds).

CONCLUSIONS

Within the conceptual framework provided for the development and utilization of biomarkers in drug development and in clinical practice, it is clear that a prolonged QTc interval represents an important biomarker for the assessment of the risk of TdP. However, the validation and qualification of this biomarker are currently incomplete in large part because of a number of complex biological and methodological issues related to the measurement of the QTc interval. A number of experimental paradigms, clinical and non clinical, have been utilized to evaluate the propensity of a drug to prolong the QTc interval (as a biomarker for an increased risk of developing

TdP). An active and fruitful discussion of these issues with academics, regulatory agencies, and the pharmaceutical industry is in the process of attempting to achieve consensus in generating guidelines for the evaluation and use of drugs associated with prolongation of the QTc interval.

REFERENCES

1. Moss AJ. Drugs that prolong the QT interval: regulatory and QT-measurement issues from the USA and European perspectives. Annals of Non-Invasive Electrocardiology, 2003, University of Rochester Medical Center. Available on www.urmc.rochester.edu
2. Biomarkers Definitions Working Group. Biomarkers and surrogate endpoints: preferred definitions and conceptual framework. Clin Pharmacol Therapeut, 2001; 69:89–95.
3. Wagner JA. Overview of biomarkers surrogate endpoints in drug development. Disease Markers 2002; 18:41–46.
4. Scandinavian Simvastatin Survival Study Group. Randomised trial of cholesterol lowering in 4444 patients with coronary heart disease: the Scandinavian Simvastatin Survival Study (4S). Lancet 1994; 344:1383–1389.
5. Mol MJTM, Erkelens DW, Gevers Leuven JA, Schouten JA, Stalenhoef AFH. Effects of synvinolin (MK-733) on plasma lipids in familial hypercholesterolaemia. Lancet 1986; 2:936–939.
6. Moss AJ. Measurement of the QT interval and the risk associated with QT interval prolongation. Am J Cardiol 1993; 72:23B–25B.
7. Torp-Pedersen C, Møller M, Bloch-Thomsen PE, et al. Dofetilide in patients with congestive heart failure and left ventricular dysfunction. N Engl J Med 1999; 341:857–865.
8. Stambler BS, Wood MA, Ellenbogen KA, Perry KT, Wakefield LK, VanderLugt JT. Efficacy and safety of repeated intravenous doses of ibutilide for rapid conversion of atrial flutter or fibrillation. Circulation 1996; 94:1613–1621.
9. Velebit V, Podrid P, Lown B, Cohen BH, Graboys TB. Aggravation and provocation of ventricular arrhythmias by antiarrhythmic drugs. Circulation 1982; 65:886–894.
10. Zhang S, Zhou Z, Gong Q, Makielski JC, January CT. Mechanism of block and identification of the verapamil binding domain to HERG potassium channels. Circ Res 1999; 84:989–998.
11. Yang T, Snyders D, Roden DM. Drug block of I(kr): model systems and relevance to human arrhythmias. J Cardiovasc Pharmacol 2001; 38:737–744.
12. Pratt CM, Ruberg S, Morganroth J, et al. Dose–response relation between terfenadine (Seldane) and the QTc interval on the scalar electrocardiogram: distinguishing drug effect from spontaneous variability. Am Heart J 1996; 131:472–480.
13. Pratt CM, et al. Risk of developing life-threatening ventricular arrhythmia associated with terfenadine in comparison with other over the counter antihistamines. Am J Cardiol 1994; 73:346–352.
14. Honig PK, et al. Changes in the pharmacokinetics and electrocardiographic pharmacodynamics of terfenadine with concomitant administration of erythromycin. Clin Pharmacol Ther 1992; 52:231–238.

15. Davies AJ, Harindra V, McEwan A, Ghose RR. Cardiotoxic effect with convulsions in terfenadine overdose. Br Med J 1989:298–325.
16. Wysowski DK, et al. Postmarketing reports of QT prolongation and ventricular arrhythmia in association with Cisapride and FDA Regulatory Actions. Am J Gastroenterol 2001; 96:1698–1703.
17. Lasser KE, Allen PD, Woolhandler SJ, Himmelstein DU, Wolfe SM, Bor DH. Timing of new black box warnings and withdrawals for prescription medications. JAMA 2002; 287:2215–2220.
18. Khongphatthanayothin A, Lane J, Thomas D, Yen L, Chang D, Bubolz B. Effects of cisapride on QT interval in children. J Pediatr 1998; 133:51–56.
19. International Conference on Harmonisation of Technical Requirements for Registration of Pharmaceuticals for Human Use. Draft Consensus Guideline: The Clinical Evaluation of QT/QTc Interval Prolongation and Proarrhythmic Potential for Non-Antiarrhythmic Drugs, E14. Released for Consultation at Step 2 of the ICH Process on 10 June 2004 by the ICH Steering Committee. http://www.fda.gov/cder/guidance/6922fnl.htm.
20. Bazett HC. An analysis of time relations of electrocardiograms. Heart 1920; 7:353–367.
21. Fridericia LS. Die Systolendauer im Elecktrokardiogramm bei normalen Menschen und bei Herzkranken. Acta Medica Scandinavia 1920; 53:469–486.
22. Sagie A, Larson MG, Goldberg RJ, Bengtson JR, Levy D. An improved method for adjusting the QT interval for heart rate (the Framingham Heart Study). Am J Cardiol 1992; 70:797–801.
23. Dmitrienko A, Smith B. Repeated-measures models for the analysis of QT interval. J Biopharm Stat 2003; 12(3):175–190.
24. Dmitrienko A, Sides G, Winters K, Kovacs R, Eisenberg P, Groh W. Electrocardiogram reference ranges derived from a standardized clinical trial population. J Cardiovasc Electrophysiol 2004. In press.
25. Malik M, Camm AJ. Evaluation of Drug-Induced QT Interval Prolongation. Drug Safety 2001; 24:323–351.
26. Browne KF, Zipes DP, Heger JJ, Prystowsky EN. Influence of the autonomic nervous system on the Q-T interval in man. Am J Cardiol 1982; 50:1099–1103.
27. Ahnve S, Vallin H. Influence of heart rate and inhibition of autonomic tone on the QT interval. Circulation 1982; 65:435–439.
28. Cappato R, Alboni P, Pedroni P, Gilli G, Antonioli GE. Sympathetic and vagal influences on rate-dependent changes of QT interval in healthy subjects. Am J Cardiol 1991; 68:1188–1193.
29. Magnano AR, Holleran S, Ramakrishnan R, Reiffel JA, Bloomfield DM. Autonomic nervous system influences on QT interval in normal subjects. J Am Coll Cardiol 2002; 39:1820–1826.
30. Morganroth J, et al. Variability of the QT interval in healthy men. Am J Cardiol 1991; 67:774–776.
31. Drici MD, Clement N. Is gender a risk factor for adverse drug reactions? The example of drug-induced long QT syndrome. Drug Safety 2001; 24(8):575–585.
32. Miller MA. Gender-based differences in the toxicity of pharmaceuticals-the Food and Drug Administration's perspective. Int J Toxicol 2001; 20(3): 149–152.

33. Wolbrette D, Naccarelli G, Curtis A, Lehmann M, Kadish A. Gender differences in arrhythmias. Clin Cardiol 2002; 25(2):49–56.
34. Bloomfield DM, Hohnloser SH, Cohen RJ. Interpretation and classification of microvolt T wave alternans tests. J Cardiovasc Electrophysiol 2002; 13(5):502–512.
35. Antzelevitch C, Nesterenko VV, Yan GX. Role of M cells in acquired long QT syndrome, U waves, and torsade de pointes. J Electrocardiol 1995; 28(suppl):131–138.
36. Jackman WM, Szabo B, Friday KJ, et al. Ventricular tachyarrhythmias related to early afterdepolarizations and triggered firing: relationship of QT interval prolongation and potential therapeutic role for calcium channel blocking agents. J Cardiovasc Electrophysiol 1990; 1:170–195.
37. Vila JA, Gang Y, Rodriguez Presedo JM, Fernandez-Delgado M, Barro S, Malik M. A new approach for TU complex characterization. IEEE Trans Biomed Eng 2000; 47:764–772.
38. Ray WA, Murray KT, Meredith S, Narasimhulu SS, Hall K, Stein CM. Oral erythromycin and the risk of sudden death from cardiac causes. N Engl J Med 2004; 351(11):1089–1096.

9

Regulatory Guidance and Validation of Toxicologic Biomarkers

Federico M. Goodsaid and Felix W. Frueh
Genomics Team, Office of Clinical Pharmacology and Biopharmaceutics, Center for Drug Evaluation and Research, U.S. Food and Drug Administration, Silver Spring, Maryland, U.S.A.

INTRODUCTION

The regulatory use of genomic biomarkers of toxicity is an important goal for the pharmaceutical industry as well as for the U.S. Food and Drug Administration (FDA) and corresponding regulatory agencies elsewhere. The application of biomarkers in general throughout drug development is specifically addressed in the Critical Path document (Innovation/Stagnation: Challenge and Opportunity on the Critical Path to New Medical Products) (1) issued by the FDA in March 2004 and The Innovative Medicines Initiative (IMI) Strategic Research Agenda (2) issued as a draft by the European Commission in July 2005. In this review, our goal is to address several questions associated with the application of genomic biomarkers of toxicity:

1. How can we enable the regulatory application of genomic biomarkers of toxicity?
2. How can the industry and the FDA overcome fears and inertia in the application of genomic biomarkers of toxicity in areas where other technologies have become gold standards over the course of several decades?

3. How can we show a compelling advantage over orthodox metho-
    dology in the application of genomic biomarkers of toxicity in
    drug development?

Definition of Genomic Biomarkers of Toxicity and Safety

The definition of what a biomarker is has provoked intense debate over the
past decade. The specific case of biomarkers of toxicity and safety adds a
layer of complexity to this definition. There is a broad overlap in the classification of genomic biomarkers of toxicity and safety. Characteristics of a
"perfect" preclinical/clinical biomarker for monitoring toxicity are outlined
in the IMI draft document (2):

1. Specific for certain types of injury.
2. Indicates injury in a variety of experimental species as well as
    humans.
3. Can be used to bridge across nonclinical/preclinical studies to
    clinical and surveillance types of studies.
4. More effective at indicating injury than any other biomarker
    currently used.
5. Used instead of classic biomarkers, not in addition.
6. Can be easily measured (in real time) even at a later stage
    (measurement is not strongly time-dependent).
7. More reproducible and sensitive than the original toxicity
    endpoint it would replace.
8. Reduces the number of individuals tested (animals or humans).

"Perfect" biomarkers are not likely to represent most biomarkers of
value in drug development and in regulatory submissions associated with
drug development. A discrepancy with one or more of the requirements in
this outline may not prevent the validation of a genomic biomarker.

A lack of consensus in the definition of a biomarker has been closely
associated not so much with the genomic, proteomic or metabolic nature of
a biomarker, but with the context of the application of a biomarker. Context in the application of a biomarker represents the most important
characterization in its definition. A broad context in the application of a biomarker requires a scientific body of evidence and a concurrent scientific consensus, which often prevent a swift and effective application of biomarkers
in drug development. Narrowing the context in the application of a
biomarker facilitates the acceptance and application of this biomarker.
For example, the application of biomarkers to better understand mechanisms of safety or efficacy is likely to require straightforward scientific
evidence for a number of examples of compounds or studies justifying the
mechanistic conclusions. At the other extreme, the acceptance of the application of the same biomarkers in surrogate testing may be expected to

include a comprehensive evidence database across multiple compounds and studies, with thorough analytical and biological support for the proposed replacement of a pre-existing test.

While we may consider more than one definition for biomarkers, it is likely that the functional definition of a biomarker will not be far from that drafted by the NIH/FDA Biomarkers Definition Working Group (3): "A characteristic that is objectively measured and evaluated as an indicator of normal biological processes, pathogenic processes, or pharmacologic responses to a therapeutic intervention." This definition captures the biological, pathological, and pharmacological contexts in which a signal such as that from changes in expression levels for gene signatures may be applied as a biomarker.

This chapter will focus on genomic biomarkers as an example of the current approaches and issues relevant to biomarker validation in general. Genomic biomarkers are subject to the same definitions and requirements for qualification (or validation) as are biomarkers defined by any other metrics or technological platforms. One of the hurdles in the application of genomic biomarkers has been a "genomic exceptionalism," a perception over the past decade that the metrics and technological platforms required in the measurement of these markers are somehow unique and not subject to the same precedents and guidance documents relevant for other biomarkers. Associated with this perception has also been a fear that data from genomic biomarkers would be overinterpreted or misinterpreted throughout the regulatory review process. The Interdisciplinary Pharmacogenomic Review Group (IPRG) (4) at the FDA is working to apply to genomic biomarkers consensus criteria for validation similar to those considered in the validation of pharmacogenomic and toxicogenomic biomarkers and to develop scientifically sound and coherent review guidelines for genomic data within the review divisions at FDA.

THE CRITICAL PATH AND GUIDANCE DOCUMENTS

The FDA released a report (1) on March 16, 2004 focusing on the significant reduction in innovative medical products submitted to the Agency over the past decade. This Critical Path document identified specific areas in the drug development process that could be improved to overcome this reduction. In this document, improvements in drug development were associated with better and more efficient application of biomarkers in general and of genomic biomarkers in particular.

Several guidance documents have been drafted in order to translate the opportunities set forth in the Critical Path document into regulatory practice. Guidance documents do not establish legally enforceable responsibilities. Instead, a guidance document describes current thinking in the FDA on a topic and should be viewed only as a recommendation. These documents do have the power to develop an intense and coherent discussion about the application of genomic biomarkers in drug development.

The submission of pharmacogenomic or toxicogenomic data to the FDA is a fundamental step in the inclusion of genomic biomarkers in drug development. Sponsors submitting or holding investigational new drug applications (INDs), new drug applications (NDAs), or biologics licensing applications (BLAs) are subject to FDA requirements for submitting to the Agency data relevant to drug safety and effectiveness as described in the Code of Federal Regulations [(21 CFR 312.22, 312.23, 312.31, 312.33, 314.50, 314.81, 601.2, and 601.12)]. Because these regulations were developed before the advent of widespread animal or human genetic or gene expression testing, they do not specifically address when such data should be submitted. Guidance is needed with recommendations to sponsors holding investigational and marketing applications on when to submit pharmacogenomic or toxicogenomic data to the Agency during the drug development processes, what format and content to provide for submissions, and how and when the data will be used in regulatory decision-making. Key information including examples of when pharmacogenomic or toxicogenomic data submissions would be required and when voluntary genomic data submissions (VGDSs) are encouraged should also provided.

The guidance document titled "Guidance for Industry: Pharmacogenomic Data Submissions" and related publications (4–11) apply to the regulatory use of genomic biomarkers of toxicity. At the core of the guidance are decision trees illustrating what type of and when this data should be submitted. This decision is critically influenced by the status of the biomarkers used for regulatory decision-making. Valid genomic biomarkers in this guidance are defined as parameters measured in an analytical test system with well-established performance characteristics and scientific framework or body of evidence that elucidates the physiologic, pharmacologic, toxicologic, or clinical significance of the test results. For example, the consequences for drug metabolism of genetic variation in the human enzymes cytochrome P450 2D6 (CYP2D6) and thiopurine methyltransferase (TPMT) are well understood in the scientific community and are reflected in certain approved drug labels. The results of genetic tests that distinguish allelic variants of these enzymes are considered to be well established and therefore valid biomarkers.

Valid genomic biomarkers are further classified in this document as either *known* or *probable* valid biomarkers. When a sponsor generates data sufficient to establish a significant association between a pharmacogenomic or toxicogenomic test result and clinical outcomes, the test result represents a probable valid biomarker. This biomarker becomes a known valid biomarker when it is broadly accepted in the scientific community. Data on known valid biomarkers need to be included in IND, NDA, and BLA submissions. Data on probable valid or exploratory biomarkers need not be included in the IND submission if they are not to be used by a sponsor to make decisions regarding specific animal safety studies or clinical trials, although sponsors or applicants will need to submit an abbreviated report or synopsis of new NDAs or BLAs (4–11).

The Critical Path document defined not only clear and measurable steps to improve the efficiency of drug development but also proposed early, intensive, and continuous communication between sponsors and the FDA throughout preclinical and clinical development stages in this process. The goal is to improve not only the technical and logistical framework associated with drug development, but also the rate, depth, and quality of information exchange between sponsors and the FDA.

An example of this improved information exchange is the VGDS. This is a novel idea for the development of genomic applications in drug development as well as early and productive interactions between the FDA and sponsors. Sponsors can submit data for genomic biomarkers that are still exploratory and for which additional data would be required to reach the level of probable biomarkers. Voluntary submissions can benefit both the industry and the FDA in a general way by providing a means for sponsors to ensure that regulatory scientists are familiar with and prepared to appropriately evaluate future genomic submissions. FDA and industry scientists alike benefit from an enhanced understanding of relevant scientific issues, for example: the types of genetic loci or gene expression profiles being explored by the pharmaceutical industry for pharmacogenomic or toxicogenomic testing; test systems and techniques being employed; problems encountered in applying pharmacogenomic or toxicogenomic tests to drug development; and the ability to transmit, store, and process large amounts of complex pharmacogenomic or toxicogenomic data streams with retention of fidelity.

The Committee for Medicinal Products for Human Use (CHMP) of the European Medicines Agency (EMEA) issued a draft guidance document for pharmacogenetics in March 2005 (12). How does the EMEA process for VGDS in this draft document compare with the process outlined in the FDA Guidance? It encouraged dialogue that may contribute to minimize risks of creating inadvertent obstacles to the use of genomic technology, as well as an opportunity to gain input from the CHMP expert group in an informal setting, i.e., without regulatory impact on the products under development as the experts would not engage in formal pre-assessment of the information provided for the briefing meeting. It also allowed applicants and regulators to share and discuss technical, scientific, and regulatory issues that arise by the inclusion of pharmacogenetics and pharmacogenomics in the development strategy and to assess their potential implications in the regulatory processes. In this document the definition for biomarkers was similar to that in the FDA Guidance, but the document made no reference to regulatory applications of genomic biomarkers or of a path with which to validate exploratory markers.

REVIEWER TRAINING AND STANDARDIZATION IN PHARMACOGENOMICS AND TOXICOGENOMICS

The analysis of VGDS DNA hybridization data requires a reproducible biological interpretation. This is a critical factor in the regulatory application of genomic data. One of the major concerns reported by the pharmaceutical industry to the docket of the draft version of the pharmacogenomic guidance was a fear that reviewers would overinterpret or misinterpret the results of DNA hybridization experiments.

The FDA has developed a pharmacogenomics and toxicogenomics reviewer training program including introductory training, a review of case studies, and training in the use of ArrayTrack (13), a hybridization data analysis tool developed at the National Center for Toxicological Research (NCTR) of the FDA. Training allowed by a sponsor with VGDS data provides reviewers an in-depth understanding of the analytical process by which biological conclusions are reached from hybridization data. It is also an opportunity to share with sponsors knowledge about analytical tools required in the review of these submissions, including those used for normalization, filtration, statistical analysis, and biological pathway analysis.

Training with VGDS data has also underscored the need for standardization throughout the generation, analysis, and interpretation of hybridization data. While VGDS data is exploratory, its analysis shows how the content of a list of genomic biomarkers that may later be proposed for validation is critically dependent on how the protocols for data generation, analysis, and interpretation are defined. There are several steps in this process where standards may be identified:

1. Laboratory proficiency in hybridization technologies
2. DNA and RNA isolation and purification
3. Chemical and enzymatic reactions required prior to hybridization
4. Hybridization sensitivity, specificity and dynamic range
5. Reader sensitivity and dynamic range
6. Data submission
7. Data analysis (gene expression or allelic discrimination result sets)
8. Biological interpretation

It is not difficult to find a consensus on the need for standards in steps 1 to 6 of this process (14). Scientists working with platform providers, pharmaceutical R&D and regulatory agencies, agree that standards need to be developed for these steps (14). Organizations such as the External RNA Controls Consortium (ERCC; Warrington J, et al. External RNA Consortium Progress Report. 2005; submitted for publication) and the Microarray Quality Control (MAQC) Project (15) have completed work leading to standards for laboratory proficiency, DNA and RNA isolation, chemical and enzymatic reactions, and hybridizations in steps 1 to 4.

The ERCC Warrington J, et al. External RNA Consortium Progress Report. 2005; Submitted for publication is an ad-hoc group with approximately 70 members from private, public, and academic organizations. The group was initiated in 2003 to develop a set of external RNA control transcripts that can be used to assess technical performance in gene expression assays. The external RNA controls will be added after RNA isolation, but prior to cDNA synthesis. They are being designed to evaluate whether the results for a given experiment are consistent with defined performance criteria. All ERCC work is intended to apply to quantitative, real-time reverse transcriptase polymerase chain reaction (QRT–PCR) assays as well as one-color and two-color microarray experiments. ERCC has worked together to define the desired properties of the transcripts, general protocols for their application, and an analysis scheme for performance assessment. In December 2003, the group developed a specification document that was discussed and refined in a public workshop at the National Institute of Standards and Technology (NIST) (16). Protocols for the use of external RNA controls in clinical applications are included in the Molecular Methods P-16 (MM16) document from the Clinical Laboratory Standards Institute (CLSI), and were developed in a formal, accredited, open, consensus forum including several ERCC members (17). The analysis approach is based on the measurement of pooled transcripts in known concentration ratios.

The purpose of the Microarray Quality Control (MAQC) project (15) is to provide quality control tools to the microarray community in order to avoid procedural failures and to develop guidelines for microarray data analysis by providing the public with large reference datasets along with readily accessible reference RNA samples. The MAQC project includes six FDA centers, major providers of microarray platforms and RNA samples, EPA, NIST, academic laboratories, and other stakeholders. The MAQC project aims to establish QC metrics and thresholds for objectively assessing the performance achievable by various microarray platforms and evaluating the advantages and disadvantages of various data analysis methods. Two RNA samples will be selected for three species, human, rat, and mouse, and differential gene expression levels between the two samples will be calibrated with microarrays and other technologies (e.g., QRT–PCR). The resulting microarray datasets will be used for assessing the precision and cross-platform/laboratory comparability of microarrays, and the QRT–PCR datasets will enable evaluation of the nature and magnitude of any systematic biases that may exist between microarrays and QRT–PCR. The availability of the calibrated RNA samples combined with the resulting microarray and QRT–PCR datasets, which will be made readily accessible to the microarray community, will allow individual laboratories to more easily identify and correct procedural failures.

The U.S. NIST has an ongoing effort to develop standards for hybridization readers in step 5 (18). The pharmaceutical industry and the FDA have been involved in efforts (19) to develop standards for the electronic submission of genomic data in general and hybridization data (step 6) in particular.

Standards in data analysis and biological interpretation have not been considered for most applications of genomic platforms. Additional experience in the analysis of exploratory hybridization data from VGDS submissions may help determine the need for data analysis and biological interpretation standards. These standards may be needed to optimize the correlation between biomarker set selection and toxicological endpoint so that the set selected may be successfully validated.

VALIDATION OF GENOMIC BIOMARKERS OF TOXICITY

VGDS generate exploratory data that accelerate development of genomic science at the FDA and in the pharmaceutical industry, but the main regulatory thrust of the Pharmacogenomics Guidance is in the application of valid genomic biomarkers. However, the Guidance does not define a process map for the validation of exploratory genomic biomarkers into the *probable* or *known* levels. The definition of this process map will be a major step in the implementation of genomic policy at the FDA.

The development of a process for validation of genomic biomarkers of toxicity requires a partnership between the FDA and the pharmaceutical industry. Collaborations between the pharmaceutical industry and the FDA are currently planned through Collaborative Research and Development Agreements (CRADAs) and the organization of industry consortia for cross-validation of genomic biomarkers. These collaborations will generate examples of validation for genomic biomarkers of toxicity in order to challenge the assumptions in proposed baseline process maps as outlined in Figure 1.

An FDA path for expert internal review in this preclinical genomic biomarker of toxicity process map proposal would be channeled through the Preclinical Toxicology Coordinating Committee (PTCC) with the technical assistance of the Genomics Team. The PTCC would be responsible for both the review and approval of both validation study protocols and final validation study results. If approved by the PTCC, next steps in this process could lead to

1. biomarker listed as *probable valid*, or
2. additional studies encouraged or planned to reach *known valid* biomarker status.

Different areas within the FDA would provide the required expert internal review for genomic biomarkers in each area. Initial steps in a validation process such as this could be started through a VGDS, where exploratory data could be discussed and debated and preliminary validation requirements may be identified. The outcome of VGDS submissions of exploratory data in this context could range from an exciting scientific

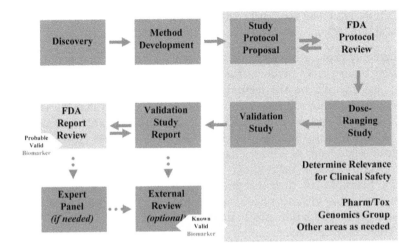

Figure 1 Process map proposal for preclinical genomic biomarkers of toxicity at the FDA.

exchange about the analytical and biological interpretations of the data to the basis for additional work leading to the validation of genomic biomarkers.

Limitations in the original assumptions of this process map proposal have already been identified. These are associated with the number of biomarkers, tissue toxicity models, positive and negative compounds, and other resources available to any one sponsor for validation studies of genomic biomarkers. These limitations underscore the need for collaboration across therapeutic areas and companies in the identification and validation of genomic biomarkers of toxicity. The FDA is working with several research institutes and sponsors on the organization of consortia to cross-validate genomic biomarkers for preclinical drug safety assessment.

Lessons learned from the specific validation examples resulting from these collaborations will refine these proposed process maps to generate information appropriate for guidance. This example is useful to assess what we should be looking for in exploratory biomarker candidates for validation. The nephrotoxicity markers in this example were

1. identified originally in exploratory studies with hybridization in whole genome chips,
2. confirmed in a second genomics platform, by quantitative PCR,
3. confirmed in a second species (nonhuman primates), and
4. included protein products with potential application as accessible bridging biomarkers.

These four observations are useful to identify genomic biomarker candidates for validation.

SELECTION OF GENOMIC BIOMARKERS OF TOXICITY FOR VALIDATION

Are there any exploratory genomic biomarkers of toxicity that may lead to validated biomarkers? Much of the work published thus far in toxicogenomics has focused on the identification of gene expression changes for which some evidence suggests a correlation between these changes and the development of specific organ toxicities, without necessarily following a path by which these findings could be formally validated (20). Some of the unpublished work in this area has been associated with the development of proprietary assays focused on ranking compounds for development (21–23). Examples of these proprietary markers are those identified by companies such as GeneLogic (21) and Iconix (22,23). We would not expect extensive public validation efforts in either of these cases.

There may be some exceptions to this observation. Genomic biomarkers of nephrotoxicity identified over the past decade may represent a good example of genomic biomarkers that may be appropriate for validation. The International Life Science Institute Health and Environmental Science Institute (ILSI-HESI) Technical Committee on the Application of Genomics to Mechanism-Based Risk Assessment started in 1999. The Nephrotoxicity Working Group within this committee published several papers (24–26) on the identification of gene expression changes associated with nephrotoxicity in the rat. These papers identified a number of gene expression changes correlating with the development of kidney proximal tubular injury that have been independently confirmed in the rat (20) and in nonhuman primates (27). The protein products of several of these genes such as kidney injury molecule (KIM-1) have been shown to be accessible biomarkers in rat (28) and human (29) urine. These findings suggest that genomic biomarkers for nephrotoxicity may be good candidates for validation.

What would make a good candidate biomarker for validation? On the basis of what we have presented in this review we can answer this question by identifying

1. value added by the biomarker,
2. context of its application (surrogate vs. mechanistic),
3. sensitivity and reproducibility of animal model,
4. sensitivity, dynamic range, and reproducibility of genomic platform, and
5. resources available for validation.

SIMILARITIES AND DIFFERENCES IN BIOMARKER VALIDATION PROCESSES BETWEEN REGULATORY AGENCIES

These criteria are consistent with current European proposals (2) for biomarker validation. While the draft guidance document from the EMEA described earlier (12) defines neither valid biomarkers nor a validation path for them, the European draft IMI document (2) proposes a validation path for biomarkers. According to this document, each new candidate biomarker would require validation in the preclinical and clinical arenas and a minimal biomarker pre-validation package prior to acceptance. To achieve general acceptance, the document considers in-house validation by a sponsor (which the FDA might consider a "probable valid" biomarker) insufficient. This document proposes creation of a European Center for Drug Safety (ECDS) that would be responsible for validation of genomic biomarkers of toxicity. In this proposal, project teams within the ECDS would

1. define transparent criteria for biomarker acceptance,
2. develop test kits for different species,
3. establish acceptable criteria in preclinical species for preclinical biomarkers,
4. validate in a sufficient number of clinical studies for clinical biomarkers,
5. provide mechanistic understanding, and
6. complete data analysis.

An essential requirement for a public process in biomarker validation is characteristic of the IMI draft (2) as well as the process defined by the European Center for Validation of Alternative Methods (ECVAM) (30). ECVAM validation consists of five main stages: test development; prevalidation; validation (involving a formal interlaboratory study with the testing of coded chemicals); independent assessment; and progression toward regulatory acceptance. In the United States, the Interagency Coordinating Committee on the Validation of Alternative Methods (ICCVAM) (31) coordinates and advises on interagency issues on development, validation, and regulatory acceptance of new, improved and alternative test methods, and the national and international harmonization of such methods. The ICCVAM process for biomarker validation closely resembles the process originally developed by ECVAM in Europe.

Congress enacted the ICCVAM Authorization Act (Public Law 106–545, December 19, 2000) "to establish, wherever feasible, guidelines, recommendations, and regulations that promote the regulatory acceptance of new or revised scientifically valid toxicological tests that protect human and animal health and the environment while reducing, refining, or replacing animal tests and ensuring human safety and product effectiveness." ICCVAM is responsible for:

1. Promotion of scientific validation and regulatory acceptance of new, improved, and alternative test methods.
2. Coordination of review/evaluation of new/revised alternative test methods of interagency interest.

3. Guidance on test method development, the validation process, validation criteria, regulatory acceptance criteria, and submission requirements.
4. Recommendations to Federal agencies on the validation status of test methods and their regulatory suitability.
5. Interagency regulatory acceptance and international harmonization and adoption of scientifically validated test methods.
6. Awareness of and training for accepted test methods (end-users, regulators).

ECVAM and ICCVAM (32) consider that the validation of toxicogenomics-based test methods may require new approaches to standardize and evaluate the scientific validity of test methods based on toxicogenomics and that the entire validation process may be different and more complex than that for classical alternatives since both the predictive test system and the applied new technology will need to be validated. Specific issues associated with these validations may include differences in platforms, impact of changes of arrays and sets of genes, quality assurance and GLP compliance, degree of acceptable variability, assessment of intra- and interlaboratory reproducibility, data evaluation and analysis procedures, reference materials and databases. All of these technical issues may be addressed for the validation of genomic biomarkers without necessarily establishing an exceptional category for this validation process.

The charter and interest of ICCVAM in the interagency validation of test methods can complement efforts of the FDA in this area. However, the application of the ICCVAM validation process for the validation and acceptance of genomic biomarkers may require a review of the ICCVAM validation process map. ICCVAM initiates a public validation process upon the direct request of private sponsors who would be eventually expected to apply the validated biomarkers in their submission of data to regulatory agencies. Its process map considers validation directly to a *known valid* level, and can require a time-consuming sequence of meetings and reviews associated with the need to assemble de novo expert external review groups and to solicit both consensus from these on their evaluation of submitted data and requests for additional data as needed.

An alternative to this process would be to have ICCVAM certify that genomic biomarker validation processes in regulatory agencies are consistent with their own validation standards while allowing the exchange of information regarding genomic biomarker validation to remain controlled by regulatory agencies within their information firewalls. This scheme, consistent with the validation process map in Figure 1, would bring closer together from the beginning of the validation process the sponsors and reviewers that would eventually be, respectively, expected to apply validated biomarkers in drug development and review results from their application in regulatory submissions. It would facilitate the assembly of internal expert review groups within regulatory agencies while protecting, where needed, intellectual property not directly required for the acceptance of validated biomarkers. A more productive path for the interaction between ICCVAM and individual regulatory agencies will facilitate guidance development for the validation of genomic biomarkers of toxicity.

REFERENCES

1. FDA whitepaper, 2004: Innovation or Stagnation, challenge and opportunity on the critical path to new medical products. http://www.fda.gov/oc/initiatives/criticalpath/whitepaper.html [accessed September 4, 2004].
2. The Innovative Medicines Initiative (IMI) Strategic Research Agenda. Creating Biomedical R&D Leadership for Europe to Benefit Patients and Society. Draft document, European Commission, July 26, 2005. http://europa.eu.int/comm/research/fp6/index_en.cfm?p=1 innomed.
3. Biomarkers Definition Working Group. Biomarkers and surrogate endpoints: Preferred definitions and conceptual framework. Clin Pharmacol Ther 2001; 69:89–95.
4. Guidance for Industry: Pharmacogenomic Data Submissions, posted on March 22, 2005. http://www.fda.gov/cder/guidance/6400fnl.pdf.
5. Salerno RA, Lesko LJ. Pharmacogenomics in drug development and regulatory decision-making: the Genomic Data Submission (GDS) proposal. Pharmacogenomics 2004; 5:25–30.
6. Salerno RA, Lesko LJ. Pharmacogenomic data: FDA voluntary and required submission guidance. Pharmacogenomics 2004; 5:503–505.
7. Leighton JK, DeGeorge J, Jacobson-Kram D, MacGregor J, Mendrick D, Worobec A. Pharmacogenomic data submissions to the FDA: non-clinical case studies. Pharmacogenomics 2004; 5:507–511.
8. Ruaño G, Collins JM, Dorner AJ, Wang S-J, Guerciolini R, Huang S-M. Pharmacogenomic data submissions to the FDA: clinical pharmacology case studies. Pharmacogenomics 2004; 5:513–517.
9. Trepicchio WL, Williams GA, Essayan D, et al. Pharmacogenomic data submissions to the FDA: clinical case studies. Pharmacogenomics 2004; 5:519–524.
10. Frueh FW, Huang SM, Lesko LJ. Regulatory acceptance of toxicogenomics data. Environ Health Perspect 2004; 112(August):A663–A664.
11. Lesko L, Woodcock J. Translation of pharmacogenomics and pharmacogenetics: a regulatory perspective. Nat Rev Drug Discov 2004; 3:763–770.
12. Guideline on Pharmacogenetics Briefing Meetings (London, March 17, 2005. EMEA/CHMP/20227/2004). http://www.emea.eu.int/pdfs/human/pharmacogenetics/2022704en.pdf.
13. Tong W, Cao X, Harris S, et al. ArrayTrack–Supporting Toxicogenomic Research at the FDA's National Center for Toxicological Research (NCTR). Environ Health Persp 2003; 111:1819–1826.
14. Cronin M, Ghosh K, Sistare F, Quackenbush J, Vilker V, O'Connell C. Universal RNA reference materials for gene expression. Clin Chem 2004; 50: 1464–1471.

15. MicroArray Quality Control (MAQC) project. 2006. http://www.fda.gov/nctr/science/centers/toxicoinformatics/maqc/.
16. External RNA Control Consortium Workshop: Specifications for Universal External RNA Spike-In Controls. National Institute of Standards and Technology. 2003. http://www.cstl.nist.gov/biotech/workshops/ERCC2003/.
17. Use of External RNA Spike-In Controls in Gene Expression Assays. 2005. http://www.nccls.org/Template.cfm?Section=Projects_in_Development8.
18. Workshop on Fluorescence Standards for Microarray Assays. 2002. http://www.cstl.nist.gov/biotech/fluormicroarray/FluorescentStdsForMicroarrays2002Notes.pdf.
19. Electronic Regulatory Submissions and Review. 2005. http://www.fda.gov/cder/regulatory/ersr/default.htm.
20. Thukral S, Nordone P, Hu R, et al. Prediction of nephrotoxicant action and identification of candidate toxicity-related biomarkers. Toxical Pathol, 2005; 33:343–355.
21. Castle A, Carver M, Mendrick D. Toxicogenomics: a new revolution in drug safety. Drug Discovery Today 2002; 7:728–736.
22. Ganter B, Tugendreich S, Pearson CI, et al. 2005. Development of a large-scale chemogenomics database to improve drug candidate selection and to understand mechanisms of chemical toxicity and action. J Biotechnol 2005; 119(3):219–244.
23. Fielden MR, Pearson C, Brennan R, Kolaja KL. Preclinical drug safety analysis by chemogenomic profiling in the liver. Am J Pharmacogenomics 2005; 5(3):161–171.
24. Thompson KL, Afshari CA, Amin RP, et al. Identification of platform-independent gene expression markers of cisplatin nephrotoxicity. Environ Health Perspect. 2004; 112:488–494.
25. Amin RP, Vickers AE, Sistare F, et al. Identification of putative gene based markers of renal toxicity. Environ Health Perspect 2004; 112:465–479.
26. Kramer JA, Pettit SD, Amin RP, et al. Overview on the application of transcription profiling using selected nephrotoxicants for toxicology assessment. Environ Health Perspect 2004; 112:460–446.
27. Davis JW II, Goodsaid FM, Bral CM, et al. Quantitative gene expression analysis in a nonhuman primate model of antibiotic-induced nephrotoxicity. Toxicol Appl Pharmacol 2004; 200:16–26.
28. Ichimura T, Bonventre JV, Bailly V, et al. Kidney injury molecule-1 (KIM-1), a putative epithelial cell adhesion molecule containing a novel immunoglobulin domain, is up-regulated in renal cells after injury. J Biol Chem 1998; 273:4135–4142.
29. Han WK, Bailly V, Abichandani R, Thadhani R, Bonventre JV. Kidney Injury Molecule-1 (KIM-1): a novel biomarker for human renal proximal tubule injury. Kidney Int 2002; 62:237–244.
30. The Validation Process at ECVAM. 2005. http://ecvam.jrc.it/index.htm.
31. The ICCVAM Test Method Evaluation Process. 2005. http://iccvam.niehs.nih.gov/about/overview.htm.
32. Corvi et al. Validation of toxicogenomics-based test Systems: ECVAM- ICCVAM/NICEATM considerations for regulatory Use. EHP. Epub ahead of print. doi:10.1289/ehp.8247.

10

Use of Biomarkers in Occupational Safety and Health

Edward V. Sargent

Global Safety and the Environment, Merck & Co., Inc., Whitehouse Station, New Jersey, U.S.A.

INTRODUCTION

A goal of all occupational safety and health programs is the prevention of adverse health effects resulting from exposure to chemical, biological, or physical agents in the work environment. The risk of adverse health effects occurring in a population of workers is dependent on three factors: (i) the inherent toxicity or hazard of the agent, (ii) the number and susceptibility of the employees handling the agent, and (iii) the uses of the agent resulting in a potential for exposure.

Biological markers or biomarkers are observed or measured events in biological systems or samples. Generally, biomarkers are classified into three types: biomarkers of prior exposures, biomarkers of early biological effects, and biomarkers of generic or individual susceptibility. A biomarker may include the measurement of a substance or its metabolite, the measurement of a product of the interaction of a substance with a cellular constituent, or the measurement of a signaling event in the biological system or sample. In occupational settings, biomarkers of exposure are often used for or equated with biomonitoring. By the same token, biomarkers of effect are commonly used in health monitoring, health surveillance, or medical surveillance programs (1).

BIOMARKERS OF EXPOSURE

The periodic measurement of biomarkers of exposure is referred to as biomonitoring. It is an industrial hygiene tool for assessing a worker's exposure to chemical, physical, or biological agents. Industrial hygiene is the science of anticipating, recognizing, evaluating, and controlling health hazards in the workplace. A classical industrial hygiene strategy (Fig. 1) for identifying, characterizing, and assessing exposures is to start with exposure modeling coupled with environmental monitoring. Exposure modeling involves an understanding of sources of emissions, fate of emissions, and the location of receptors, which in this case are employees, in space and time. Environmental monitoring involves the measurement of agents in air, water, and other media.

Biological monitoring examines biomarkers of exposure in body fluids as well as skin, hair, teeth, breath, and cells. The major determinants of the usefulness of biomonitoring to estimate exposure are validated sampling and analytical methods, cost, availability of technical resources, and the invasiveness of the procedure for obtaining a sample. There are still few validated, cost-effective, and noninvasive measurement techniques available for routine biomonitoring. For example, the use of K-X-ray fluorescence to measure bone lead (2) has been proposed as a noninvasive monitoring technique; however, cost, the availability of technical know-how, and lack of validation make this technique questionable for routine use.

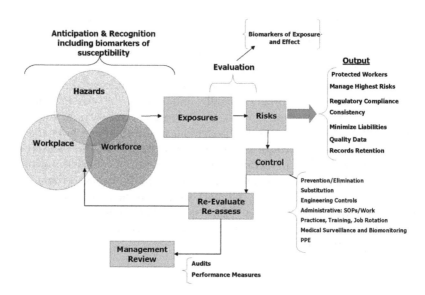

Figure 1 An industrial hygiene strategy for exposure assessment.

Analysis of urine and exhaled air has shown some promise as a non-invasive and cost-effective tool for assessing exposure to certain metals, volatile solvents, and cholinesterase-inhibiting pesticides; however, validated sampling procedures along with biological exposure indices (BEI) have been established for only five solvents in exhaled air and approximately 25 other compounds or their metabolites in urine (3).

Biomonitoring is thought to be superior to air monitoring because it is a measure of internal dose rather than an estimate of the quantity of chemical presented to a worker. Biomonitoring might also be considered in order to assess workplace exposures through the dermal route or inadvertent ingestion. Biomonitoring can be further expanded to a determination of a biologically effective dose by determining the quantity of material that interacts subcellular, cellular, or tissue constituents.

BIOMARKERS OF BIOLOGICAL EFFECT

Biological effects have been defined as: (i) recognized disease or health impairment, (ii) early precursors of the disease process indicating potential for health impairment, or (iii) an indicator event peripheral to but correlated with the disease process (1).

In the occupational setting, health or medical surveillance is conducted for employees who work with hazardous agents, with markers of early precursors in the disease process an obvious preference. Health surveillance is generally needed: (i) to confirm adequacy of workplace controls (engineering work practices or personal protective equipment), (ii) to support the appropriateness of an occupational exposure limit, and (iii) to reduce uncertainty in the exposure assessment process.

Biological markers of effect must be attributable to specific environmental exposures in order to be useful, as the guiding purpose of any biomarker program in any occupational setting is the prevention of workplace exposure, which results in adverse health. Health effects or disease characteristics that occur within a short period of time after exposure are more easily linked to that xenobiotic exposure. Diseases or disease processes occurring many years after exposure are very difficult to associate with exposure to specific agents, unless the disease or its consequences have been causally or mechanistically related to exposure to specific agents, i.e., aplastic anemia and benzene or asbestos and mesothelioma. Biomarkers of exposure and effect primarily assess more recent exposures, and are especially problematic when applied to the assessment of carcinogen exposure (4). In epidemiological research, biomarkers of both exposure and effect have been used to overcome the many limitations encountered with existing exposure data. This is especially so in conducting retrospective studies where exposure estimates are crudely estimated using work histories, job titles, qualitative exposure assessment, and exposure monitoring and modeling (5).

BIOMARKERS OF SUSCEPTIBILITY

Biomarkers can indicate individual or population differences in response to exposure to environmental agents (1,5). In toxicology and risk assessment, much effort is given to identifying and accounting for sensitive or susceptible individuals and subpopulations.

Biomarkers that reflect some intrinsic genetic characteristic or pre-existing condition that alters the susceptibility of the individual in response to environmental exposures, can be useful; however, the ethical issues with the use of biomarkers to single out hypersusceptible employees continues to be of concern and has prevented its more widespread use. While many of the recent ethical issues stem from advances in genetic screening and the identification of hypersusceptibility, the issues have been discussed for many years as a function of different diseases such as breast cancer and diabetes, and for exposures such as lead.

Use of biomarkers is thought to have some benefit in certain standard occupational health programs such as preplacement examinations, medical surveillance programs incorporating biomonitoring, and in illness investigations and epidemiological studies aimed at determining whether disease or symptoms are causally related to work (6). The ethical considerations of using biomarkers in occupational health vary considerably depending on whether they are examined to identify exposures, identify clinical effects resulting from exposure, or to identify susceptible individuals. Preplacement or fitness for duty examinations are conducted on employees to determine the presence or absence of a physical or psychological condition that could interfere with the safe performance of a job. For example, employees who are required to wear a respirator undergo preplacement and periodic medical monitoring to confirm that the employee can perform the job in a safe manner, that the respirator will not cause any physiological problems, and that the employee is psychologically able to wear a respirator.

The incorporation of markers of genetic susceptibility into preplacement examinations of workers could identify individuals at increased risk of the consequences of exposure and thus raise questions about the suitability of employment in certain exposing operations. While confidentiality is one concern with susceptibility, it is not the only concern. Communication of increased susceptibility to disease is not a trivial matter. Finally, the most significant concern is likely to be the impact on the susceptible employees' future employment. One classic ethical dilemma that occurred in the United States was when several women working in a lead plant chose to undergo tubal ligation rather than risk losing their jobs. The reason was concern on the part of the company management with fetal hypersensitivity to lead exposures (7).

The need for guidelines for the use of biomarkers, particularly to identify susceptibility, has been recommended, but up until now not acted upon (8). Generally, proponents of biomonitoring offer that identifying susceptible individuals will allow for the identification of needed improvement in occupational exposure levels (OELs). A simpler and more practical approach has been to simply incorporate an additional margin of safety or uncertainty factor (UF) into the determination of the occupational exposure limit (9). Recent improvements in the use of toxicokinetic and toxicodynamic data to better define interindividual differences have led to significant refinement of UFs and improvement of risk estimates (10).

PRACTICAL ISSUES IN THE APPLICATION OF BIOMARKERS IN OCCUPATIONAL HEALTH PROGRAMS

Selection and Validation of Biomarkers

Many potential biomarkers may exist, including measurement of parent compound or its metabolites in body tissues, blood, expired air, and excretory products. Biomarkers should ideally be sensitive, i.e., they should vary consistently and quantitatively with the extent of exposure or effect, and also be specific for the environmental exposure or adverse health effect of concern. An approach to determining the validity of a biomarker proposed by the NRC Committee on Biological Markers is to develop a matrix of data from acute and chronic animal studies and clinical studies that allows for the comparison of markers of effect in animals to effects in exposed human populations (1). The selection of a biological marker of exposure, effect, or susceptibility, however, requires a significant amount of experimental research in animals and clinical studies in humans in order to understand the basic underlying events resulting in an adverse health effect. Such research has only been conducted on a rare few chemicals handled in workplaces. Further, it is highly unlikely that resources will be devoted to conducting the research necessary for the broad scale use of biomarkers in routine occupational health programs.

Sampling and Analytical Methodology

Under Haber's Rule, dose is considered to be a function of contaminant concentration and exposure time. In an occupational setting, however, exposure is impacted by many variables such as body size, personal hygiene, work practice, level of fitness, smoking, alcohol and drug usage, and nutritional status. Dose is further impacted by inter- and intraindividual variability in pharmacokinetics and pharmacodynamics. Biological monitoring has an advantage in that it can take into account all of these variables while providing a more accurate estimate of internal dose, thus serving as a useful adjunct to workplace air monitoring.

The major limitation for the widespread use of biomonitoring in occupational settings is the limited number of substances for which there are suitable, definitive, and validated tests as well as values to assist in the interpretation of results. The American Conference of Governmental Industrial Hygienists (ACGIH) has established BEI for a little over 40 substances (3), while the U.K. Health and Safety Executive has established 10 biological monitoring guidance values (BMGV) and the German Deutsche Forschungsemeinschaft has established values for 63 chemicals (11,12). For many more chemicals, an appropriate biological parameter is known but an acceptable exposure index cannot be established because toxicological and clinical studies to define the relationship between exposure, uptake, and quantitative changes in the measured biological parameter have not been conducted (13). Analytical methods exist for a relatively few biomarkers that could be applied in a general workplace biomonitoring program. These consist primarily of the measurement of adducts or metabolites. Cytogenetic measurements of chromosome aberrations and micronuclei have been occasionally used in routine applications. Other methods such as the incorporation of immunochemistry to detect adducts, noninvasive measurement of bone lead using K-X-ray fluorescence (14), and toxicogenomics and proteomics have found use in research epidemiological investigations but will require significant development before they can be applied in routine occupational health programs (15).

Blood, urine, and exhaled air are the most likely sources of specimens for examining biomarkers in an occupational setting largely because they are the least invasive sampling matrices. Other specimens such as tissue samples, hair and nails, and feces are not suitable for routine testing because they are either invasive, sensitive to external contamination, or inconvenient, respectively (3). Variables affecting the measurement of a biomarker are shown in Table 1. Each type of specimen has certain variables, which must be considered when interpreting results of samples. Measurement of urinary contaminants must consider variability in urinary output/volume, blood sample analysis must consider plasma:erythrocyte ratio and protein binding, and exhaled air concentrations rapidly change during the course of expiration (3).

Quality Assurance

Generally, when animal or human studies are conducted, certain quality control or quality assurance procedures are required. This is especially so for testing conducted for occupational health purposes, where decisions related to employee health and safety require a full understanding of exposure and risk. Good Laboratory Practices have been developed by any number of organizations such as the OECD (17), ISO (17), and FDA (18), which could be applied to human biomonitoring. However, the majority of studies conducted to date have been for research purposes; few are likely to meet such GLP standards (15). Table 2 from the ACGIH

Table 1 Variables Affecting Determinant Levels in Biomonitoring

Variable	Effect
Time	
Exposure duration	Levels increase with exposure duration
Repeated exposures	Levels increase if $t_{\frac{1}{2}} > 5$ hours
Sampling time	Vary with length of exposure to sample interval
	Chemical-dependent differences
Sampling period	Blood samples generally reflect recent exposure
	Urine samples reflect average of the sample duration
Physiological	
Physical activity	Increases absorption during exposure, accelerates elimination postexposure
Metabolism	Decreased concentration of parent compound, increased concentration of metabolites. Multiple metabolites of concern produced
Plasma protein binding	Decreased levels of total determinant in urine and free determinant in blood samples
Nutrition	
Body fat	Effect on lipophilic compounds
Fasting	Effect on lipophilic compounds
Diet	Potential source of background determinant, may change pH and thus levels of weak electrolytes
Water intake	Can affect urine concentration significantly
Disease state	
Pulmonary disease	Significant effect on blood determinant levels
Renal disease	Significant effect on blood and urine samples
Liver disease	Significant effect for metabolized chemicals
Medications	May affect metabolism, protein binding, or elimination of determinant
Environment	
Chemical mixtures	Can alter metabolic activity if codeterminants are at high concentration
Temperature	Minimal affect

Source: From Ref. 16.

presents some methodological considerations necessary in order to meet GLP requirements.

Program Administration

In published biomonitoring or epidemiological studies of workers, there are very few, if any, discussions around program administration. For that reason, there is little written on issues regarding informed consent, employee communications, consequences of the results, and recordkeeping.

Table 2 Methodological Considerations in Biomonitoring

Sampling	*Analytical*
Physicochemical properties of determinants	Cleanup procedures
Volatility	Possible interferences
Reactivity	Good laboratory practices
Photolability	Sensitivity and specificity of method
Specimen characteristics	Acceptable criteria
Sample collection period	
Qualified health personnel	*Administrative*
Biohazard protection	Recordkeeping
Proper timing of sample	Medical confidentiality
Sources of contamination	Employee communications
Chemical mixtures	Administrative controls
Sample collection materials	Exposure control
Sample volume	Medical removal
	Medical follow-up
Transportation and storage	Training
Eliminate contamination	
Source of deterioration	
Storage temperature	

Source: From Ref. 16.

SPECIFIC EXAMPLES OF BIOMARKER APPLICATION IN OCCUPATIONAL HEALTH

Lead

For more than three decades, the scientific community has been accumulating evidence of adverse health effects associated with lead exposure. This has led to a number of regulatory initiatives aimed at the elimination of lead from products such as paint, solder, and gasoline. Lead remains a significant component in many products manufactured, including radiators, batteries, ceramics, and ammunition, and as such is a significant occupational exposure hazard.

The U.S. Occupational Safety and Health Administration (OSHA) established standards for a number of workplace contaminants (19) including several for which biological monitoring is recommended or required, including cadmium, benzene, methylene chloride, and lead. The OSHA lead standard includes a permissible exposure level (PEL) of $50\,\mu g/m^3$ (eight-hour time weighted average, TWA) and an action limit (AL) of $30\,\mu g/m^3$ (eight-hour TWA) and requires employers to conduct biological monitoring of all employees exposed to lead above the AL for more than 30 days in a single year. The standard specifies that the biological monitoring should consist of tests for blood lead and blood zinc protoporphyrin levels. Samples must be taken every six months, unless the employee has exposure resulting in a blood lead level above 40 µg/100 g of whole blood, in which case the biomonitoring must be conducted every two months and continued until two consecutive tests are below the 40 µg/100 g criterion. The standard further defines requirements for blood test accuracy and quality assurance and outlines requirements for employee notification of results and removal from the workplace until normal blood lead levels are reached. All these point to the level of complexity necessary to conduct biomonitoring as part of an occupational surveillance program.

Blood lead levels are a good indicator of current or recent lead exposure, but are not necessarily representative of the total body burden of lead and do not adequately reflect past exposures. The majority (up to 90%) of the body burden of lead accumulates in skeletal bone (20,2) and this accumulated level is not reflected by blood lead levels. Urinary lead levels can also be measured; however, like blood lead levels, urinary lead is also a measure of recent exposure and it also is not considered as a reliable measure due to variability in urinary lead excretion and difficulty in collecting 24-hour urine samples. Lack of convenient and noninvasive methods for determining bone lead have made the determination of cumulative lead body burdens difficult. Techniques involving use of K-X-ray fluorescence have been developed, which have allowed for the noninvasive in vivo measurement of bone lead levels (14,21); however, these techniques are not used in routine lead biomonitoring, but rather in epidemiologic research.

The toxicity of lead has been well studied but, while not completely understood, has resulted in further refinement of biomarkers of the effects. Lead toxicity includes the induction of anemia, neurotoxicity evidenced by behavioral changes, cognitive effects and central nervous system changes, renal toxicity leading to hypertension, and reproductive toxicity. Anemia, one of the earliest effects of lead, results from the inhibition of two enzymes in the heme synthesis pathway. Delta-aminolevulinic acid dehydrase, which catalyzes the conversion of delta-aminolevulinic acid to protoporphyrin, is inhibited at blood lead levels less than 20 µg/100g whole blood. Ferrochelatase is also inhibited at low blood levels, which leads to increased production of zinc protoporphyrin (ZPP). ZPP has also been used (and is required by OSHA) as a biomarker of exposure and effect. More recent studies in Korean lead workers have demonstrated associations between blood and bone lead and poor renal function (22) and between blood lead and poorer neurobehavioral test scores (23). In examining the implications for biomarker selection, it is interesting to note that in the latter study, blood lead was found to be a better predictor of neurobehavioral performance.

Propylene Oxide

Biomonitoring of exposure to or effect of genotoxic carcinogens continues
to be a major research interest for biomarker development (15). Biomarkers
of exposure and effect have been developed, which reflect what is currently
known about the sequence of molecular and cellular events leading to cancer, starting with early evidence of exposure such as DNA and protein
adducts, to DNA damage, chromosomal aberrations, mutations, and ultimately cancer (24). The earliest biomonitoring for genotoxic carcinogens
was conducted to determine internal dose and to refine risk estimates of
human exposure. A large body of research evidence in cells and animals
has linked DNA damage and mutations to carcinogenesis (25–27). Increasing knowledge of the chemistry of nucleic acids lead to an understanding of
a mechanism whereby electrophilic compounds (either direct acting or metabolic products) reacted with nucleophilic centers in both DNA and proteins.
It quickly became apparent that protein adducts and specifically hemoglobin protein adducts provided significant advantages over DNA adducts
for human biomonitoring (28–30).

DNA adducts have proven difficult to correlate with dose due to the
fact that they are repaired, with the rate and extent of repair dependent
on the type of adduct, tissue, and age. On the other hand, blood, being
one of the only readily available tissues for biomonitoring, is an abundant
source of protein for adduct determination (31). Serum albumin is the most
abundant blood protein; however, it is subject to turnover and therefore
adducts have a relatively short half-life of approximately 20 days (5). Hemoglobin (Hb) is the next most abundant protein, and since adducts do not
affect the stability of hemoglobin, the consequent removal of adducts is
dependent on the lifetime of the red blood cell, which is approximately
120 days. Hemoglobin adducts are thus an excellent biomarker to assess
internal dose resulting from repeated low-dose exposures most likely seen
in occupational or environmental settings. The cumulative effects of such
repeated low-dose exposures, whether they be by inhalation or the dermal
route, are most difficult to evaluate and quantify by traditional industrial
hygiene exposure assessment methods.

Ehrenberg and his colleagues originally examined histidine adducts
in hemoglobin of workers exposed to ethylene oxide or propylene oxide
(32–35). However, since then hemoglobin adducts have been used to study
worker populations with occupational exposure to a number of genotoxic
chemicals, including aromatic amines (36), acrylamide (37), acrylonitrile
(38) 1,3-butadiene (39), and benzene (40). The earliest methods utilized
gas chromatograph–mass spectrometer (GC–MS) in order to obtain the sensitivity needed (41); however, tedious and complicated sample preparation
methods hampered more widespread use in routine biomonitoring (31). A
more recent modification of an Edman-degradation method by Tornqvist

et al. (42) led to a more reliable determination of the N-terminal valine adducts to hemoglobin and improved greatly their suitability for use as a routine biomonitoring tool (43).

The use of hemoglobin adducts as a biomonitor of propylene oxide (PO) provides an excellent example of the usefulness of biomarkers in occupational health. Hemoglobin adducts have been incorporated into bio-monitoring programs for propylene oxide, which allow for the reliable quantification of chronic, intermittent, and low-level airborne exposures (31). Such exposures are often the most difficult to assess using standard ambient air monitoring. Correlation between personal breathing zone data and PO:Hb adduct levels allowed for the derivation of a biological exposure limit (BEL) for PO. For example, at the Dutch OEL for PO of 10 mg/m^3, the corresponding BEL for PO is 5.3 nmol HOPrVal/g globin (43). Finally, measurement of PO:Hb adducts following inhalation exposure in multiple animal species has allowed for improved interspecies comparisons based on internal dose (44) and for suggested refinement of the human carcinogenic potency factor for PO (45).

Polycyclic Aromatic Hydrocarbons

Polycyclic aromatic hydrocarbons (PAHs) are a class of highly lipophilic, persistent compounds ubiquitous in the environment. PAHs are found naturally in crude oils, mineral oils, coal, and tars and are formed during the incomplete combustion of hydrocarbons, particularly fossil fuels. PAHs are widely distributed in the environment and in all environmental media (i.e., air, water, and soil), largely due to combustion and spills. Within the class of PAHs are many individual chemicals; however, exposure to these chemicals is never to individual chemicals but to complex mixtures in the form of tobacco smoke, air pollution, dietary sources, and by dermal contact with oils, soot, and tars (46). The International Agency for Research on Cancer (IARC) has conducted several reviews of polyaromatic compounds and concluded that there was sufficient evidence of carcinogenicity for a number of them (46). IARC further concluded there was sufficient evidence of carcinogenicity for the subclass of PAHs (46).

PAH exposure has been associated with a number of occupations, some of which have excess rates of cancer. These include coke oven workers, asphalt pavers, roofers, aluminum smelters, foundry workers, boilermakers, carbon black workers, and coal tar painters. Worker exposures to PAHs have primarily been assessed through area and breathing zone sampling of the workplace or ambient air. In many of these assessments it was necessary to sample for an individual surrogate, either coal tar pitch volatiles or benzo[a]pyrene, to represent total PAH exposure (47). While industrial exposure assessment largely has focused on the inhalation route, increasing evidence suggests that the dermal route may account for as much as 90%

of exposure for some workers (48). Given that occupational exposures are generally to mixtures of PAHs and that exposures by the dermal route are significant, major research efforts have focused on the development of PAH biomarkers suitable for the biomonitoring of workers.

PAH absorption and uptake has been monitored by several different biomarkers, including urinary metabolites, protein adducts, and DNA adducts. Urinary mutagenicity and urinary thioethers have also been used in studies of workers but, because they are nonspecific indicators of PAH exposure and subject to confounding exposures, they are not suitable for routine biomonitoring (47). The most widely used biomarker of human exposure to PAH is the measurement of urinary 1-hydroxypyrene (1-OHP), a metabolite of pyrene (49). Pyrene is relatively abundant in PAH mixtures and metabolized and excreted as a glucuronide in urine. Half-lives for urinary formation of 1-OHP are relatively long, ranging from 6 to 48 hours, allowing for the collection of spot urine samples at the end of a work shift and end of a work week (47). Other data suggest that a sampling strategy where urine is collected over a 24-hour period gives a better estimate of the relationship between PAH dose and 1-OHP metabolite levels (50,51). In general, published occupational health studies using the urinary 1-OHP marker have used the spot sample protocol and include workers in asphalt paving (52), aluminum smelting (53), coke oven refineries (54), coal tar painting (55), and steel manufacturing (56). In each of these studies, urinary 1-OHP was demonstrated as a useful measure of recent PAH exposure, which had occurred by multiple routes. These studies also demonstrate, however, that cigarette smoking, diet, nonoccupational environmental exposures, and genetic polymorphisms of cytochrome P450 1A1 and glutathione transferases can all affect urinary concentration of 1-OHP.

No international organization or agency has proposed any BEL for 1-OHP. Lauwerys (57) provided a tentative limit of $27\,\mu g/g$ (1.4 umol/mol). Jongeneelen (47) proposed a three level benchmark guideline for urinary 1-OHP. In this system, the first level is based on the 95th percentile reference values of 0.24 and $0.76\,\mu gmol/mol$ creatinine for nonoccupationally exposed nonsmoking and smoking workers, respectively. The second level is based on the no-biological-effect-level of $1.4\,\mu gmol/mol$ of 1-OHP in urine of PAH exposed workers, and the third is based on the correlation between 1-OHP levels of 2.3 and 4.9 umol/mol creatinine measured in coke oven workers and aluminum smelters, respectively, with the OEL for PAHs.

DNA adducts have been studied as a biomarker of PAH exposure in a large number of occupational epidemiology studies. Reactive metabolic products of PAHs form adducts with DNA in many target tissues including skin, lungs, liver, and bladder, however, circulating white blood cells are the only readily available tissue for biomonitoring. Sensitive methods developed to measure PAH:DNA adducts including ^{32}P-postlabeling, immunochemical assays, and GC–MS have been extensively reviewed (58,27). The major difficulties with using DNA adducts in biomonitoring programs are that the techniques are relatively complex and costly and measure a wide range of adducts, thus limiting their usefulness in quantitative measurement. Some studies have shown unsatisfactory correlations between DNA adducts measured in white bloods cells and workplace PAH exposures (59), thus designating them more suitable for qualitative exposure assessment. Finally, it is uncertain what if any relationship exists between exposure, DNA adducts in peripheral white blood cells, and cancer risk, making the ultimate communication of results to workers a potential problem.

Antineoplastic Drugs

An extensive body of literature on biological markers of genetic damage or exposure in human populations has been developed since the 1960s (60). Biomarkers most widely applied to occupational exposure assessment studies have been the measurement of chromosome aberrations in circulating lymphocytes and the testing of urine mutagenicity. Other markers have been studied, however, most have not been subjected to use in large occupational cohort investigations. Attention must also be given to the genotoxic mode of action as well as the target tissue when attempting to select biomarkers to monitor worker exposure to genotoxic agents.

Early techniques for enumerating chromosomal aberrations were labor-intensive and in some instances, not sufficiently sensitive for use in routine biomonitoring (61,62). Methodological improvements have resulted in more efficient analytical procedures, however, cytogenetic testing is not routinely used and remains limited to epidemiologic research and study.

Two large cohort studies, the Nordic Study Group on the Health Risk of Chromosome Damage (63) and the European Study Group on Cytogenetic Biomarkers and Health (64), as well as numerous collaborative evaluations of the data (65–67), have shown clear and consistent evidence of an association between high levels of chromosome aberrations in circulating lymphocytes and increased total cancer incidence and mortality (68). Similar associations were not observed for sister chromatid exchanges and micronuclei in circulating lymphocytes, suggesting these endpoints might not be appropriate or relevant biomarkers of effect (69). Direct testing of urine for the presence of a specific mutagenic chemical or its metabolite(s) is useful when exposures are known. When identification of a specific mutagenic agent is not possible, simple, direct testing of urine mutagenicity has proven very useful in a number occupational exposure investigations (70,71). Again the relevance of elevated urine mutagenicity to risk of subsequent occupationally related disease is unknown.

Occupational exposure of health care workers to pharmacologically active compounds was first observed in the late 1970s when Falck et al. (72) demonstrated that the urine of nurses handling antineoplastic agents was mutagenic in the Ames microbial mutagenicity assay. Over the next 25 years, this early work has led to hundreds of studies of the exposure of health care workers to cytotoxic and/or antineoplastic drugs using biological monitoring for either urinary mutagenicity or cytogenetic analysis of circulating white blood cells (73). This effort has culminated in the recent publication by the U.S. National Institute for Occupational Safety and Health of an Alert for Preventing Occupational Exposures to Antineoplastic and other Hazardous Drugs in Health Care Settings (74).

Health care workers are potentially exposed to a large and myriad number of different drugs during the course of the work day and exposures may occur through one or more routes, including inhalation, dermal absorption, inadvertent ingestion, or injection (74). Genetic toxicity is often the basis of pharmacologic activity for many antineoplastic agents and a number have been shown to cause cancer and/or reproductive or developmental toxicity in laboratory animals. In a meta-analysis of published occupational epidemiologic studies, an association was found between exposure to antineoplastic drugs and adverse reproductive outcomes in health care workers (73). Further, Skov et al. (75) reported an increased risk of leukemia in Danish oncology nurses. Attempts to characterize exposures to antineoplastic drugs have been limited due to the lack of availability of sampling and analytical methods as well as OELs (76–78), however, such attempts generally show surface contamination to be consistently measurable while airborne concentrations to be either nondetectable or of very low concentration. It is for these reasons that so many investigations have employed biomonitoring to assess worker exposure. While no single marker has been routinely employed, the majority have examined urinary mutagenicity followed by sister chromatid exchange and analysis of chromosome aberrations in peripheral lymphocytes (73). Some of these studies conducted follow-up testing after appropriate handling precautions and other exposure control measures were implemented and clearly demonstrated a reduction in exposure (79). Sessink et al. (80) utilized data on urinary excretion of the antineoplastic drug cyclophosphamide along with evidence of increased chromosome aberrations in peripheral lymphocytes to estimate the risk of cancer in exposed oncology nurses and pharmacy technicians. They estimated that a 70 kg individual working 200 days/yr for 10 years would have a mean daily uptake of 3.6 to 18 μg. This resulted in additional cancer risk of 1.4 to 10 cases per million workers per year for pharmacy technicians and 7 to 50 cases per million workers per year for oncology nurses. The development of OELs by manufacturers of pharmaceutically active compounds has somewhat reduced the reliance on biomonitoring for purposes of exposure assessment (81,82).

SUMMARY

A review of biomarker methods written over a decade ago concluded that "although some of the more optimistic aspirations for human biomonitoring studies envisaged a decade ago have not been realized thus far, some considerable advances have been made" (58). The authors went on to discuss a number of methodological advances leading to a further conclusion that "the feasibility of biomonitoring has been clearly established." It is clear that in the intervening years we have seen even greater advances in the understanding of molecular mechanisms of disease, advances in the identification of relevant biomarkers for many of those diseases, and increasing sensitivity and specificity of chemical analyses. However, it would appear that many of the aspirations for the use of biomonitoring in occupational health remain unrealized. Biomarkers of susceptibility to toxicants and gene–environment interactions are expected to contribute to significant improvements in risk assessment and the prevention of disease, particularly cancer (83). However, until the many ethical, legal and sociological, and scientific issues identified earlier are addressed, biomonitoring to identify susceptible workers will not become a routinely used tool in occupational health practice. More likely possibilities are that biomonitoring will continue to be used to (i) establish whether workplace exposures have occurred, (ii) aid in the classification of exposures for occupational epidemiology studies, and (iii) determine an internal dose for medical surveillance purposes. Even still, the practical circumstances under which biomonitoring data will be validated, compared, communicated, and otherwise used must be clarified.

REFERENCES

1. National Research Council. Biological markers in environmental health research. Environ Health Perspect 1987; 74:3–9.
2. Hu HR, Kim R, Fleischaker G, Aro A. Measuring bone lead as a biomarker of cumulative lead dose. In: Mendelsohn ML, Mohr LC, Peeters JP, eds. Biomarkers: Medical and Workplace Applications. Washington: Joseph Henry Press, 1998:71–86.
3. American Conference of Governmental Industrial Hygienists. Biological Exposure Indices, Cincinnati: ACGIH, 2001.
4. Lauwerys RR. Occupational toxicology. In: Amdur MO, Doull J, Klaassen CD, eds. Toxicology—The Basic Science of Poisons. 4th ed., New York: McGraw-Hill, 1983.
5. Mutti A. Biological monitoring in occupational and environmental toxicology. Toxicol Lett 1999; 108:77–89.
6. McCunney RJ. Use of biomarkers in occupational medicine. In: Mendelsohn ML, Mohr LC, Peeters JP, eds. Biomarkers: Medical and Workplace Applications. Washington: Joseph Henry Press, 1998:377–386.

7. Bingham E. Ethical issues of genetic testing for workers. In: Mendelsohn ML, Mohr LC, Peeters JP, eds. Biomarkers: Medical and Workplace Applications. Washington: Joseph Henry Press, 1998:415–422.
8. Schulte PA, Rothman N. Epidemiological validation of biomarkers of early biological effect and susceptibility. In: Mendelsohn ML, Mohr LC, Peeters JP, eds. Biomarkers: Medical and Workplace Applications. Washington: Joseph Henry Press, 1998:23–32.
9. Naumann BD, Weidemann PA. Scientific basis for uncertainty factors used to establish occupational exposure limits for pharmaceutical active ingredients. Hum Ecol Risk Assess 1995; 5:590–613.
10. Naumann BD, Weideman PA, Dixit R, Grossman SJ, Shen CF, Sargent EV. Use of toxicokinetic and toxicodynamic data to reduce uncertainties when setting occupational exposure limits for pharmaceuticals. Hum Ecol Risk Assess 1997; 3:555–565.
11. Health and Safety Executive (UK) Laboratory Methods for Biological Monitoring. London: HMSO, 1985.
12. Deutsche Forschungsgemeinschaft (DFG). List of MAK and BAT values. Report No. 30; Commission for the Investigation of Health Hazards of Chemical Compounds in the Work Area. Weinheim: UCH Verlagsgesellschaft mbh, 1994.
13. Lauwerys RR. Industrial Chemical Exposure: Guidelines for biological monitoring. Davis: Biomedical Publications, 1983.
14. Hu HA, Aro A, Rotnitzky A. Bone lead measured by x-ray fluorescence: Epidemiological methods and a new biomarker. Environ Health Perspect 1995; 103(suppl 1):105–110.
15. Watson WP, Mutti A. Role of biomarkers in monitoring exposures to chemicals: present position, future prospects. Biomarkers 2004; 9:211–242.
16. American Conference of Governmental Industrial Hygienists (ACGIH). The Documentation of the TLVs and BEIs with Other Worldwide Occupational Exposure Values. Cincinnati: ACGIH, 2004.
17. Organization for Economic Cooperation and Development (OECD). Decision of the Council Concerning the Mutual Acceptance of Data in the Assessment of Chemicals. Paris: OECD, 1981.
18. International Standards Organization (ISO). Guide 25; General Requirements for the Competence of Calibration and Testing Laboratories, 3rd ed., Geneva: ISO, 1989.
19. U.S. Food and Drug Administration (FDA). Good laboratory practice for nonclinical laboratory studies, Code of Federal Regulations 1986; 21:227–240.
20. Occupational Safety and Health Administration. Lead. 29 CFR Part 1910.1025, Washington: U.S. Department of Labor, Government Printing Office, 1999.
21. Schroeder HA, Tipton IH. The human body burden of lead. Arch Environ Health 1968; 17:965–978.
22. Todd AC, McNeill FE, Palethorpe JE, et al. In vivo X-ray fluorescence of lead in bone using K X-ray excitation with [109]Cd sources: radiation dosimetry studies. Environ Res 1992; 57:117–132.
23. Weaver VM, Jaar BG, Schwartz BD, et al. Associations among lead dose biomarkers, uric acid and renal function in Korean lead workers. Environ Health Perspect 2005; 113:36–42.

24. Schwartz BS, Lee B, Lee G, et al. Association of blood lead, dimercaptosuccinic acid-chelatable lead and tibia lead with neurobehavioral test scores in South Korean lead workers. Am J Epidemiol 2001; 153:453–464.

25. Collins AR. Molecular epidemiology in cancer research. Mol Aspects Med 1998; 19:359–432.

26. Hemminki K, Dipple A, Shuker DG, Kadluber F, Segerbäck D, Bautsch H. DNA Adducts: Identification and Biological Significance. In: IARC Publication No. 125. Lyon: International Agency for Research on Cancer, 1994.

27. Hemminki K. DNA adducts, mutations and cancer. Carcinogenesis 1993; 14: 1007–1012.

28. Hemminki K. DNA adducts in biomonitoring. J Occup Environ Med 1995; 37: 44–51.

29. Ehrenberg L, Osterman-Golkar S, Segerbäck D, Svensson K, Calleman CJ. Evaluation of genetic risks of alkylating agents III. Alkylation of hemoglobin after metabolic conversion of ethene to oxide in vivo. Mutat Res 1977; 45: 175–184.

30. Ehrenberg L, Osterman-Golkar S. Alkylation of macromolecules for detecting mutagenic agents. Teratogen Carcinogen Mutagen 1980; 1:105–127.

31. Boogaard PJ. Use of hemoglobin adducts in exposure monitoring and risk assessment. J Chromatogr B 2002; 778:309–322.

32. Calleman CJ, Ehrenberg L, Jansson B, et al. Monitoring and risk assessment by means of alkyl groups in hemoglobin in persons occupationally exposed to ethylene oxide. J Environ Pathol Toxicol 1987; 2:427–442.

33. Osterman-Golkar S, Bergmark E. Occupational exposure to ethylene oxide: relation between in vivo dose and exposure dose. Scand J Work Environ Health 1988; 14:372–377.

34. Van Sittert NJ, De Jong G, Clare MG, et al. Cytogenetic immunological and hematological effects in workers in an ethylene oxide manufacturing plant. Br J Ind Med 1985; 42:19–26.

35. Czene K, Osterman-Golkar S, Yun X, et al. Analysis of DNA and hemoglobin adducts and sister chromatid exchanges in a human population occupationally exposed to propylene oxide: a pilot study. Cancer Epidemiol Biomarkers Prev 2002; 11:315–318.

36. Skipper PL, Tannenbaum SR. Molecular dosimetry of aromatic amines in human populations. Environ Health Perspect 1994; 102(suppl 6):17–21.

37. Bergmark E, Calleman CJ, He F, Costa LG. Hemoglobin adducts in humans occupationally exposed to acrylamide. Toxicol Appl Pharmacol 1993; 120:45–54.

38. Bergmark E. Hemoglobin adducts of acrylamide and acrylonitrile in laboratory personnel, smokers, and non smokers. Chem Res Toxicol 1997; 10:78–84.

39. Osterman-Golkar S, Peltonen K, Anttinen-Ylemetti T, Landin HH, Zorcec V, Sorsa M. Hemoglobin adducts as biomarkers of occupational exposure to 1,3-butadiene. Mutagenesis 1996; 11:145–149.

40. Yeowell-O'Connell K, Rothman N, Waidyanatha S, et al. Cancer Epidemiol Biomarkers Prev 2001; 10:831–838.

41. Farmer PB. Studies using specific biomarkers for human exposure assessment to exogenous and endogenous chemical agents. Mutat Res 1999; 428:69–81.

42. Tornqvist MJ, Mowrer J, Jensen S, Ehrenberg L. Monitoring of environmental cancer initiators through hemoglobin adducts by a modified Edman degradation method. Anal Biochem 1986; 154:255–266.

43. Boogaard PJ, Rocchi PSJ, VanSittert NJ. Biomonitoring of exposure to ethylene oxide and propylene oxide by determination of hemoglobin adducts: correlations between airborne exposure and adduct levels. Inter Arch Occup Environ Health 1999; 72:142–150.

44. Segerback D, Osterman-Golkar S, Molholt B, Nilsson R. In vivo tissue dosimetry as a basis for cross-species extrapolation in cancer risk assessment for propylene oxide. Regul Toxicol Pharmacol 1994; 20:1–14.

45. Nilsson R, Molholt B, Sargent EV. Quantitative assessment of a human carcinogenic potency for propylene oxide. Regul Toxicol Pharmacol 1991; 14:229–244.

46. International Agency for Research on Cancer (IARC). IARC Monographs on the Evaluation of Carcinogenic Risks to Humans, No. 35: Polynuclear aromatic compounds, Lyon: IARC, 1985.

47. Jongeneelen FJ. Benchmark guideline for urinary 1-hydroxy pyrene as biomarker for occupational exposure to polycyclic aromatic hydrocarbons. Ann Occup Hygiene 2001; 1:3–13.

48. Vanrooij JG, Van Lieshout M, Rodelier-Bade E, Jongeneelen FJ. Effect of the reduction of skin contamination on the internal dose of creosote workers exposed to PAH. Scand J Work Environ Health 1993; 19:200–207.

49. Jongenellen FJ, Anzion RB, Leijdekkers M, Bos RP, Henderson PT. 1- Hydroxypyrene in human urine after exposure to coal tar and coal tar derived product. Int Arch Occup Environ Health 1985; 57:47–55.

50. Grimmer G, Dettbaur G, Naujack KW, Jacob J. Relationship between inhaled PAH and urinary excretion of phenanthrene, pyrene and benzo[a]pyrene metabolites in coke plant workers. Polycyclic Arom Comp. 1994; 5:269–277.

51. Lafontaine M, Gendre C, Morele Y, Laffitte-Rigeaud G. Excretion of urinary 1-hydroxypyrene in relation to the penetration routes of polycyclic aromatic hydrocarbons. Polycyclic Arom Hydrocarbons 2002; 22:579–588.

52. McClean MD, Rindhart RD, Ngo L, et al. Urinary 1-hydroxypyrene and polycyclic aromatic hydrocarbon exposure among asphalt paving workers. Ann Occup Hygiene 2004; 48:565–578.

53. Ny ET, Heederik D, Kromhout H, Jongeneelen F. The relationship between polycyclic aromatic hydrocarbons in air and in urine of workers in a Soderberg pot room. Am Ind Hygiene Assoc J 1993; 54:277–284.

54. Kuljukka TR, Vaaramrinta R, Veidebaum T, Sorsa M, Deltonen K. Exposure to PAH compound among cokery workers in the oil shale industry. Environ Health Perspect 1996; 104(suppl 3):539–554.

55. Lee KH, Ichiba M, Zhang JS, et al. Multiple biomarkers study in painters in a shipyard in Korea. Mutat Res 2003; 540:89–98.

56. Kang D, Rothman N, Cho SH, et al. Association of exposure to polycyclic aromatic hydrocarbons (estimated from job category) with concentration of 1-hydroxypyrene glucuronide in urine. Occup Environ Med 1995; 52:593–599.

57. Lauwery RR. Occupational toxicology. In: Cassarett M, Doull J, eds. Toxicology—The Basic Science of Poisons. New York: Pergamon Press, 1997:947–969.

58. Strickland PT, Routledge MN, Dipple A. Methodologies for measuring of carcinogenic adducts in humans. Cancer Epidemiol Biomarkers Prev 1993; 2:607–619.
59. Brandt HCA, Watson WP. Monitoring human occupational and environmental exposures to polycyclic aromatic compounds. Ann Occup Hygiene 2003; 47:349–378.
60. Macgregor JT, Claxton LD, Lewtas J, Jensen R, Lower WR, Pesch GG. Monitoring environmental genotoxicants. In: Brusick DJ, ed. Methods for Genetic Risk Assessment, Boca-Raton: Lewis Publishers, 1994. .
61. DeJong G, VanSittert NJ, Natarajan AT. Cytogenetic monitoring of industrial populations potentially exposed to genotoxic chemicals and of control populations. Mutat Res 1988; 204:451–464.
62. Hagmar L, Bellander T, Hogstedt B, et al. Biological effects in a chemical factory with mutagenic exposure. I. Cytogenetic and haematological parameters. Int Arch Occup Environ Health 1988; 60:437–444.
63. Nordic Study Group on the Health Risk of Chromosome Damage. A Nordic data base on somatic chromosome damage in humans. Mutat Res 1990; 241:325–337.
64. Hagmar L, Bonassi S, Stromberg U, et al. Cancer predictive value of cytogenetic markers used in occupational health surveillance programs: a report from an ongoing study by the European Study Group on Cytogenetic Biomarkers and Health. Mutat Res 1998; 405:171–178.
65. Bonassi S, Abbondandolo A, Camurri L, et al. Are chromosome aberrations in circulating lymphocytes predictive of future cancer onset in humans? Preliminary results of an Italian cohort study. Cancer Gen Cytogen 1995; 79:133–135.
66. Hagmar LA, Brogger IL, Hansteen S, et al. Cancer risk in humans predicted by increased levels of chromosomal aberrations in lymphocytes: Nordic study group on the health risk of chromosome damage. Cancer Res 1994; 54:2919–2922.
67. Bonassi S, Hagmar L, Stromberg U, et al. Chromosomal aberrations in lymphocytes predict human cancer independently of exposure to carcinogens—European Study Group on Cytogenetic Biomarkers and Health. Cancer Res 2000; 60:1619–1625.
68. Hagmar L, Stromberg U, Bonassi S, et al. Impact of types of lymphocyte chromosomal aberrations on human cancer risk: results from Nordic and Italian cohorts. Cancer Res 2004; 64:2258–2263.
69. Hagmar L, Brogger A, Hansteen IL, et al. Cancer risk in humans predicted by increased levels of chromosomal aberrations in lymphocytes: Nordic study group on the health risk of chromosome damage. Cancer Res 1994; 54:2919–2922.
70. Albertini RJ, Robison SH. Human population monitoring. In: Li AP, Heflich RH, eds. Genetic Toxicology. Boca Raton: CRC Press, 1990.
71. Hagmar L, Bellander T, Persson L, et al. Biological effects in a chemical factory with mutagenic exposure. III. Urinary mutagenicity and thioether excretion. Int Arch Occup Environ Health 1988; 60:453–456.
72. Falck K, Grohn P, Sorsa M, Vaino H, Heinoren E, Holsti LR. Mutagenicity in urine of nurses handling cytostatic drugs. Lancet 1979; 1(8128):1250–1251.
73. Harrison BR. Risks of handling cytotoxic drugs. In: Perry MC, ed. The Chemotherapy Source Book. 3rd ed. Williams and Wilkins: Philadelphia, Lippincott, 2001.

74. National Institute of Occupational Safety and Health (NIOSH). Preventing occupational exposures to antineoplastic and other drugs in health care settings. Washington: U.S. Department of Health and Human Services, 2004.

75. Skov TB, Maarup B, Olsen J, Rorth M, Winthereik H, Lynge E. Leukaemia and reproductive outcome among nurses handling antineoplastic drugs. Br J Ind Med 1992; 49:855–861.

76. McDiarmid MA, Egan MA, Furio T, Bonacci M, Watts SR. Sampling for air-borne fluorouracil in a hospital drug preparation area. Am J Hosp Pharm 1986; 43:1942–1945.

77. Connor TH, Anderson RW, Sessink PJ, Broadfield L, Power LA. Surface con-tamination with antineoplastic agents in six cancer treatment centers in Canada and the United States. Am J Hosp Pharm 1999; 56:1427–1432.

78. Larson RR, Khazaeli MB, Dillon HK. A new monitoring method using solid sorbant media for evaluation of airborne cyclophosphamide and other antineo-plastic agents. Appl Occup Environ Hygiene 2003; 18:120–131.

79. Anderson RW, Puckett WH, Dana WJ, Nguyen TV, Theiss JC, Matney TS. Risk of handling injectable antineoplastic agents. Am J Hosp Pharm 1982; 39:1881–1887.

80. Sessink PJM, Wittenhorst BJ, Anzion RBM, Bos RP. Exposure of pharmacy technicians to antineoplastic agents. Arch Environ Health 1997; 52:240–244.

81. Sargent EV, Kirk GD. Establishing airborne exposure control limits in the pharmaceutical industry. Am Ind Hygiene Assoc J 1988; 49:309–313.

82. Sargent EV, Naumann BD. Occupational exposure limits. In: Alaimo RJ, ed. Handbook of Chemical Health and Safety. Washington: Oxford University Press, 2001:75–80.

83. Garte S. Metabolic susceptibility genes as cancer risk factors. Cancer Epidemiol Biomarkers Prev 2001; 10:1233–1237.

11

Toxicogenomic and Toxicoproteomic Approaches for Biomarkers

Joshua W. Hamilton

Department of Pharmacology and Toxicology and Center for Environmental Health Sciences, Dartmouth Medical School, Hanover, New Hampshire, U.S.A.

INTRODUCTION

This chapter will discuss the use of genomics and proteomics to identify and develop biomarkers in toxicology, focusing in particular on genomics. Such investigations are referred to by toxicologists as "toxicogenomics" and "toxicoproteomics" studies, but these two subareas are often referred to generically as toxicogenomics studies. As with other molecular tools of toxicology, genomics- and proteomics-based studies can be used both for mechanistic investigations, which typically involve both hypothesis testing and hypothesis generation, and for biomarker-based research and its application. While biomarkers are the focus of this discussion, it is important to keep in mind that mechanistic studies critically inform and overlap with biomarker studies and vice versa. Indeed, many biomarkers are discovered in the process of understanding basic mechanisms, and the best biomarker studies have mechanistic underpinnings that allow us to distinguish among the different types of biomarkers, to validate specific biomarkers across platforms and species, and to choose those biomarkers that are most informative and diagnostic.

As with other areas of toxicologic biomarker research, these global toxicogenomics approaches can be used to identify biomarkers for assessing exposure, biological effects, disease processes, altered phenotypes, disease states, and individual susceptibilities (Fig. 1). Toxicogenomics and toxico-proteomics have enormous potential as new biomarker tools, both by providing a means to quantitatively examine global changes in gene and protein expression, and by their simultaneous ability to identify and validate new individual candidates as biomarkers for each of the specific steps in the toxicology paradigm. This allows a more comprehensive investigation into patterns of alterations that can also link new biomarkers to underlying mechanisms of action.

It has become apparent that toxicogenomics, in particular, can provide highly sensitive biomarkers that respond to very low levels of toxicants, well below the threshold for toxicity, allowing the use of such tools for diagnostic and other applications within the population at environmentally relevant concentrations reflecting typical exposures. Interestingly in this regard, there has been concern expressed by several recent reviews that such sensitive alterations in gene expression may be misinterpreted as being of toxico-logical significance when they may simply reflect adaptive responses of the target cells that do not have pathophysiological consequences (1,2).

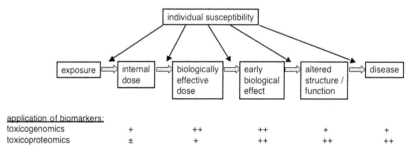

Figure 1 The toxicology paradigm and the application of toxicogenomics and toxicoproteomics tools for the development of biomarkers. The toxicology paradigm of an exposure leading to a pathophysiological state can be modeled in its simplest form as a series of linked and progressive steps. Exposure to a toxicant can lead to an internal dose. For a toxicological or pathophysiological process to occur, the internal dose must be sufficient to produce a biologically effective dose. The biologically effective dose can then initiate or contribute to early biological events such as alterations in gene and protein expression and early alterations in cell phenotype, which may be of toxicological consequence. If these, in turn, are sufficient, they can lead to more sustained and more profound alterations in structure and function, which in turn can lead to development or progression of a disease state. An individual's unique genetic makeup and phenotypic status (e.g., occupational and lifestyle influences) contribute to individual susceptibility, which can influence each of these steps. Toxicogenomics and toxicoproteomics have potential usefulness in identifying and validating biomarkers for each of these steps or processes, as well as in providing underlying mechanistic information.

Nonetheless, such low level responses may still be useful for determining exposures to low levels of environmental chemicals of concern, and may also provide information about "no effect" levels and/or thresholds of response. Understood in the context of the biological responses they represent, such low level responses are of potential value in risk assessment models and in determining the extent to which individuals within the population respond heterogeneously to a given exposure, thereby assisting in identifying and defining potentially sensitive subpopulations.

A second important issue for the use of toxicogenomics in biomarker research will be to determine the specificity of response. Classic biomarkers of exposure have typically measured parent compounds or their metabolites in matrices such as blood or urine, or have examined specifically altered macromolecules such as DNA or protein adducts in target tissues (3). Such biomarkers provide a high degree of specificity for individual exposures but also typically require specific assays for each chemical or end point of concern. In environmental exposures that often involve complex mixtures, toxicogenomics has the advantage that it can measure altered gene expression patterns that not only reflect individual chemicals but also the combined responses to complex mixtures, with the sum total of the response reflecting the entire exposure. Moreover, one can measure responses at the genomic level without knowing anything about the exposure. However, such gene expression changes may not provide specificity because many different exposures might yield the same or similar gene alterations. A challenge then will be to determine the extent to which individual agents produce distinct patterns of alteration, and also to determine how complex mixtures alter gene expression patterns in comparison to those of the individual constituents.

One can imagine a combination of two different chemicals producing a pattern of response that is the simple additive of the individual responses, is synergistic or antagonistic, or represents a complex and entirely new pattern of gene alterations that is not easily predicted from knowing the individual responses. Although current data are very limited, there are some examples for each of these interactions occurring depending on the mixture and biological context. However, most recent reports examining toxicogenomic effects of mixtures have reported either additive or subadditive responses. For example, two recent studies of gene induction by combinations of chemicals failed to observe synergy (4,5). A recent review on the topic by researchers at the U.S. Environmental Protection Agency noted that "A substantial effort has been spent over the past few decades to label toxicologic interaction outcomes as synergistic, antagonistic, or additive. Although useful in influencing the emotions of the public and the press, these labels have contributed fairly little to our understanding of joint toxic action." (6). Regulatory agencies currently assume additivity of responses for chemical carcinogens in their risk assessment models.

Toxicogenomics may provide a very sensitive and systematic means of determining the patterns of response for particular combinations, but as with other aspects of genomics-based studies, it will be important to correlate such effects at the toxicological level. However, this may also yield interesting biomarkers that could be used to more globally assess effects of complex mixtures when monitoring populations.

Proteomics may offer even greater potential for identification of new biomarkers for each of the steps in the paradigm shown in Figure 1. Individual protein biomarkers identified in this manner may or may not have greater sensitivity than genomic markers with respect to exposure assessment or biologically effective dose. However, certain protein biomarkers, particularly those involving covalent modifications, will likely have greater specificity, much like traditional biomarkers. In addition, because protein biomarkers are likely to have longer half-lives than the typically more transient alterations in gene expression, they may be of greater utility in monitoring environmental exposures where it is usually not possible to sample immediately after exposure or where a specific exposure may not be known. Serum or urinary proteins and protein fragments in particular have great potential utility because they will not require invasive techniques for sample acquisition, and provide a more systemic picture than genomics approaches that sample a particular tissue or cell type (2).

An ancillary field to genomics is the use of these and other molecular biology tools to investigate individual genetic susceptibilities, which is currently one of the major areas of emphasis in the field of molecular epidemiology (7–9). Discussion of the genetics of disease susceptibility is beyond the scope of this review, but is worth mentioning with respect to toxicogenomics tools. Advances in this field have been particularly fruitful in the development of single polynucleotide polymorphism (SNP) tools. SNPs represent allelic differences in individual genes within the population, which are potentially useful as biomarkers of disease risk. Genetic differences may influence each of the steps shown in Figure 1, contributing to the overall susceptibility of an individual to chemically induced disease. The recent development of the so-called "SNP chips" has provided a means to screen individuals within the population for allelic differences using the information from the human genome project and the power of microarray technology (10). Such tools have great promise and will eventually provide a rich source of information on the role of genetics in individual risk.

A major challenge will be to link the occurrence of SNPs in individuals and their frequencies within the population with specific degrees of susceptibility. The most useful and desirable SNPs will be those where a particular allelic difference is functionally linked to a biochemical step that is causal or contributes to the pathophysiological process of interest. However, given the multistep nature of most diseases and the fact that most genetic susceptibilities are likely to involve combinations of genes rather than a single allelic difference, it will be challenging to develop a comprehensive picture of the role of individual SNPs in disease risk. It will also require the accumulation of a large database of observations before the field will be able to examine systematically the various combinations of SNPs that are of greatest predictive value for increased or decreased risk.

GENOMICS AND PROTEOMICS

The genome can be defined as the entire complement of genetic information in an organism. Genomics has sometimes been defined simply as the study of genes and their function. However, such a definition does not distinguish genomics from the more classical field of genetics, which is also defined as the study of genes and their function. Genomics is more properly defined as the comprehensive study of sets of genes, their interactions, and their functional dynamics; in most cases when we are discussing genomics studies, we are specifically focusing on the expressed genome, i.e., the complement of expressed genes in a particular cell or tissue at a given time under a given set of conditions, which is sometimes referred to as the transcriptome to distinguish it from the genome. Thus, while the genome itself is fixed (barring mutations), the transcriptome is fluid and reflects changes in conditions, which inform us both about the basic biology of a given cell or tissue and its response to changes in the environment, which includes responses to toxicants and other chemicals. It is in this latter context that toxicogenomics becomes a powerful tool for assessing toxicological responses. We now have the ability, with the advent of the new generation of gene microarray chips, to literally investigate the entire expressed genome of a cell under a given set of conditions.

We can define the proteome as the protein equivalent to the transcriptome, i.e., the entire complement of expressed proteins in a cell or tissue at a given time under a given set of conditions. Unlike genomics, the tools of proteomics do not yet give us the ability to investigate the entire expressed proteome of a cell, nor is the throughput such that we can perform the types of experiments currently feasible with genomics tools. Nonetheless, proteomics holds great promise for toxicology, particularly in the area of biomarkers research. Ultimately what toxicologists want to know is how a given chemical treatment affects the expression and function of proteins leading to altered phenotype, rather than or in addition to, information about the messenger RNAs (mRNAs) that code for them. Moreover, it is now clear that there is typically an indirect relationship, at best, between mRNA expression and protein expression. It is useful to review why this is not a more direct relationship to understand how genomics and proteomics can be used as biomarker tools in toxicology.

In most cases, genomics is used to examine the steady-state expression of mRNAs at a given point in time, giving us essentially a snapshot of the cell.

The human genome has now been sequenced to 99% completion within the euchromatic region (11). There are approximately 20,000 to 25,000 protein-coding genes in the human genome (11), and likely an equal or greater number of pseudogenes (incomplete but currently numbered at over 20,000), as well as an unknown but large number of noncoding RNAs, including tRNAs, rRNAs, snRNAs, snoRNAs, and microRNAs (11). It should be noted that although the entire human genome has now been sequenced, there has until recently been considerable debate about just how many genes there are in the human genome, with estimates ranging from less than 20,000 to more than 70,000; to a large extent, this has centered on a revived discussion of precisely how one defines a gene, and how one characterizes a gene based on genomic sequence alone, but was also based on an incomplete first draft of the human genome. Interestingly, only about 1.5% of the approximately three billion base pairs of the human genome encode expressed genes. Only a fraction of the total available genes are expressed at any one time or by a particular cell type, with estimates on the order of 10% to 15% of the total, or about 2000 to 3800 genes per cell (12). There is often a presumption that changes in mRNA levels reflect changes in gene transcription, and indeed, some genes are transcriptionally regulated such that steady-state mRNA levels directly reflect alterations in transcription rate.

However, mRNA expression is also regulated at several other steps, including attenuation of transcription, processing of nascent RNAs to mature transcripts, transport of mature mRNAs to the cytoplasm, sequestering, availability for translation, and mRNA turnover or half-life. Moreover, these steps are not necessarily directly linked. For example, one could have a change in mRNA half-life, which may not result in a change in its translational efficiency, at least in the short term, such that measuring an increase or decrease in steady-state mRNA levels may not be predictive of a change in protein levels in the cell as measured by Western blotting or other quantitative techniques. Indeed, in many cases where candidate genes have been identified as potential biomarkers by polymerase chain reaction (PCR) analysis of mRNA, there has not been a corresponding change in protein expression or activity; and in the few cases where both the transcriptome and the proteome have been examined for diagnostic patterns in the same system, there is often a poor correlation between changes in mRNA expression and changes in protein expression (13).

Likewise, even in cases where mRNA expression is closely linked to cellular protein levels, the expression and function of a protein is far more complicated than its mere translation from mRNA. It is now clear that there can be multiple transcripts produced from a single gene, each yielding a different protein product. Recent estimates have suggested that there are an average of two to three alternative transcripts per gene across the genome, with alternative splicing being the most widespread mechanism for transcript diversity (12,14,15). Thus, at the transcript level alone, there are potentially many more proteins being produced than the number of expressed genes.

Moreover, each transcript from a gene can be differentially regulated, so that the ratio can change under different conditions. On a practical level, if a particular microarray sequence cannot distinguish among different transcripts (e.g., it is based on an oligonucleotide sequence that is common to all transcript forms), this differential expression will not be captured in the toxicogenomics experiment, yet it may be crucial to understanding the toxicant response.

Proteins can also undergo a myriad of cotranslational and/or post-translational processing steps, including proteolytic cleavage and disulfide bridge formation to go from pre- and proprotein forms to one or more mature forms. Most proteins undergo several posttranslational modifications, including phosphorylation and glycosylation, the latter of which can profoundly change a protein's structure, function, processing, trafficking, and cellular localization (16). Proteins can undergo sequestration, alterations in cellular localization and compartmentalization, and alterations in half-life, among other modifications. Many of these posttranscriptional changes can profoundly change their activity or other biological properties. Thus, there could be tens of thousands of different individual forms of proteins in a cell, which are expressed from a far smaller number of active genes, and there may be profound alterations in their expression or function, which are not reflected by changes in mRNA expression. Finally, one can have direct or indirect modification of proteins as a result of chemical exposures or other environmental factors, such as generation of protein adducts (2,3).

Because ultimately it is the proteome of the cell that gives it its phenotype, it is important to characterize these proteomic level alterations. Unfortunately, the tools of proteomics do not currently allow us to fully survey and characterize the entire proteome at this level of complexity, which includes the added dimensions of spatial and functional complexity. Thus, at the current time, we have a full suite of tools for toxicogenomics but only an incomplete set of tools for toxicoproteomics, with which to investigate toxicant responses. However, both approaches are already providing a rich resource for toxicologic biomarkers, and these approaches are expected to continue their rapid evolution and improvement over the next decade.

DEVELOPMENT OF GENOMICS TOOLS IN TOXICOLOGY

Some of the earliest applications of the new genomics tools were in the field of toxicology. For example, almost 20 years ago, our laboratory began a series of studies examining the effects of chemical carcinogens on gene expression as one approach to understanding their toxicological properties and mechanisms of action (17–26). At the time we began these studies, Northern blotting and slot blotting were the only tools available to measure changes in mRNA expression. However, these methods were slow, labor intensive, and semiquantitative at best, such that it was difficult to examine changes in more than a few genes at a time and with only limited sampling of treatment conditions. To increase throughput, we developed a solution hybridization assay that provided a means to quantitatively measure expression of individual genes in a higher throughput manner, with great precision and at very low levels of expression (17,27). We then used this assay to examine alterations in gene expression by various carcinogens, including a series of organic mutagen-carcinogens (19,20,22,24,28) and the toxic and carcinogenic metals, chromium(VI) and arsenic (17,21–23,25,26,29).

We had hypothesized that each agent would uniquely alter a characteristic pattern of genes that was related to its underlying mechanism of toxicity and carcinogenesis. Using solution hybridization, we demonstrated both in cell culture and in an in vivo animal model that relatively low doses of chromium or arsenic, which were administered at levels well below a threshold dose that would cause overt signs of toxicity such as growth arrest or global changes in RNA and protein expression, preferentially and strongly altered a subset of highly inducible genes while not affecting the expression of a set of constitutively regulated genes (17,22,25). Moreover, detailed time course and dose–response studies revealed subtle differences in the patterns of gene expression changes, which correlated with other biological effects and suggested a mechanism of action for each metal. The effects of chromium(VI), which is genotoxic and mutagenic, were most closely correlated with its pattern of DNA damage and repair in the same systems, suggesting that these effects were related (17).

In contrast, arsenic did not cause overt DNA damage in these systems, but its effects on gene expression were closely correlated with its effects on nuclear receptor signaling (25,26,29). A limitation of these early gene expression studies using Northern blotting or solution hybridization was that one needed to choose the individual genes of interest in advance, and then design hybridization probes that were specific for those genes (17,27). This limited the number of genes that could be studied, and also required one to know— or guess—"a priori" which genes would be of most interest to examine from either a mechanistic or biomarkers identification standpoint. However, it also seemed likely, given the limited knowledge of the genome at the time, that there would be other, as yet undiscovered genes that would be important in understanding the effects of a particular metal and the underlying mechanism for those effects.

Subsequently, other methods were developed to allow a more global examination of the biological response to a given treatment. One early approach was the development of subtractive hybridization of expression libraries, in which RNA pools isolated from control and treated samples were hybridized to each other to subtract out mRNAs that were expressed at equal levels in the two samples (30). The goal of this design was to enrich for those RNAs that were differentially expressed in the two samples, which would allow subsequent cloning and sequencing to reveal those genes that were of greatest interest. One of the first published experiments to apply this technique examined the effects of cadmium on gene expression in mammalian cell culture (31). The majority of the sequenced clones coded for the same mRNA, metallothionein, which is a moderately expressed mRNA and protein known to be strongly upregulated in response to cadmium, zinc, and other divalent metals. Thus, while identification of metallothionein as the major cadmium-inducible gene in this study validated this overall experimental approach, it also pointed out two major drawbacks to its use in identifying novel responsive genes. First, by its very design, this technique strongly favors the selection of those mRNAs that are most abundantly expressed, and second, it tends to select for those mRNAs whose expression is most dramatically altered in response to a given treatment.

While the genes such as metallothionein are often useful as biomarkers, it is rare that the gene discovery experiments using these prior techniques yielded new information or led to identification of a previously uncharacterized gene that turns out to be highly responsive to and diagnostic of a given treatment. It has long been thought that many of the genes of potential interest for understanding the overall response to a specific toxic agent such as cadmium are likely to be expressed at much lower levels than are captured in these screens and might also exhibit a smaller magnitude of change. Such genes would almost certainly be excluded or poorly represented in the clonal pool resulting from the subtractive hybridization method without screening thousands, perhaps tens of thousands, of clones. Initially, this method was extremely labor-intensive, slow, and expensive because cloning and DNA sequencing were in their early days. Thus, it was not practical to screen and identify more than a few dozen clones at a time and this took upward of one to two years to accomplish. The rare clone representing a less abundant and more subtly altered mRNA was therefore unlikely to be discovered using this approach. However, with the advent of cheaper and higher throughput screening and sequencing approaches, differential hybridization has remained a useful tool for generating expression libraries because it removes highly redundant populations, biasing the resulting pool toward differentially expressed genes.

The advent of the PCR technique was revolutionary to the field of molecular biology in many ways. Initially, its most obvious application was that it provided a higher throughput means of measuring expression of individual genes than solution hybridization. Subsequently, PCR has provided a means to "multiplex" the analysis by simultaneously amplifying several different mRNAs in the same sample with a pool of specific primers, producing different-sized products that could be visualized on the same gel. A variation of the multiplex PCR approach using different dyes is still employed in quantitative real-time PCR (Q-RT-PCR) for experiments that focus on a specific subset of genes (32).

Another method called the RNase protection assay (RPA) combined the basic steps of solution hybridization with the concept of multiplexing to quantify multiple mRNAs in the same sample. In this method, a specific subset of mRNAs are simultaneously analyzed by using different-length radioactive probes to create different-sized products that are visualized on a gel (30). Typical results from this approach are shown in Figure 2. The RPA technique provided a useful way to examine several different genes simultaneously and with high specificity, both expediting the analysis and providing a means of internally normalizing across samples. Prior to the

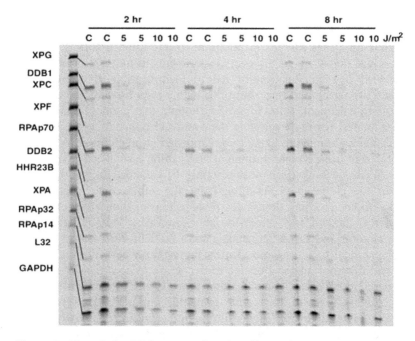

Figure 2 Use of the RPA to examine the effects of an agent on simultaneous mRNA expression of a suite of DNA genes. In this example, human EJ-138 bladder cancer cells in culture were exposed to UV irradiation at 0, 5, or 10 J/m^2 and allowed to recover for two, four, or eight hours as indicated on the *top axis* labels. The mRNA from these cells was analyzed for steady-state mRNA levels of 12 different genes as indicated on the *left axis*; 11 of these genes are involved in different aspects of DNA repair and were compared to the expression of a control gene, GAPDH. Note the strong dose- and time-dependent suppression of these DNA repair genes. These images can then be digitally quantified and analyzed as in Figure 3 below. *Abbreviations*: RPA, RNase protection assay; UV, ultraviolet. *Source*: From Warren AJ, Hamilton JW (unpublished results).

introduction of Q-RT-PCR and microarrays, this was considered the method of choice for analysis of multiple genes, but like solution hybridization, it requires choosing the genes of interest in advance and knowledge of the genetic sequences.

Figure 3 illustrates the application of this technique to analysis of a complex experiment that examined a suite of 10 different DNA repair genes in human lung epithelial cells treated with arsenic alone, benzo(a) pyrene diolepoxide [the mutagenic metabolite of the carcinogen benzo(a) pyrene] alone, or a combination of the two agents. Interestingly, although each agent alone only modestly increased a similar subset of these 10 genes, the combination produced a striking pattern of synergy where the mRNA expression levels of these same four DNA repair genes were substantially upregulated in response to this chemical mixture. Because arsenic and cigarette smoke [which contains benzo(a) pyrene and other polycyclic aromatic hydrocarbons] have been shown to be synergistic for increasing the risk of lung cancer, these results may provide important clues as to the mechanistic basis for this interaction, as well as specific candidate genes that may serve as biomarkers for

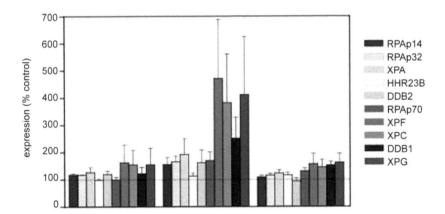

Figure 3 Use of the RPA technique to examine combinations of agents on expression of DNA repair genes. In this example, human lung BEAS-2B cells in culture were exposed to 0.2 μM BPDE for six hours, 10 μM sodium arsenite for 24 hours, or the combination (arsenite for 18 hours prior to addition of BPDE for an additional 6 hours). The steady-state mRNA expression of 10 different DNA repair genes (shown by *shaded bars left* to *right* as in the legend going *top* to *bottom*) was analyzed in total RNA by RPA analysis as shown in Figure 2. Note that either agent alone had little or no effect on the expression of these genes, whereas the combination appeared to be synergistic and caused a substantial increase in expression of nine of these genes by up to fivefold (*bars* represent the mean ± SD, $n = 4$ per group). *Abbreviations*: RPA, RNase protection assay; BPDE, benzo(a)pyrene diol epoxide; SD, standard deviation. *Source*: From Warren AJ, Andrew AS, Hamilton JW (unpublished results).

this effect. Such studies would be impractical and extremely tedious and expensive if one had to examine each gene in this set on an individual basis, but indicated the promise of more genomically based studies that could assess patterns of response.

The powerful PCR technique rapidly became incorporated into other genomic approaches in addition to its direct use for analyzing expression of individual genes. One of these applications was in a method called differential display of mRNA expression (33). This approach to genomic screening exploited a variation of multiplex PCR and was used both to globally examine patterns of altered gene expression and for direct gene discovery. The technique is based on use of short random hexamer primers that simultaneously amplify numerous segments of complementary DNA (cDNA) in the entire isolated RNA pool. Parallel amplification of RNAs from control and treated samples is followed by running out the PCR products on a sequencing gel for a side-by-side pattern comparison of the two samples. Typically, it was observed that most bands were identical in the two samples, indicating that most mRNAs were not differentially expressed (Fig. 4). This observation also provides a means for normalizing the treated to the control pattern, such that the altered band intensities are more apparent, and represent only those products that are substantially up or downregulated by a given treatment. The mRNA segment of interest can then be identified by subsequent isolation of the band from the gel, followed by reamplification, subcloning, and sequencing of the product. Figure 4 shows an example of the results of a differential display experiment from our laboratory, examining the effects of cadmium on gene expression in the zooplankton, *Daphnia pulex*. Using this method, we identified several candidate mRNA fragments that were up- or downregulated in response to nonovertly toxic exposures of *Daphnia* to cadmium. As expected, one of these fragments turned out to represent the mRNA for *Daphnia* metallothionein, but several other cadmium-responsive mRNAs were also identified.

One interesting application of this technique was a study examining the effects of cadmium on gene expression in the roundworm, *Caenorhabditis elegans* (34). As we had observed for *Daphnia*, one of the most prominently cadmium-altered *C. elegans* mRNAs was for metallothionein. In fact, these investigators had purposely added short primers that were based on the metallothionein mRNA sequence and which were expected to specifically amplify this mRNA; these amplified sequences served as a useful positive control in these experiments. However, in addition to metallothionein, many other cadmium-altered genes were also identified in this study, indicating the utility of examining gene expression in a more global, open-ended manner (34). Because one could visually examine all amplified bands and then determine which products to isolate and further characterize, in theory this method was not as prone to selection bias as the previous subtractive hybridization libraries. However, in this method, there is still an unavoidable bias toward

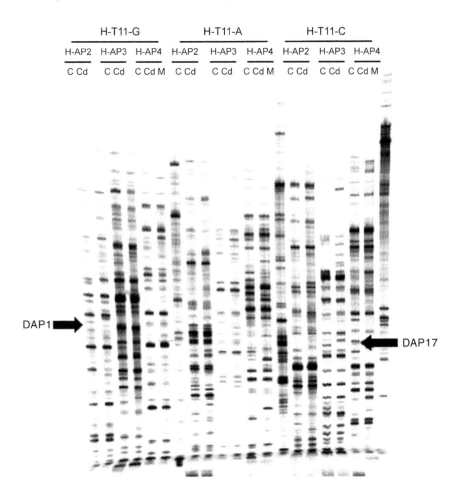

Figure 4   Use of the Differential Display technique to examine global alterations in mRNA expression. In this example, a population of *Daphnia pulex* were exposed in the laboratory to cadmium chloride for 24 hours prior to isolation of total RNA and analysis of mRNA expression using nine different combinations of primers in the PCR-based differential display assay and comparing control to cadmium-treated animals as shown in the *top axis* labels. An example of an observed difference in the level of a particular amplified band is indicated by the DAP1 and DAP17 labels and *arrows*. Seventeen such unique bands showing differential expression were cut from this gel, reamplified, and sequenced to determine their identities, leading to the identification of a putative *Daphnia* metallothionein sequence that is cadmium responsive. *Abbreviation*: PCR, polymerase chain reaction. *Source*: From Sillett C, Hamilton JW (unpublished results).

mRNAs that are of greater abundance and those whose expression is most dramatically changed by treatment conditions.

As with subtractive libraries, this approach also relies on subsequent subcloning and sequencing of individual bands to identify the specific mRNAs. It also requires amplification and comparison of treated versus control using 24 to 48 different combinations of specific primers to theoretically cover all possible mRNAs. And it has an additional drawback that, because short products are produced by the random primer PCR step—and in fact the sequencing gel is optimal for visualizing bands in the 300 to 1000 base pair range—one often finds that the same mRNA is represented in multiple bands on the gels. As a result, it is possible to pick and sequence several differentially expressed bands and find that they are different PCR products of the same gene. Thus, this approach has now largely been replaced by DNA microarrays for studies in humans and several other major model organisms. However, it is still a potentially valuable approach in species for which there is little or no genomic information, to be used in lieu of or in addition to sequencing of expression libraries.

The development of DNA microarray methodologies was clearly a major leap forward in the analysis of differential gene expression. Not only can this approach simultaneously examine large numbers of individual genes—or in some cases the entire expressed genome—but it also provides a means to simultaneously test existing hypotheses of the investigator, as well as generate entirely new hypotheses. The power of this latter capability cannot be underestimated. While much of recent experimental biology has been dominated by hypothesis-driven research—and, in fact, some scientists refer to hypothesis-generating or discovery-driven experiments pejoratively as "fishing expeditions"—the history and foundation of modern empirical biology is fundamentally that of observational science. Indeed, the history of biological research demonstrates that the biological systems we study are far more complex than typical reductionist models that drive hypothesis testing can predict. DNA microarrays provide the ability to globally assess the mRNA expression of a biological system in response to a stimulus without external bias from the investigator as to what the predicted response might be. Moreover, it provides a means to examine patterns of gene expression, rather than, or in addition to, examination of individual genes. Nonetheless, the best genomics and proteomics experiments combine both aspects, i.e., testing of a specific hypothesis and subsequent analysis of novel patterns or individual genes of interest which generate new hypotheses (35).

The early use of microarrays to examine effects of various toxicants on gene expression has demonstrated both the power of, and some of the difficulties inherent in, this approach. The field of genomics is still developing rapidly, and the tools have changed quickly over these first several years of its use. Parallel to, but lagging behind, the generation of microarray data has been the development, standardization, and application of statistical and bioinformatics tools for accurately analyzing the results. Experimental design of microarray studies has also evolved rapidly. The result is that one must often evaluate previously published studies in the historical context of the tools available at the time. For example, many early genomics studies had an *n* of 1, examining only a single, often pooled sample of treated versus control RNA due to the cost and difficulty of array experiments and the difficulty in obtaining sufficient RNA for analysis.

However, it has become increasingly clear that one must compare data from multiple individuals to see consistent patterns of alteration. Moreover, to understand the nature of a toxicant response at the genomic level, one must typically perform dose–response and time course studies, and also compare acute versus chronic treatments, as is routine in other areas of toxicology. With the rapid evolution of this field has come an exponential increase in the publication of microarray and other toxicogenomic data. Lagging behind has been any standardization of techniques or data-reporting protocols. It has been recommended by several journals that all current toxicogenomics studies adhere to the Minimum Information About Microarray Data Experiments (MIAME) standards and also that authors submit their data to one of two genomics databases so that others can examine and reanalyze the raw data from these studies (36). Hopefully, this will soon be a requirement of all scientific journals rather than a recommendation or individual journal decision.

A limitation of early toxicogenomics studies is that the first available microarrays contained probes representing only a few hundred to a few thousand individual genes. In contrast, with the completion of the human, mouse, and other genomic sequencing projects, and the rapid evolution in array technology, gene arrays are now available, which contain from several thousand genes to the entire expressed genome. The early studies were therefore limited by definition to examining only those identified genes present on the array, which was often a small and nonrandom subset of all the possible genes that might have responded to a given treatment. The genes chosen for these arrays were often those that had previously been studied in some other context, and so while there was often some indication that these would be toxicant responsive, by definition, discovery of new candidate genes that had not previously been characterized was unlikely. The larger arrays now provide a much richer and less biased source for evaluating patterns of expression. This has allowed a process of gene discovery, often producing surprising results that have generated new hypotheses. On the other hand, because almost half of the putative genes in the human genome have unidentified function and little or nothing is known of their regulation; the relevance of alterations in such genes to toxicological processes is unknown and will require additional follow-up investigations to determine.

The physical media used for arraying genes has also evolved rapidly, from DNA spotted onto nylon membranes (Fig. 5) or glass slides to DNA

Control   Treated

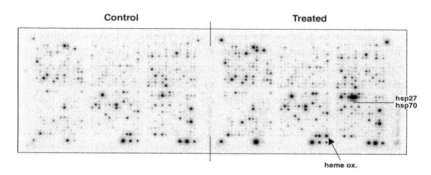

hsp27
hsp70

heme ox.

Figure 5 Use of one-color membrane-based microarrays for toxicogenomic analysis of gene expression. Unique cloned sequences derived from a human cDNA library were spotted in a microarray on nylon membranes in duplicate panels and used to compare control and treated animals. In this example, human lung BEAS-2B cells in culture were exposed to 5 µM sodium arsenite for four hours prior to isolation of total RNA. RNA from control or treated cells was radiolabeled and hybridized separately to individual membrane arrays. The data were digitized from autoradiogaphs such as shown in this figure, and levels of mRNA expression for individual genes were compared following normalization to positive and background control signals. Examples of three genes that were clearly differentially expressed are shown by the labels and *arrows* in the figure. Results from these experiments were published in Ref. 37. *Source*: Courtesy of Warren AJ, Andrew AS, Hamilton JW (unpublished figure).

oligonucleotide arrays on "chips" such as those produced by Affymetrix. Although the membrane-based arrays are no longer widely used, glass slide arrays are still employed, particularly for arraying of genomes from "orphan" animal species that are not commercially available and/or because individual laboratories or university core facilities can readily print these in abundance. These include genomic arrays for species such as *Cholera, Arabidopsis* and *Daphnia*, which are of importance to specific researchers, as well as custom arrays produced to specifically contain subsets of genes that are of particular interest.

Such custom arrays typically use a two-color competitive hybridization scheme where control and treated RNA samples are labeled with two different fluorescent dyes, cohybridized, and then analyzed by color emission for their relative and absolute intensities. In contrast, the membrane arrays such as those shown in Figure 5 and the Affymetrix-type gene chip arrays are a "one color" system where separate control or treated arrays are hybridized with radioactive (Fig. 5) or fluorescent probes, the images are scanned and analyzed, and the data are then compared by bioinformatics techniques to assess relative expression. These different types of physical arrays require different methodological approaches and will also provide different levels of response and reproducibility.

Another major complication in evaluating and comparing results among previous published studies is that they often use entirely different biological models that make comparisons among them—for example, immortalized cancer cells or transformed cells versus normal primary cells, cell culture versus whole animal, rat versus mouse versus human, etc.— highly problematic. As discussed in more detail below, it is now quite clear that there can be strain, sex, and tissue and developmental age differences in genomic level responses, even within the same species, which suggest caution in making such direct comparisons. Moreover, different studies have used different types of arrays, containing different sets of genes, and often use different statistical packages to analyze and report the results. Thus, much of the available literature does not allow a direct comparison of results, nor are we yet able to compile many of these studies into a common database format that would allow facile comparison across studies. Hopefully, this will become far less of a problem with the advent of standards for study design, methodology, data analysis, and data reporting (36), but in the meantime, it can be difficult to translate the results of a given study to other applications. A major impediment to broad applicability of study results has been the considerable lag in the development of standardized and validated statistical and bioinformatics tools for toxicogenomics studies, discussed below.

STATISTICAL AND BIOINFORMATICS-BASED ANALYSES OF TOXICOGENOMICS RESULTS

The use of different statistical methods in data analysis can lead to highly variable results when determining which genes are "significantly" altered following a given treatment (37a,38). As methods and experimental approaches have matured, the data being generated have become increasingly valuable as a primary source of information that can be catalogued and archived, allowing subsequent researchers to reanalyze previous studies for new insights. A fairly standardized way of analyzing gene array data is the use of statistical analysis of microarrays (SAM) or a similar statistical package (39). Basically, following several normalization techniques, one is generating the equivalent of a series of *t*-tests that provide statistical comparisons between control and treated groups. Our own reanalysis of these approaches has indicated that while similar but nonoverlapping gene lists can be generated by these various approaches (37a,38), they may all be missing key data because of the basic assumptions that are made about microarray results. These issues are only briefly discussed here but may provide insight into the biological nature of transcriptome level responses and their validity as biomarkers.

Following correction and normalization for background, which is an important first step, many software packages do two additional normalizations. Imagine that we are comparing two groups in which there is no alteration in gene expression from our treatment, i.e., our data supports the null hypothesis, and we graph the levels of individual gene expression comparing group 1 to group 2. If one considers the data from such arrays as falling along a diagonal axis, we see that genes distributed along this axis reflect their individual levels of expression from low (lower left) to high (upper right) and also fall across the diagonal in a scatter from upper left to lower right (e.g., the central axis in Fig. 6).

The first assumption of many standard normalization approaches is that the level of expression of the individual genes should be distributed normally along the axis, and the second is that they should be distributed normally, with respect to scatter, orthogonal to the axis. As shown in Figures 6 and 7 and in numerous other array experiments, neither of these assumptions is directly supported by biological data, and we believe that basic biology would argue strongly against the first normalization in particular. More importantly, these normalizations overmanipulate the

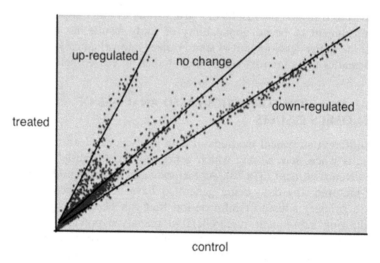

Figure 6 Graphical representation of data from a large two-color microarray experiment (*Daphnia pulex*) where the treated group [lethal concentration 1% (LC1) treatment with sodium arsenite, 1.4 mg/L, 48 hr] shows a variation in expression of a subset of genes. The microarray data have been minimally normalized: each gene signal has been corrected against its local background fluorescence, and the average relative fluorescence of one color has been adjusted to the other to balance the two signals (to account for slight variations in labeling efficiency). Each gene has been plotted based on its control and treated fluorescence values. Note that most genes lie along the central diagonal axis, indicating no change in expression. However, one subset of genes demonstrated a higher level of expression in the treated group, as indicated by the upper grouping ("upregulated"), and another subset demonstrated a lower level of expression as indicated by the lower grouping ("downregulated") *Source*: Shaw JR, Davey JC, Hampton TH, Hamilton JW (unpublished results).

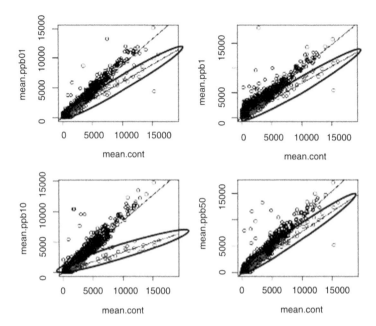

Figure 7 Use of nonparametric statistical analysis of gene expression from micro-array experiments in toxicogenomics studies. Mice were treated with sodium arsenite in drinking water at concentrations of 0.1, 1, 10, and 50 ppb (μg/L) as shown in each *panel* for five weeks (note that the current U.S. drinking water standard for arsenic is 10 ppb), and mRNA expression was examined using one-color microarrays (Affyme-trix Gene Chips) in the lungs of individual animals ($n = 6$ for each treatment). Mini-mal normalization of data was performed analogous to the process described in Figure 6, and control versus treated groups were compared. Nonparametric statisti-cal analysis identified those genes (indicated by open circles within the oval cluster) that were differentially expressed in treated versus control in all six of six treated ani-mals. Note the apparent dose-dependent increase in the magnitude of the altered gene expression from the lower to the higher dose of arsenic. More than 90% of the genes in each of these subsets overlapped among the four doses, in contrast to the dose-response results shown in Figure 9. *Abbreviation*: ppb, parts per billion.

data and are likely to obscure real experimental differences, such that one will have far more false negatives than false positives. From our perspective, there is far less concern about potential false positives (or "false discovery rates") because these will be sorted out when one confirms, as it is always critical to do, whether these genes are altered by a given treatment using a complementary and more quantitative approach such as Q-RT-PCR. How-ever, false negatives are more problematic because one misses the opportu-nity for gene discovery, which is the greatest inherent power of the toxicogenomics approach, and the available alternative techniques are unli-kely to reveal this loss of information.

Rather than normalizing the distribution of the data as described above, if one simply corrects for background and plots the results, it typically looks like the data shown in Figure 6. We see that there is clearly not a normal distribution of the individual genes along the length of the diagonal axis. What is the basis for this non-normal distribution? Clearly, each gene is expressed at its own unique level, which is not the result of a stochastic process, but rather is dictated by its biological role and its degree of regulation and is a result of its own biological history of evolutionary selection pressure.

Moreover, because each gene is specifically and uniquely designed to perform its own task, there is no reason to assume that genes, as a group, will distribute normally with respect to their relative levels of expression. One could imagine, instead, that genes might cluster into subgroups based on common functional characteristics. For example, transcription factors are typically expressed at similar low copy numbers, and their regulation at the mRNA level often does not fluctuate extensively in a given cell type. Other genes that are highly responsive to changes in environmental stimuli, such as certain metabolic proteins, might be expressed, on average, at higher levels but might also be highly variable in their expression from cell to cell or organism to organism depending on the precise time of sampling. Genes for structural proteins, such as the actins or tubulins, are typically expressed at very high levels and are also typically refractory to temporal or environmental influences in a given cell type—in fact, they are often used as normalization controls in such experiments for this reason. Thus, statistically forcing the normal distribution of the gene expression data will skew the actual patterns of expression and may also mask subtler changes produced by a given treatment.

Likewise, if we look at the scatter of data perpendicular to this diagonal axis, we see that the data appear to be evenly distributed (and may or may not be normally distributed) orthogonal to the axis, but they have not been "corrected" in any way. Examining the central axis in Figure 6, for example, it may not be obvious why it should matter whether the data are forced into a normal distribution along this orthogonal axis. However, if we compare control samples to treated samples (e.g., arsenic treatment of *Daphnia* and mice, respectively in Figs. 6 and 7), we observe a distinct shift in the distribution of genes between control and treated groups, producing a "pigeon toe" pattern of a subset of genes that are clearly separated from the central axis in a highly clustered manner. In other words, there are distinct groups of genes that are substantially overexpressed in treated versus control ("toe" in upper left quadrant) and those that are clearly underexpressed ("toe" in lower right quadrant). By not normalizing the data in either axis, these clusters are readily apparent in this visual representation. The genes in each of these toes are consistently displaced in the treated group, i.e., they are represented in that cluster in all five of five replicates, whereas those same genes lie along the central axis (and are randomly distributed above or below the axis) in the orthogonal direction in all five control samples.

Based on our interpretation of such minimally corrected and graphed results, we have developed a nonparametric statistical approach to analyzing these gene patterns for statistical significance. The more traditional parametric SAM-type statistical approach is based on the assumption that the absolute magnitude of alteration in a given gene's expression will be consistent with a given treatment, and conversely, that genes with a highly variable response, as reflected by a large standard deviation and a high, nonsignificant p value, are not statistically—and presumably not biologically—different from controls. However, let us alternatively consider that a given gene is, in fact, biologically responsive to a treatment such as arsenic, but that its absolute level of expression is highly variable from individual to individual, resulting in a large standard deviation. Traditional parametric statistical approaches such as SAM would not identify this gene on a list of statistically significant, arsenic-responsive candidates.

But assuming this gene is arsenic responsive, we would want to have a method for identifying such a gene. A nonparametric statistical approach will allow us to do so. What might explain such biological variation? One possibility is that the gene's temporal response to arsenic is highly transient, e.g., increasing rapidly but also returning to control levels rapidly. In this scenario, it would be difficult to obtain reproducible results because individual samples might reflect slightly different time points in this steep temporal response curve. A second possibility is that the absolute level of expression of the gene may be inherently variable from individual to individual, but the quantal response itself is highly consistent. If, for example, the cell regulates the level of the protein product from that mRNA at a posttranscriptional level—e.g., at the level of translational efficiency—the cell may not tightly regulate the absolute amount of mRNA. It may be sufficient to simply ensure that the gene is "on" when needed and "off" when not needed because the absolute level of the mRNA pool may be less important than the speed and robustness of the response leading to altered protein levels or function.

As discussed previously, there is a relatively poor correlation between steady-state mRNA levels and cellular protein levels for many, perhaps most, genes and thus such a scenario might be very common. Using nonparametric statistics, we should be able to observe such a gene's change in mRNA expression as being highly statistically significant if we simply ask what the probability is that a given gene would consistently be found in a particular cluster (i.e., in the "up" toe or "down" toe of the pigeon foot) in all replicates based on random chance. Analyzing the genes in the clusters shown in Figures 6 and 7 in that way, we observed that many of the p values for individual genes approached 10^{-6} (i.e., $p < 0.000001$). In fact, almost all of the genes shown in the labeled clusters in Figure 6 and 7 were highly significant by this nonparametric approach, whereas many of these same genes were not identified as being statistically significant using the standard SAM parametric method because of the variability in their absolute level of expression among replicates, even with individual replicates of five or more per group. SAM appears to have a particular bias against downregulated genes, and identified only a few of the dozens of genes in the downregulated toes in Figures 6 and 7. For a compound like arsenic, where the majority of affected genes decrease in expression, this is problematic and results in far too many false negatives.

Conversely, analyzing the genes shown in Figures 6 and 7, which are in the "heel" of the pigeon foot (lower left), the clustering/nonparametric approach becomes a little more problematic because of the tight juxtapositioning of data at these lower levels of absolute expression and the much lower signal-to-background ratio. In this region, more traditional SAM-based parametric statistics provide an appropriate analysis of potential gene candidates. Thus, these methods are not mutually exclusive, and we currently favor using a combination of parametric and nonparametric approaches. But in all cases, we perform only the minimal normalization required to subtract background signal on the array and, in the case of two-color arrays, we also balance the relative fluorescence signals from the two different dye wavelengths used in the experiment for each array before combining the results of the multiple replicates.

The use of a nonparametric approach and understanding its underlying biological basis have important implications not only in the identification of candidate genes that might be useful biomarkers but also in the application of such biomarkers to population studies. First, as with all candidate genes, it is important to use Q-RT-PCR or similar methods to confirm that the gene is consistently altered by a given response. However, in this nonparametric model, one must carefully define what is meant by "consistently altered." Second, one must also develop nonparametric approaches in developing such a gene for subsequent application as a useful biomarker for laboratory, field, or epidemiology studies, particularly if the gene is to be used for diagnostic purposes. Most diagnostic tests are based on absolute quantitation of an end point, whereas a gene that is consistently changed but highly variable in absolute expression will be problematic in the standard methodologies of such an application. This does not negate the potential value of these nonparametric gene responses, but it will require the development of different analytical and statistical approaches for such genes to be useful as biomarkers.

As mentioned previously, we began our own differential gene expression studies before the advent of modern genomics tools with the hypothesis that different toxicants would selectively and preferentially alter gene expression in patterns that were both unique and characteristic of each agent, but which would also provide insights into their mechanisms of action. We have generally taken an iterative approach in these studies, using solution hybridization, differential display, RPA, multiplex PCR, and DNA microarrays to both test and validate hypotheses and to generate new hypotheses, and also using more classical individual gene expression tools such as solution hybridization and Q-RT-PCR to further validate these hypotheses and generate new hypotheses for testing at the genomic level. This is also the general approach taken by the field in such toxicogenomics studies, which typically have focused on one compound or a series of related compounds to understand mechanism and to generate candidate biomarkers that reflect exposure, effect, pathophysiological process, disease end point, or genetic susceptibility.

The results shown in Figure 8 illustrate one of the central hypotheses of toxicogenomics, that individual toxicants will display characteristic but

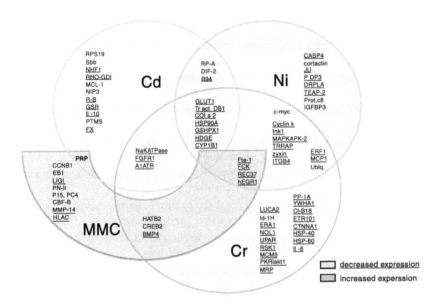

Figure 8 Venn diagram showing characteristic and unique patterns of altered gene expression using five different treatments in the same system. Human lung BEAS-2B cells in culture were treated for four hours with toxicologically equivalent (highest noncytotoxic) doses of either cadmium chloride (Cd, 3 μM), nickel subsulfide (Ni, 3 μg/cm²), sodium dichromate (Cr, 10 μM), and mitomycin C (MMC, 1 μM), and microarray analysis of gene expression was performed using one-color 1200 gene microarrays as shown in Figure 5. Genes that were differentially regulated by Cd, Ni, Cr, and MMC are listed in each enclosed area for each treatment, and genes that were similarly affected by more than one treatment are shown by the overlapping areas. Downregulated genes are shown with an underline; the other genes were upregulated. No gene was significantly altered by all four treatments and there was little overlap among the treatments. *Source*: From Ref. 37.

different patterns of altered gene expression. In this example, a microarray similar to the one shown in Figure 5 and containing approximately 1200 different gene probes was used to assess alterations in gene expression in a human lung epithelial cell line in response to various individual treatments. Unique patterns of altered gene expression were observed in response to arsenic, chromium, cadmium, nickel, and mitomycin C treatments in the same system, at the same time point, and at comparable "toxic equivalent" doses (37). This illustrates how genomic information may be able to be used diagnostically to characterize a biological response, as well as generate potential biomarkers for use in subsequent basic research and translational studies. Similar results have been reported for other groups of toxicants (40,41), supporting the idea that toxicogenomics can reveal signature patterns of response that may be able to "fingerprint" a chemical or closely related class of chemicals in a diagnostic manner.

Surprisingly, different patterns emerge even among chemicals that might be expected to produce similar patterns. Each agent mentioned in Figure 8 was observed to produce a strikingly different pattern of gene alterations, with little overlap, even though several of these ostensibly have similar mechanisms of action (37). For example, chromium and nickel are both genotoxic and mutagenic metals (and mitomycin C is also a genotoxic and mutagenic agent), whereas cadmium and arsenic are nongenotoxic metals that both attack sulfhydryl groups and cysteines in particular. Yet the patterns suggest little overlap among these genes. For the five agents tested, there were between 16 and 63 differentially expressed genes out of 1200, or a response of between 1% and 5% of the total genes. Yet among those, not a single gene was altered by all five treatments, and, in fact, only seven genes were commonly altered by three or more agents. Although some early researchers had predicted that the predominant gene expression response of such treatments would be an induction of stress-related genes and other acute phase response pathways, there was little evidence of this and, in fact, the majority of genes were actually decreased in response to these noncytotoxic treatments. Moreover, while many of the altered genes were well known to the toxicology field and might have been predicted to respond based on other information, an equal number of genes were altered, which had not previously been characterized as being toxicant responsive, at least with respect to these agents (37).

These results illustrate another important concept of toxicogenomics. While the resulting gene lists appear small in comparison to the total genes investigated, it would still be impractical for a single laboratory to do follow-up studies on all of the more than 160 genes of interest (13% of the total genes on the array) that were generated by this one experiment. More recent experiments, using microarrays with over 45,000 features that represent the entire human or mouse genome, routinely generate lists that contain hundreds of potentially interesting genes—a 1% response rate on such an array would still represent approximately 450 candidate genes. Thus, it is critical to go back to first principles for such experiments, similar to the process used in large epidemiology studies that measure hundreds of parameters in hundreds or thousands of individuals. First, one can examine the data to determine whether there is information relevant to the testing of the central hypothesis that was used to drive the experimental design. The data may or may not be informative in this regard, and this may lead to confirmatory studies and/or a repeat of the experiment with an altered experimental design.

Second, one can examine the data for other interesting features, which may lead to the generation of new hypotheses and the identification of new candidate genes for subsequent study. However, testing these new hypotheses will require additional experimentation with a design that focuses specifically on those observations, both genomic level analyses and other more traditional toxicological approaches. And it may be misleading to select only those genes that had the "highest" response or the most statistically significant response as analyzed by SAM or similar statistical approaches. Finally, while it is not practical for a single lab to examine all the potentially interesting observations in detail, conducting the experiments using the MIAME standards and publishing the entire raw data set in a publicly accessible genomics database will allow others to examine the data for patterns of interest, compare the results to other studies, and otherwise glean useful information that greatly enhances the value of such large-scale and expensive experiments.

Indeed, it is likely that useful biomarkers will be developed only after analysis of many different data sets from many different toxicogenomics studies. However, meta-analysis of these data sets is likely to yield important information about mechanism of action, toxicological relevance of specific end points, structure–activity relationships among different toxicants, and other critical information that will allow more rapid development and validation of useful biomarkers from these data. In this latter regard, it is becoming increasingly important to develop, disseminate, and adhere to certain standards in experimental design, data collection and storage, annotation, statistical analysis, and data presentation so that collective results can be accumulated in toxicogenomics databases that allow others to appropriately analyze this information. This will also allow the field to avoid costly and time-consuming repetition of studies, while also being able to systematically and collectively determine data gaps for future experimentation.

Another important point is illustrated by the results shown in Figure 9 in which two different doses of arsenic are compared in the same system. Surprisingly, there is almost no overlap between these gene lists, despite the fact that this is the same chemical and there is only a 10-fold change in dose (37). As discussed above, the lower dose of arsenic, comparable to the doses of the treatments shown in Figure 8, was the highest nonovertly

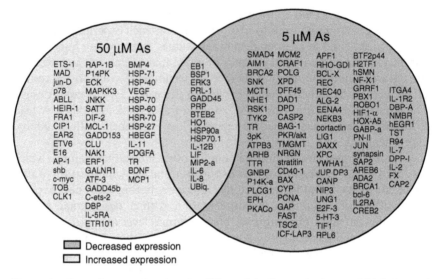

Figure 9   Venn diagram showing the differential effects of a low and high dose of arsenic on gene expression in the same system. The experiments were performed as described in Figure 8, using either a noncytotoxic (5 μM) or cytotoxic (50 μM) concentration of sodium arsenite (As). Downregulated genes are shown with an underline; the other genes were upregulated. *Source*: From Ref. 37.

toxic dose to these cells. This treatment produced a pattern that consisted of an approximately equal number of genes that were increased as were decreased. Moreover, while differential expression of many of these genes might have been predicted from other toxicological information, many of these genes were not previously known to be arsenic-responsive. And only a small subset of altered genes were part of a general stress pathway, most of which were also common to the higher dose. Also surprisingly, a greater number of genes were altered at the lower dose (37).

At the higher arsenic dose, which is cytotoxic to these cells over a 24- to 48-hour period, virtually all the differentially expressed genes were upregulated (one exception out of 65 genes), and virtually all of them were known to be involved in stress and apoptotic response pathways. Historically, the general paradigm of toxicology has been that individual responses or end points are progressively dose-dependent, i.e., lower doses may cause a lower effect, and higher doses are expected to cause the same effect but to a greater magnitude. There are clearly many examples in toxicology of such changes occurring over relatively narrow dose ranges, such as was observed in the experiments shown in Figure 7 in which essentially the same subset of genes was altered by arsenic, but the magnitude of change differed with dose. However, the results shown in Figure 9 clearly indicate that, at least for these treatments, there was a fundamental difference in the biological response to a lower, noncytotoxic arsenic dose as compared to the higher, cytotoxic dose, suggesting a qualitative, threshold-based shift in response resulting in a nontraditional dose–response relationship. It is not yet clear whether this is more generally true for other agents and over other dose ranges. However, this could have profound implications for use and interpretation of biomarkers in toxicology, particularly with respect to the use of such data in risk assessment extrapolations over large dose ranges, and also has important mechanistic implications.

As discussed previously, some concern has been expressed regarding the use of toxicogenomics results in toxicology (1,2). One concern is that gene expression may be "too" sensitive to very low levels of exposure, and a related concern is that such responses may not be of toxicological relevance, but rather they may simply reflect adaptive responses that are typical for many other environmental stimuli. It will clearly be important to understand the biological basis—and potential toxicological implications—of such low level responses. However, there is likely to be great utility in such responses regardless of their toxicological impact. First, such responses may be sensitive indicators of very low level exposures within the population at concentrations far below those required to alter more traditional toxicological end points. So long as such sensitive responses are clearly defined as biomarkers of exposure only, they will still have utility. Second, such highly sensitive responses may provide a means of surveying the population to determine the variability in responses of individuals, with the aim of determining and defining sensitive subpopulations. Third, such responses may allow a determination of a true "no effect" level for a given chemical, which may be extremely useful for risk assessment modeling and for cross-species extrapolations.

Toxicogenomics approaches provide a unique means of investigating and comparing the specificity of biological responses in different systems that are beyond the scope of many traditional biomarkers. For example, we recently completed a series of toxicogenomics studies in mice given arsenic in drinking water, comparing different concentrations of arsenic, different exposure periods, and responses of different tissues within the same individuals. Interestingly, there were profound dose-, time point-, and tissue-specific differences in gene expression profiles in these animals (37a,42). This example illustrates the complex dynamics that can occur at the transcriptome level in response to a given agent but also suggests both the diagnostic and mechanistic potential of such patterns.

It has long been recognized that individual toxicants can induce pathophysiological effects that are highly tissue- and disease-specific, although the mechanistic basis for this is often poorly understood or may even appear to be counterintuitive based on cell culture or other mechanistic studies. For example, aflatoxin B1 is one of the most potent mutagen-carcinogens known based on laboratory studies, yet it does not produce a complex pattern of cancers in humans, but rather is highly specific in inducing liver cancer and is also highly synergistic with hepatitis B viral infections for cancer risk (43). Although there are clearly metabolic pathways in the liver that are important for aflatoxin activation, these alone cannot explain this remarkable tissue specificity. Why is aflatoxin so organ-specific in cancer induction given its potent genotoxic potential? Toxicogenomics approaches are now being applied to this problem (40) and may now be able to provide some answers to this long-standing puzzle.

Conversely, arsenic is known from human epidemiology studies to increase the risk of a wide variety of diseases, including several different types of cancer, vascular and cardiovascular disease, type 2 diabetes, and reproductive and developmental effects, yet clearly influences different disease risks in different tissues (44–47). How is one chemical able to influence so many different pathophysiological processes, and why does arsenic cause disease in one tissue but not another or different diseases in different tissues? One hypothesis is that arsenic selectively, but differentially, alters patterns of gene expression in different tissues and cell types, leading in turn to different phenotypic changes that influence disease processes specific to those cell types. As discussed above and as shown in Figures 8 and 9, toxicogenomics experiments in cell culture and animal models support this model of tissue-specific alterations, and further suggest that there are time- and dose-dependent alterations that may also play a causal role in the pathophysiological effects of arsenic.

Recent gene expression studies in people exposed to arsenic indicate that toxicogenomics will be able to provide valuable information that is directly relevant to disease processes and risk. Genomic profiling of lymphocytes from people who are exposed to various levels of arsenic in their drinking water have demonstrated a striking inverse correlation between levels of individual arsenic exposure, as measured by arsenic concentrations in toenails, and the level of mRNA expression of certain key DNA repair genes in their lymphocytes (48). Based on these and other studies, it has been hypothesized that arsenic may influence cancer risk in exposed individuals, at least in part, by suppressing DNA repair, thereby making people susceptible to DNA damage and mutations by other agents such as ultraviolet irradiation, cigarette smoke, and other environmental carcinogens (48).

Toxicogenomics will be an important tool for investigating such hypotheses as well as in identifying and validating new biomarkers. In particular, one or more of these affected DNA repair genes may represent an excellent candidate for a biomarker of arsenic-related cancer risk in exposed individuals. The hallmark of a good biomarker is a high degree of both sensitivity and specificity. These DNA repair genes are clearly highly sensitive to effects of arsenic at concentrations in drinking water that are directly relevant and of widespread concern throughout the United States. Whether these gene responses are also highly specific to arsenic exposure still remains to be determined, but the strong correlation with arsenic exposure, in a population that is otherwise heterogeneous with respect to other risk factors, suggests that this is likely to be the case. Moreover, given the important role of DNA repair in cancer risk, these genes not only represent biomarkers of exposure but are also likely to be linked mechanistically to processes that are central to the pathophysiological pathway of greatest concern, i.e., carcinogenesis.

DEVELOPMENT OF TOXICOPROTEOMICS AS A BIOMARKERS TOOL

As discussed above, proteomics has emerged as a potentially more relevant and specific tool than genomics for biomarker development in toxicology. As with genomics, the field of proteomics did not develop de novo but grew progressively out of an increasing interest and need to examine protein expression and its diversity at a more global level than previous biochemically based experiments. There are two basic types of proteomics applications in toxicology. The first is the use of the tools of proteomics—particularly two-dimensional (2-D) separations and analysis of proteins by mass spectrometry—in the characterization of individual proteins that are potential biomarkers of the pathophysiological pathway illustrated in Figure 1. These applications are essentially an extension of more classical biochemical techniques in toxicologic biomarkers research, and such individual biomarkers are also discussed in detail in other sections of this book. The second application is the use of true proteomics approaches to characterize alterations in proteins at a more global level within the proteome, with the aim of discovering new mechanisms of action and/or new candidate biomarkers for further detailed investigation. This latter area is still in its infancy and will be reviewed briefly with respect to its potential use as well as some of the remaining challenges in applying it to biomarkers development.

Proteomics is ultimately of even greater interest than genomics in toxicology, given that we are most interested in toxicant-induced changes in protein expression and function, which result in sustained alterations in the phenotype of a cell and which ultimately contribute to pathophysiological consequences. Other advantages of proteomics are that body fluids can be readily sampled for alterations in protein patterns, particularly blood and urine, and that alterations in the proteome are likely to be sustained over a longer period of time and be more reflective of long-term alterations in tissue phenotype than the more transient alterations in mRNA expression, which transcriptome profiling normally reflects. Moreover, because many proteins are covalently modified by toxicant exposures, either directly or indirectly as a consequence of toxicant response, proteomics offers a higher degree of agent specificity than alterations in gene expression, which may reflect many different biological stimuli and may be simple adaptive responses rather than of direct toxicological significance.

Ideally, we would like to be able to survey the entire proteome of a given matrix or tissue to fully characterize the toxicant-induced alterations. Unfortunately, because of the enormous complexity of the proteome and the current lack of adequate tools to investigate cellular alterations at the true proteomic level, it is not yet possible to perform such analyses. There are several important methodological barriers to analysis of the proteome in an analogous manner as the transcriptome. First, there is no protein equivalent to Taq polymerase and PCR amplification, which would enable us to systematically amplify the quantities of proteins in a sample, and so the amount of individual proteins in a given sample is usually limiting. And as discussed previously, this is further hampered by the complexity of the proteome as compared to the transcriptome, and the fact that a single protein can be present in many different forms in the same cell, including different phosphorylation and glycosylation states, different covalent and noncovalent processing variants, and different multimeric complexes. Proteins can also be found as structural components or as integral parts of membranes, further complicating their purification and analysis. We also do not have adequate and consistent separation technologies to fully distinguish the various protein species completely in two or three dimensions for subsequent analysis. Finally, we do not yet have the equivalent of complete microarrays for proteins that will adequately and quantitatively analyze the proteome should we be successful in amplifying and separating the components.

Nonetheless, the field is progressing rapidly on most of these technological fronts, and most importantly, the evolving tools of proteomics do provide a means to more selectively analyze subsets of proteins within the proteome, much as in the early days of genomics, when arrays with sub-sets of genes yielded important preliminary information. The ongoing development of new instrumentation and methodologies for examining the proteome has already yielded powerful new tools for biomarkers research. These include improvements in classical gel-based 2-D separations of proteins, as well as development of newer liquid-based 2-D and 3-D separation technologies (49). There have also been important advances in high-resolution mass spectrometry instrumentation, and new methods are rapidly developing for use in systematically examining posttranslational modifications to proteins, such as complex phosphorylation patterns (50–53).

One way that the proteome can change in response to a toxicant exposure is by alterations in expression of specific proteins or protein species within the cell. The majority of such alterations would likely involve altered expression of existing species, rather than new proteins or protein species. For example, a protein's total cellular levels could be altered, and/or the ratio of particular posttranslationally modified species could be altered. Both circumstances are frequently encountered in toxicology and pharmacology, and given the identity of the protein of interest, one could use either traditional biochemical techniques such as Western blotting or the tools of proteomics to characterize such alterations. The use of proteomics is particularly advantageous when the protein(s) of interest is not known, and also has the advantage that many, perhaps most, changes could be observed for a given treatment. A disadvantage of such toxicant-induced alterations with respect to biomarkers is similar to that of genomics, i.e., lack of specificity. One could imagine many different treatments altering the expression of a particular protein, or altering its species ratio, e.g., by altering the pattern or extent of its phosphorylation. Moreover, if this involves a common pathway, such as a kinase-signaling pathway, such an end point will not necessarily provide a good candidate biomarker but may be highly informative for understanding the mechanism of action.

A second way that proteins can be altered in response to toxicants is by undergoing various covalent alterations, which may be direct targets (e.g., protein adducts) or indirect targets (e.g., specific proteolytic products of targeted proteins, or alterations in secretion of such products into blood or urine). These types of modifications have great potential as biomarkers because they may be highly specific for a particular toxicant or class of toxicants with similar mechanisms of action. Again, previous knowledge of a given target (e.g., adduction of serum albumin or hemoglobin) can allow one to use more traditional approaches for isolating and characterizing such alterations. However, the tools of proteomics can greatly increase the ability to look at multiple alterations of targeted proteins simultaneously, and is also invaluable for the identification of new candidate biomarkers in a more global fashion, e.g., by characterizing all soluble serum proteins. This proteomics-based biomarkers approach has been applied with increasing success in recent years as proteomics methodologies have advanced.

One of the first applications of a more proteomics-based approach was the use of 2-D gels to investigate alterations in expression of specific subsets of proteins simultaneously. For example, 2-D gels have been used successfully to examine different phosphorylation states of a given protein in response to specific chemical treatments (54). A distinct disadvantage of this approach, analogous to the differential hybridization and differential display approaches of genomics, is that one typically can only observe proteins that are of high abundance and whose expression is changed by a substantial (usually > two- to threefold) level. Moreover, many proteins can still comigrate on 2-D gels, and so individual spots on these gels, when cut out and further separated, can often reveal many different underlying proteins, which complicates the analysis. Nonetheless, such an approach has provided useful insights into the responses to certain toxicants. The use of 2-D gels or other multidimensional separation technologies in combination with mass spectrometric analysis of the isolated fractions has been successful in examining patterns of toxicant-induced protein adducts

(49). The use of tailored liquid chromatographic separations in combination with tandem mass spectrometry analysis is particularly fruitful for analysis of specific targets such as albumin or hemoglobin adducts (55).

With the advent of instrumentation and methodology improvements, it is now possible to combine several different proteomics approaches for a more comprehensive survey of the proteome following a given toxicant treatment. For example, a recent review discusses the potential application of these combined proteomics approaches specifically with respect to investigations in the field of neurotoxicology (56), but clearly these same approaches could be used in any area of toxicology with equal effect (57,58).

The clinical cancer research field has been at the forefront of using proteomics approaches to investigate basic differences between specific cancer states and between normal and cancer patients for particular diseases, with the principal aim of providing better diagnostic tools as well as identifying biomarkers that could be used for early detection. Many cancers, such as pancreatic and kidney cancer, for example, would have a high rate of treatment success if they could be detected at an early stage, but unfortunately by the time they are detected clinically, these cancers are usually highly advanced and these diseases are almost uniformly fatal. Successes have been reported for the detection of specific serum markers for prostate cancer and several other neoplasms (59–61). Some technical advances have been targeted specifically at the clinical arena; for example, a moderate throughput platform called surface-enhanced laser desorption ionization has been developed, which enables a more global, proteomic level screening of protein differences among samples, is being increasingly used to screen clinical patients (57).

As with toxicogenomics, one of the principal challenges to proteomics studies beyond the technical aspects of the experiments is the lag in the development of appropriate statistical and bioinformatics tools. Proteomics, like genomics, can generate enormous volumes of data that require careful analysis, which can take many times longer than the experiment itself. Mass spectrometers equipped with 2-D separation technology can accumulate thousands of spectra in a single run, and each of these requires analysis and comparison against one or more protein databases using complex algorithms and a high level of computing power. Supercomputers and massively parallel multiprocessor arrays are required to process these data in a timely manner. Thus, there is a great need for advancing the area of bioinformatics and computer science support for both toxicoproteomics and toxicogenomics. This will become further exacerbated when databases accumulate sufficient data to perform cross-experiment meta-analyses. However, as with toxicogenomics, there is also enormous potential for subsequent data mining of the information in these databases across experiments that may reveal new patterns leading both to new mechanistic insights and to the identification of useful biomarkers for subsequent translational studies.

SUMMARY

Toxicology studies over the past 20 to 30 years have clearly demonstrated that gene and protein expression is almost always altered in response to toxicant exposures of concern, through either direct or indirect mechanisms. Advances in genomics and proteomics technologies have led to these approaches being increasingly used in toxicology, both for mechanistically based studies and for identifying and characterizing candidate biomarkers. Toxicogenomics and toxicoproteomics approaches can now accurately measure alterations in gene and protein expression at very low, often nonovertly toxic concentrations prior to overt pathophysiological changes. Thus, these tools can be used to assess both low level toxicant exposures and toxicologically relevant exposures. Moreover, these same approaches can be used to investigate early biological responses to toxicant exposure, specific pathophysiological pathways of concern, early- and late-stage disease states, and individual host susceptibility factors. Significant technical and analytical challenges remain, the most important being the need to develop mature bioinformatics tools for appropriate analysis of the results from genomics and proteomics studies.

There is also a need to better understand the mechanistic basis for alterations in gene and protein expression in response to toxicant exposure, particularly at the lower dose levels where it is not yet clear whether such responses represent an adaptive response or an important toxicological response that is directly linked to a pathophysiological outcome. Nonetheless, toxicogenomics- and toxicoproteomics-based approaches have enormous potential for identifying, validating, and applying sensitive and specific biomarkers for basic and translational toxicology research, and may have particular utility for the assessment of low level environmental exposures of concern, as well as for risk assessment modeling of such exposures.

REFERENCES

1. Smith LL. Key challenges for toxicologists in the 21st century. Trends Pharmacol Sci 2001; 22:281–285.
2. Barlow T, Battershill J, Jeffery BR, Pollitt FD, Tahourdin CSM. Report of a symposium on the use of genomics and proteomics in toxicology. Mutagenesis 2003; 18:311–317.
3. Watson WP, Mutti A. Role of biomarkers in monitoring exposures to chemicals: present position, future prospects. Biomarkers 2004; 9:211–242.
4. Tully DB, Collins BJ, Overstreet JD, et al. Effects of arsenic, cadmium, chromium, and lead on gene expression regulated by a battery of 13 different promoters in recombinant HepG2 cells. Toxicol Appl Pharmacol 2000; 168:79–90.

5. Mumtaz MM, Tully DB, El-Masri HA, De Rosa CT. Gene induction studies and toxicity of chemical mixtures. Environ Health Perspect 2002; 110:947–956.
6. Hertzberg RC, MacDonell MM. Synergy and other ineffective mixture risk definitions. Sci Total Environ 2002; 288:31–42.
7. Bonassi S, Ugolini D, Kirsch-Volders M, Stromberg U, Vermeulen R, Tucker JD. Human population studies with cytogenetic biomarkers: review of the literature and future prospectives. Environ Mol Mutagen 2005; 45:258–270.
8. Au WW, Salama SA. Use of biomarkers to elucidate genetic susceptibility to cancer. Environ Mol Mutagen 2005; 45:222–228.
9. Warren AJ, Shields PG. Molecular epidemiology: carcinogen-DNA adducts and genetic susceptibility. Proc Soc Exper Biol Med 1997; 216:172–180.
10. Syvanen AC. Toward genome-wide SNP genotyping. Nat Genet 2005; 37.
11. Consortium IHGS. Finishing the euchromatic sequence of the human genome. Nature 2004; 431:931–945.
12. Schadt EE, Edwards SW, GuhaThakurta D, et al. A comprehensive transcript index of the human genome generated using microarrays and computational approaches. Genome Biol 2004; 5:R73.
13. Heijne WHM, Steirum RH, Slijper M, van Bladeren PJ, van Ommen B. Toxicogenomics of bromobenzene hepatotoxicity: a combined transcriptomics and proteomics approach. Biochem Pharmacol 2003; 65:857–875.
14. Nekrutenko A. Reconciling the numbers: ESTs versus protein-coding genes. Mol Biol Evol 2004; 21:1278–1282.
15. Sorek R, Shamir R, Ast G. How prevalent is functional alternative splicing in the human genome? Trends Genet 2004; 20:68–71.
16. Aguiar M, Masse R, Gibbs BF. Regulation of cytochrome P450 by posttranslational modification. Drug Metab Rev 2005; 37:379–404.
17. Hamilton JW, Wetterhahn KE. Differential effects of chromium (VI) on constitutive and inducible gene expression in chick embryo liver in vivo and correlation with chromium (VI)-induced DNA damage. Mol Carcinogen 1989; 2:274–286.
18. Hamilton JW, Bloom SE. Correlation between induction of xenobiotic metabolism and DNA damage from chemical carcinogens in the chick embryo in vivo. Carcinogenesis 1986; 7:1101–1106.
19. Hamilton JW, Louis CA, Doherty KA, Hunt SR, Reed MJ, Treadwell MD. Preferential alteration of inducible gene expression in vivo by carcinogens that induce bulky DNA lesions. Mol Carcinogen 1993; 8:34–43.
20. McCaffrey J, Hamilton JW. Comparison of effects of direct-acting DNA methylating and ethylating agents on inducible gene expression in vivo. Environ Mol Mutagen 1994; 23:164–170.
21. Alcedo JA, Misra M, Hamilton JW, Wetterhahn KE. The genotoxic carcinogen chromium (VI) alters the metal-inducible expression but not the basal expression of the metallothionein gene in vivo. Carcinogenesis 1994; 15:1089–1092.
22. Hamilton JW, McCaffrey J, Caron RM, et al. Genotoxic chemical carcinogens target inducible genes in vivo. Ann NY Acad Sci 1994; 726:343–345.
23. McCaffrey J, Wolf CM, Hamilton JW. Effects of the genotoxic carcinogen chromium (VI) on basal and hormone-inducible phosphoenolpyruvate carboxykinase gene expression in vivo: correlation with glucocorticoid- and developmentally-regulated expression. Mol Carcinogen 1994; 10:189–198.

24. Caron RM, Hamilton JW. Preferential effects of the chemotherapeutic DNA crosslinking agent mitomycin C on inducible gene expression in vivo. Environ Mol Mutagen 1995; 25:4–11.
25. Hamilton JW, Kaltreider RC, Bajenova OV, et al. Molecular basis for effects of carcinogenic heavy metals on inducible gene expression. Environ Health Perspect 1998; 106:1005–1015.
26. Kaltreider RC, Pesce CA, Ihnat MA, Lariviere JP, Hamilton JW. Differential effects of arsenic (III) and chromium (VI) on nuclear transcription factor binding. Mol Carcinogen 1999; 25:219–229.
27. Hamilton JW, Bement WJ, Sinclair PR, Sinclair JF, Wetterhahn KE. Expression of 5-aminolaevulinate synthase and cytochrome P-450 mRNAs in chicken embryo hepatocytes in vivo and in cell culture: effect of porphyrinogenic drugs and haem. Biochem J 1988; 255:267–275.
28. Ihnat MA, Lariviere JP, Warren AJ, et al. Suppression of P-glycoprotein expression and multidrug resistance by DNA cross-linking agents. Clin Cancer Res 1997; 3:1339–1346.
29. Kaltreider RC, Davis AM, Lariviere JP, Hamilton JW. Arsenic alters the function of the glucocorticoid receptor as a transcription factor. Environ Health Perspect 2001; 109:245–251.
30. Calvet JP. Molecular approaches for analyzing differential gene expression: differential cDNA library construction and screening. Ped Nephrol 1991; 5:751–757.
31. Griffith JK, Enger MD, Hildebrand CE, Walters RA. Differential induction by cadmium of a low-complexity ribonucleic acid class in cadmium-resistant and cadmium-sensitive mammalian cells. Biochemistry 1981; 20(16):4755–4761.
32. Coen DM. The polymerase chain reaction. In: Ausubel FM, Brent R, Kingston RE, et al., eds. Current Protocols in Molecular Biology. Vol. 2. New York: John Wiley & Sons, Inc., 2005:15.10.11–15.17.18.
33. Liang P, Pardee AB. Differential display of eukaryotic messenger RNA by means of the polymerase chain reaction. Science 1992; 257:967–971.
34. Liao VH-C, Freedman JH. Cadmium-regulated genes from the nematode *Caenorhabditis elegans*. Identification and cloning of new cadmium-responsive genes by differential display. J Biol Chem 1998; 273:31962–31970.
35. Dmitrovsky E. Tissue microarrays for hypothesis generation. J Natl Cancer Inst 2004; 96:248–249.
36. Bradfield CA. Genomics and proteomics. Chem Res Toxicol 2004; 17:2.
37. Andrew AS, Warren AJ, Barchowsky A, et al. Genomic and proteomic profiling of responses to toxic metals in human lung cells. Environ Health Perspect 2003; 111:825–835.
37a. Bernardo V, Andrew AS, Ihnat MA, Warnke LA, Daney JC, Hamilton JW. Integrated computational analysis of microarray data applied to a dose response experiment. J Biomed Informatics 2005. In press.
38. Davey JC, Andrew AS, Barchowsky A, et al. Toxicogenomics of drinking water arsenic in vivo: effects of replicates on microarray analysis. Toxicol Sci 2004; 78(S1):60.
39. Draghici S. Data Analysis Tools for DNA Microarrays. Boca Raton: Chapman & Hall/CRC, 2003.

40. Ellinger-Ziegelbauer H, Stuart B, Wahle B, Bomann W, Ahr HJ. Characteristic expression profiles induced by genotoxic carcinogens in rat liver. Toxicol Sci 2004; 77:19–34.

41. Hamadeh HK, Bushel PR, Jayadev S, et al. Gene expression analysis reveals chemical-specific profiles. Toxicol Sci 2002; 67:219–231.

42. Andrew AS, Barchowsky A, Davey JC, et al. In vivo exposure to drinking water arsenic modifies expression of genes in the mouse lung. Toxicol Sci 2004; 78(S1):145.

43. Wogan GN, Hecht SS, Felton JS, Conney AH, Loeb LA. Environmental and chemical carcinogenesis. Semin Cancer Biol 2004; 14:473–486.

44. ATSDR. Toxicological Profile for Arsenic (Update). Washington: Agency for Toxic Substances and Disease Registry, USDHHS, PHS, 1999.

45. NRC. Arsenic in Drinking Water. Washington: National Research Council, 1999.

46. NRC. Arsenic in Drinking Water: 2001 Update. Washington: National Research Council, 2001.

47. Abernathy CO, Thomas DJ, Calderon RL. Health effects and risk assessment of arsenic. J Nutr 2003; 133:1536S–1538S.

48. Andrew AS, Karagas MR, Hamilton JW. Decreased DNA repair gene expression among individuals exposed to arsenic in United States drinking water. Intl J Cancer 2003; 104:263–268.

49. Liebler DC. Introduction to Proteomics: Tools for the New Biology. Totowa: Humana Press, 2002.

50. Denison C, Rudner AD, Gerber SA, Bakalarski CE, Moazed D, Gygi SP. A proteomic strategy for gaining insights into protein sumoylation in yeast. Mol Cell Proteomics 2005; 4:246–254.

51. Kirkpatrick DS, Gerber SA, Gygi SP. The absolute quantification strategy: a general procedure for the quantification of proteins and post-translational modifications. Methods 2005; 35:265–273.

52. Ballif BA, Roux PP, Gerber SA, MacKeigan JP, Blenis J, Gygi SP. Quantitative phosphorylation profiling of the ERK/p90 ribosomal S6 kinase-signaling cassette and its targets, the tuberous sclerosis tumor suppressors. Proc Natl Acad Sci USA 2005; 102:667–672.

53. Gerber SA, Rush J, Stemman O, Kirschner MW, Gygi SP. Absolute quantification of proteins and phosphoproteins from cell lysates by tandem MS. Proc Natl Acad Sci USA 2003; 100:6940–6945.

54. Hartigan JA, Green EG, Mortensen RM, Menachery A, Williams GH, Orme-Johnson NR. Comparison of protein phosphorylation patterns produced by adrenal cells by activation of cAMP-dependent protein kinase and Ca-dependent protein kinase. J Steroid Biochem Mol Biol 1995; 53:95–101.

55. Badghisi H, Liebler DC. Sequence mapping of epoxide adducts in human hemoglobin with LC-tandem MS and the Salsa algorithm. Chem Res Toxicol 2002; 15:799–805.

56. LoPachin RM, Jones RC, Patterson TA, Slikker W Jr, Barber DS. Application of proteomics to the study of molecular mechanisms in neurotoxicology. Neurotoxicology 2003; 24:761–775.

57. Petricoin EF, Rajapaske V, Herman EH, et al. Toxicoproteomics: serum proteomic pattern diagnostics for early detection of drug induced cardiac toxicities and cardioprotection. Toxicol Pathol 2004; 32:122–130.

58. Gillespie JW, Gannot G, Tangrea MA, et al. Molecular profiling of cancer. Toxicol Pathol 2004; 32:67–71.
59. Wright ME, Han DK, Aebersold R. Mass spectrometry-based expression profiling of clinical prostate cancer. Mol Cell Proteomics 2005; 4:545–554.
60. Xiao Z, Prieto D, Conrads TP, Veenstra TD, Issaq HJ. Proteomic patterns: their potential for disease diagnosis. Mol Cell Endocrinol 2005; 230:95–106.
61. Kuruma H, Egawa S, Oh-Ishi M, Kodera Y, Maeda T. Proteome analysis of prostate cancer. Prostate Cancer Prostatic Dis 2005; 8:14–21.

12

Biomarkers of Chemical Warfare Agents

William J. Smith

Cell & Molecular Biology Branch, U.S. Army Medical Research Institute of Chemical Defense, Aberdeen Proving Ground, Aberdeen, Maryland, U.S.A.

Harry Salem

Research and Technology Directorate, U.S. Army Edgewood Chemical Biological Center, Aberdeen Proving Ground, Aberdeen, Maryland, U.S.A.

INTRODUCTION

As can be judged from the variety of definitions and uses seen in this volume, the term biomarkers is applied to a broad array of biological phenomena from normal cellular activity through disease states through toxicant-induced cell and tissue changes. Depending on the primary focus of one's research, the selection of a working definition of a biomarker may vary. As a good general starting definition, the National Academy of Science in 1989 defined a biomarker as "a xenobiotically-induced variation in cellular or biochemical components or processes, structures, or functions that is measurable in a biological system or sample" (1). The Biomarkers Definition Working Group has provided a working definition as applied to drug development, "a characteristic that is objectively measured and evaluated as an indicator of normal biological processes, pathological processes or pharmacological responses to a therapeutic intervention" (2). In applying a toxicological interpretation to biomarkers, Mayer et al. (3) defined biomarkers as "quantifiable biochemical, physiological, or histological measures that relate in a dose- or time-dependent manner the degree of dysfunction that the contaminant has produced." In a chapter on risk assessment and risk management, Olajos and Salem (4) defined the critical aspects of biomarkers to be reliability, sensitivity and specificity (chemical and biological), validity, and relevance. They further pointed out that biomarkers can be general (e.g., stress proteins) or specific (i.e., organ-specific or toxicant-specific), and that biomarkers can be classified as markers of exposure, markers of effect, or markers of susceptibility. Biomarkers of exposure can be a xenobiotic agent or its metabolite or the product of an interaction between the xenobiotic and its cellular target molecule. Biomarkers of effect are measurable biochemical, physiological, or histological alterations that signal cell, tissue, or organ dysfunction. Biomarkers of susceptibility are indicators of decreased ability to respond to challenge by a chemical, biological, or physical stressor. The purpose of this chapter is to point out the unique applications of biomarker determination to the study of chemical warfare agents (CWA), a current threat to military and civilian personnel, and a subject of much interest to laboratory managers in the homeland defense community.

CWA: DEFINITIONS AND CLASSIFICATION

CWA are chemicals designed for use in military operations to kill, injure, or incapacitate humans through physiological actions. CWA are usually classified as nerve agents, vesicating (blistering) agents, respiratory agents, or blood agents. For a more comprehensive treatment of the chemistries and toxicological properties of the CWA, the reader is referred to any number of texts currently on the market due to the heightened interest in this subject. The principal medical textbook in this area is the *Textbook of Military Medicine* published by the Surgeon General of the U.S. Army (5). Table 1 lists the agents discussed in the following text.

The predominant nerve agents of historical note are the "G-agents" (GA-tabun, GB-sarin, GD-soman, GF-cyclo-sarin) and the "V-agents" (VX and, more recently, VR). Many of these nerve agents are related to common pesticides and function through inhibition of the enzyme acetylcholinesterase (AChE). AChE is a critical regulatory enzyme in the conduction of neuromuscular activity in that it breaks down the neurotransmitter acetylcholine (ACh). When the nerve agent binds to the active site of AChE, the enzyme can no longer function in destroying ACh. As ACh builds up in the neuromuscular junction, it causes continual nerve impulse generation and organ stimulation. Organs with cholinergic receptors include smooth muscle, skeletal muscle, central nervous system, and exocrine glands. The effects of nerve agent exposure vary based on dose and route of exposure but can range from miosis through increased secretions,

Table 1 Chemical Warfare Agents

Agent class	Military designation	Common name	Chemical name
Nerve agents	GA	Tabun	Ethyl *N,N*-dimethylphosphor-amidocyanidate
	GB	Sarin	Isopropyl methylphosphono-fluoridate
	GD	Soman	Pinacolyl methylphosphono-fluoridate
	GF	Cyclo-sarin	Cyclohexyl methylphosphono-fluoridate
	VX	—	*O*-Ethyl *S*-(2-diisopropylami-noethyl) methylphosphono-thiolate
	VR	Russian VX	*O*-Isopropyl *S*-(2-diethylaminoethyl) methylphosphono-thiolate
Vesicant agents	H or HD	Sulfur mustard	Bis-(2-chloroethyl) sulfide
		Mustard gas	
	L	Lewisite	β-Chlorovinyldi-chloroarsine
Respiratory agents	CG	Phosgene	Carbonyl chloride
Blood agents	AC	Cyanide	Hydrogen cyanide
	CK		Cyanogen chloride

bronchoconstriction, muscle fasciculations, to convulsions, seizures, loss of consciousness, and death at the higher exposures.

Among the vesicating or blistering agents, the most well-documented is sulfur mustard or mustard gas. The other weaponized blistering agent is Lewisite. These agents are not usually considered lethal, but can be at high doses. Exposure to skin results in debilitating blisters with long periods of healing. The vesicants also cause severe eye and lung injuries. The mechanisms of chemical vesication are complex and not completely understood even though many of the pathological sequelae to mustard exposure have been defined. Mustard is an alkylating agent, meaning that it takes part in chemical interactions with critical cellular and tissue molecules. When these molecules become alkylated by mustard, their biological function is modified and pathological processes are set in motion. Lewisite, as organoarsenic compound, disrupts normal cellular functions by chemical interactions with key cellular enzymes. It may react with numerous enzymes but is believed to specifically cause the inhibition of pyruvate dehydrogenase in the citric acid cycle. Whatever mechanisms are involved, the vesicants sulfur mustard and Lewisite cause similar pathologies with separation of epidermis and dermis at the basement membrane zone, followed by infusion of serous fluid to produce frank blisters of the exposed skin.

The respiratory agents usually include phosgene, chlorine, or combustion products of Teflon , the organofluoride polymers. Of these, only phosgene appears on current threat lists. Many of the chemical weapons (nerve agents, vesicants, cyanide, etc.) can produce respiratory injuries, but they are usually discussed under their primary categories. Phosgene inhalation exposure results in coughing, choking, or dyspnea. High dose exposures can result in pulmonary edema within two to six hours, which indicates severe injury.

The principal chemical agent among the blood agents is cyanide, a well-known, historical poison. While the toxicity of cyanide has been attributed to the inhibition of cytochrome oxidase and subsequent blockage of aerobic cellular metabolism resulting in histotoxic anoxia, it also causes a rapid disruption of neuronal mechanisms controlling consciousness and breathing. Cyanide is acutely toxic at high doses and gives rise to serious neurological problems following chronic low-level exposures.

USE OF BIOMARKER DETERMINATIONS IN CWA RESEARCH

Biomarkers of CWA consist of numerous classes depending on the ultimate goals of the studies being undertaken. Medical diagnosis of a casualty to determine if a chemical exposure has taken place requires the detection of unaltered CWA in biofluids of victims. Since many of these compounds are highly reactive, the unaltered forms do not stay around the body for long periods of time. It therefore becomes necessary to detect metabolic products of CWA. In the case of sulfur mustard, this might be thiodiglycol (TDG) or conjugates of glutathione. For nerve agents, it might be hydrolyzed or conjugated organophosphate residues. Detection of CWA exposure can be complicated by the fact that some of the target molecules for medical diagnosis of CWA exposure can exist in the body as residues of non-CWA compounds.

When forensic diagnosis is the goal, as in late stage verification of prior exposures for confirmation of CWA use in treaty verification or for concerns of low-level exposure to storage depot workers, the possibility of detecting unaltered agent is nil and metabolic products are the only available targets. Their long-term presence will be dose- and time-dependent. In 2002, Noort et al. wrote a comprehensive overview of the methods and chemistries involved for detection of exposure to CWA (6).

If the studies underway are attempts to define mechanisms of toxic action of the CWA, the biomarkers of interest will potentially be unrelated to the actual CWA and be physiological receptors or macromolecules altered by the toxic action of the CWA. These biomarkers then become signal markers to the pathogenic process taking place on the target cells and tissues. For example, nerve agents specifically target the active site of AChE. The single most reliable biomarker of nerve agent exposure is blood level of AChE as measured by assays such as the Ellman assay for AChE activity (7). When the CWA has a diverse array of pathological sequelae, as with sulfur mustard, the biomarkers of toxicity may be cellular structural proteins, or reduction of certain cell types, or inflammatory responses.

If the studies of interest are focused on developing medical countermeasures against the toxic actions of CWA, the same biomarkers defined as pathological correlates to CWA exposure may become the bioparameters used to define countermeasure efficacy. While the CWA causes a marked change in a given biomarker, effective medical intervention should reduce the extent of the biomarker alteration.

As we learn more about the pathologies created by different CWA, we see that while the agent toxicities are often unique, frequently there are commonalities in the physiological processes induced by exposure to different CWA. There are attempts to define these commonalities and exploit medical interdiction strategies against these common manifestations such as inflammation induced by a variety of CWA (8). Unfortunately, it is also true that many of the clinical manifestations of CWA exposure are not unique to threat agents and can be seen with normal disease processes, nonchemical toxicants, stress, xenobiotic agents, and other undefined physiological stressors. The more clearly defined the biomarkers, the better the diagnosis and response to CWA exposure.

BIOMARKERS OF SPECIFIC CWA EXPOSURE

Nerve Agents

Exposure to nerve agents usually consists of either vapor exposure to the eyes or respiratory tract or liquid on the skin. The clinical effects of exposure are related to the dose and route of exposure. Low amounts of vapor result in miosis, rhinorrhea, or mild breathing difficulties. Large doses of vapor can result in loss of consciousness, convulsions, apnea, flaccid paralysis, and copious secretions. With liquid exposures, small doses can lead to localized sweating, nausea, vomiting, and weakness. Large liquid exposures can give rise to sudden loss of consciousness, convulsions, apnea, flaccid paralysis, and copious secretions. Many of these symptoms can be confused with symptoms of numerous other clinical conditions. The only clinical laboratory value useful in differential diagnosis is a reduced level of red blood cell cholinesterase (RBC-ChE) levels.

Medical Diagnosis

In order to establish validated assays for verification of exposure to certain CWA, the U.S. Army has published a Technical Bulletin #Med 296 (TB MED 296) containing specific assay techniques for monitoring levels of RBC-ChE, and for detection of specific inhibitors of ChE, sarin (GB), soman (GD), and cyclo-sarin (GF) in biological fluids (9). This technical bulletin and other valuable information related to medical chemical defense can be found on the website of the Army's Medical Research Institute of Chemical Defense (USAMRICD) http://usamricd.apgea.army.mil. For monitoring RBC-ChE, TB MED 296 recommends using the Test-Mate^{TM} OP Kit (EQM Research Inc, Cincinnati, Ohio, U.S.A.). This technology is based on the classic Ellman chromogenic assay procedure in which thiocholine, produced by esteratic cleavage of ACh, is detected by the chromogen DTNB (6).

For verification of specific nerve agent exposure, TB MED 296 describes gas chromatographic/mass spectrometry (GS–MS) techniques for measuring alkylmethylphosphonic acids in urine. The nerve agents sarin, soman, and GF are organophosphorous compounds that upon entry into the body are hydrolyzed to their corresponding phosphonic acids: isopropyl methylphosphonic acid (IMPA) for sarin, pinacolyl methylphosphonic acid (PMPA) for soman, and cyclohexyl methylphosphonic acid (CMPA) for cyclo-sarin. These can be readily analyzed in environmental samples, but their presence in biological samples adds a level of complexity to quantification of these polar acids. These metabolites can be detected in urine by the GC/MS method in TB MED 296 for four to seven days after exposure.

Forensic Diagnosis

For forensic, or retrospective, analysis of human exposure to chemical agents, the native agent will have disappeared from the biological samples as will most of the immediate metabolic products. The inhibited esterases, however, remain in the circulation for extended periods of time with half-lives for butyrylcholinesterase (BuChE) up to 16 days. If one could release an identifiable portion of the toxicant from these biomolecules, it could potentially be detectable by standard analytical procedures. Polhuijs et al. (10) developed a procedure known as fluoride reactivation that converts the bound phosphoryl moiety to its corresponding phosphono- or phosphofluoride. Using gas chromatographic techniques, the product can be detected in a specific and quantifiable manner. These data translate to the toxicant of origin and extent of poisoning. While subject to some limitation imposed by the chemistry of the inhibited esterases, such as spontaneous reactivation and aging, the method has proven highly useful in retrospective studies. Jakubowski et al. (11) utilized fluoride reactivation for detection of VX exposure. The reader is referred to the July to August 2004 issue of the *Journal of Analytical Toxicology* that is a special issue on current analytical methods for CWA for full reporting of the current methodologies in this area (12–14).

Vesicant or Blistering Agents

Exposure to vesicating agents comprises either mustard ("mustard gas," sulfur mustard) or Lewisite (an arsenical). A third vesicant, phosgene oxime (CX), is listed among the chemical threat agents, but information concerning it is sparse other than its ability to generate early, severe pain. Phosgene oxime will not be further discussed. Mustard and Lewisite generate similar final-stage pathologies, but the clinical sequelae immediately following exposure are different between the two agents.

Following exposure to mustard, there is a latent period with no overt clinical signs and symptoms. The duration of the latent period can vary from hours to a couple of days depending on dose of exposure. High dose cutaneous exposure can demonstrate erythema within two to four hours, whereas low dose exposure may not be evident for 24 hours. Other organs, besides the skin, known to be pathological targets of exposure to mustard are the eyes and the respiratory tract. Within one to two hours, following high vapor exposure to the eyes, the victim can experience tearing, itching, and burning followed quickly by swelling of the eyelids, corneal damage, and severe pain. Even at low levels of exposure that would fail to evidence any other organ pathology, the eyes can demonstrate tearing, itching, and burning. Respiratory involvement can range from low dose exposures having rhinitis, sneezing, and hoarseness over a 12- to 24-hour period up to severe productive coughing and shortness of breath within two to four hours of high-dose vapor exposures. Once the overt pathology (in the skin, small blisters, or groups of blisters) begins to develop, differential diagnosis is difficult because these symptoms mimic other blistering conditions such as poison ivy or poison oak or reactions to drugs. No clinical laboratory findings aid the diagnostic process, especially early in the post-exposure course, but severe exposures might demonstrate initial leukocytosis followed by a neutrophil-based leukopenia seen several days after the exposure.

While mustard exposures have a latency to their pathology, exposure to Lewisite causes an immediate pain along with irritation to the skin and mucous membranes. Erythema and blisters on the skin or eye and respiratory damage similar to that seen with mustard appear later.

Medical Diagnosis

Because of its high reactivity, mustard cannot be directly detected in biological materials such as urine. A major metabolic product of mustard (bis[2-chloroethyl] sulfide) is TDG. In the detection method published in TB MED 296, TDG is derivatized with heptafluorobutyric anhydride and detected in a GS–MS procedure (9). Using deuterated TDG as an internal standard along with spiked urine samples, a linear regression plot is used to quantify TDG levels in suspect urines. Using this technique, trace levels of TDG could be determined up to one week following mustard exposures in rats.

Many laboratories, including the USAMRICD, Aberdeen Proving Ground, Maryland, U.S.A. the TNO Prins Maurits Laboratory, Rijswijk, The Netherlands, and DSTL, Porton Down, Salisbury, U.K., are working on more accurate and reliable tests for markers of mustard exposure. Robin Black et al. from the United Kingdom reported on the identification of numerous metabolites of mustard in rat urine following exposure to sulfur mustard (15). Of the metabolites studied, TDG was found to be only a minor component of the hydrolysis of mustard. Much more significant levels of the products of β-lyase mediated metabolism were seen.

Forensic Diagnosis

Given the highly reactive nature of sulfur mustard, neither native mustard nor its metabolic products would be expected to remain in the circulation or in tissues for extended periods of time (15). While Black and Read (16,17) detected the β-lyase metabolites of mustard as late as 13 days after exposure, most of the efforts for retrospective detection of mustard exposure have focused on isolation and detection of mustard-altered biomolecules. With the knowledge that a primary biomolecular target of mustard is the N7-position of guanine in cellular DNA, Fidder et al. (18) developed techniques for detection of the mustard adduct, N7-(2-hydroxyethylthioethyl) guanine (N7-HETE-Gua). Eventual modifications of these techniques to use liquid chromatography and tandem mass spectrometry analysis (LC–MS–MS) led to successful detection of mustard exposure in urine, skin, and blood (19). Immunochemical detection of the N7-HETE-Gua adduct in cells using a monoclonal antibody-based enzyme-linked immunosorbent assay (ELISA) proved useful in retrospective analysis of mustard exposure using blood samples from casualties of the Iran–Iraq war collected 26 days after the exposure (20,21).

While DNA adducts have proven useful for forensic diagnosis, they have a limited window of applicability due to repair of DNA damage and cellular turnover rates. Researchers at the TNO in the Netherlands and Porton Down in the United Kingdom realized that proteins also are targets of mustard alkylation and, given the long transit time of hemoglobin (up to

120 days), they began developing analytical techniques to detect mustard-adducted amino acids. Initial successes were obtained identifying histidine, glutamic acid, and valine adducted residues (22,23). Price et al. (24) showed the potential of using MALDI-TOF/MS to confirm the presence of adducted hemoglobin following exposure to sulfur mustard. Human serum albumin has also been used as a biomolecular target useful in retrospective analysis. Noort et al. (25), using a tryptic digest of albumin, developed an LC–MS–MS technique to identify the adducted cysteine-34 residue. While not having the extended biological half-life of hemoglobin, albumin analysis proved successful in confirming mustard exposure of an Iranian casualty in serum collected nine days after the exposure. Since the skin is a primary target of mustard, van der Schans (26) developed a rapid detection method for mustard adducts of dermal keratins. This technique employs monoclonal antibodies against 2-hydroxyethylthioethyl modified glutamine or asparagine and can be used on easily obtained tape-stripped samples from suspected exposure victims. Again, the reader is referred to the special issue of the *Journal of Analytical Toxicology* for specific techniques currently being employed for sulfur mustard detection (27–34).

Lewisite, being an organoarsenical, works through mechanisms not involving alkylation. Therefore, analytical developments have focused on detection of hydrolysis products of Lewisite formed in blood such as 2-chlorovinylarsonous acid (CVAA). Fowler et al. (35) developed a GC-based assay for CVAA derivatized with 1,2-ethanedithiol (CVAA-EDT). Logan et al. (36) showed that CVAA-EDT could be detected in urine of animals up to 24 hours after subcutaneous exposure to Lewisite. Wooten et al. (37) employed derivatization of CVAA with 1,3-propanedithiol, solid-phase microextraction and GC–MS to develop an automated assay for CVAA with a limit of detection down to 7.4 pg/mL of urine. Using British Anti-Lewisite (BAL; 2,3-dimercaptopropanol) to bind to CVAA associated with globin and extracting the CVAA-BAL, Lewisite exposure in animals could be confirmed by GC–MS in blood samples taken 10 days after exposure (38).

Respiratory Agents

Many chemicals can produce respiratory injury. All of the other chemical threat agents discussed in this chapter, i.e., nerve agents, vesicants, and cyanide, can have a respiratory component to their toxicity. Ammonia, chlorine, oxides of nitrogen, and combustion products of Teflon (PFIB) produce severe pulmonary edema. The prototypic respiratory edemogen, however, is phosgene. The United States alone produces over a billion pounds of phosgene for use in industrial processes. While it has been considered a military threat, phosgene is not stockpiled as a military weapon. The principles of phosgene toxicity and therapy can be applied to a wide spectrum of pulmonary agents. Since these agents are gases, they readily penetrate down to the bronchioles and the alveoli. Following exposure to phosgene, there is a latent period preceding clinical signs and symptoms. This period is related to the amount of exposure and the extent of physical activity of the victim. The earliest effects may be those of mucous membrane irritation such as burning sensation in the eyes, conjunctivitis, mild coughing, or substernal pressure. The most common symptom following the latent period usually is dyspnea (shortness of breath). As fluid buildup continues in the lungs, oxygen delivery is disrupted resulting in hypoxemia and cyanosis. Eventually oxygen is not delivered to the brain and other critical organs. Death results from respiratory failure, hypoxia, and hypotension.

No clinical laboratory tests specifically identify or quantify phosgene exposure. Arterial blood gas studies, expiratory flow rates, and other indicators of lung compliance indicating fluid buildup in the lungs are not specific for phosgene exposure. Sciuto et al. have conducted numerous studies on changes in bioparameters following phosgene exposure in mice. They have seen alterations in cytokine profiles (39), antioxidant enzymes (40), electrolyte levels (41), and bronchoalveolar lavage parameters (42). Noort et al. (43) have reported the detection of adducts formed in vitro by phosgene with albumin and hemoglobin. Hopefully, one or more of these parameters will lead to an analytical procedure for diagnosis of phosgene exposure.

Cyanide

Cyanide is a rapidly acting, lethal agent capable of interacting with sulfur compounds and metallic complexes. It interferes with the body's ability to utilize oxygen. With the interruption of aerobic processes, the tissues switch to anaerobic metabolism resulting in buildup of lactic acid and creation of metabolic acidosis. Death can occur within six to eight minutes following absorption of toxic levels of cyanide. Following acute exposure to low or moderate levels of cyanide, the victim can experience increased rate and depth of breathing, dizziness, nausea, vomiting, and headache. If exposure continues, the signs and symptoms can quickly progress to convulsions, cessation of respiration, cardiac effects, and death. Cyanide casualties may appear similar to nerve agent casualties but will not evidence miosis, copious secretions, or fasciculations. Immediate laboratory findings may include elevated blood cyanide levels, metabolic acidosis with high lactate levels, or elevated arterial oxygen levels. The latter two findings may reflect disease states other than cyanide poisoning.

Medical Diagnosis

The published method for cyanide detection in TB Med 296 (9) incorporates an automated fluorometric assay (44). Many methods have been published for direct detection of cyanide in biological fluids and have been reviewed by Troup and Ballantyne (45).

Forensic Diagnosis

Direct detection of cyanide for retrospective confirmation of exposure is limited because of factors related to the analyte, such as volatility and rapid metabolic detoxification. Even the metabolic product of cyanide, thiocyanate, suffers from difficulties in its detection in biological fluids. Baskin et al. (46) proposed a more useful diagnostic target molecule in the cyanide metabolite 2-aminothiazoline-4-carboxylic acid (ATCA). Lundquist et al. (47) developed an assay for ATCA using a high-performance liquid chromatography (HPLC) technique for quantitation of derivatized ATCA. Recently, Logue et al. (48) showed the validity of ATCA detection as a forensic test for cyanide exposure.

SUMMARY

In the Introduction, we pointed out the diversity of definitions of biomarkers, yet for the study of CWA exposure, aspects of all the diverse definitions can be applied. We also see organ-specific markers (e.g., reduction of AChE) and numerous toxicant-specific markers (e.g., fluoride reactivation, mustard metabolites). As for the different types of biomarkers mentioned, markers of exposure (metabolites) and markers of effect (loss of AChE, immunohistochemical detection of altered keratins) have been applied to the evaluation of CWA exposure. As one explores the toxicological sequelae to CWA exposure, markers of susceptibility, especially immune susceptibility, become evident. For all the varied types of biomarkers employed in evaluation of CWA exposure and effects, the critical aspects of biomarkers as defined by Olajos and Salem (4) remain inviolable—they must be reliable, sensitive, specific, valid, and relevant.

REFERENCES

1. National Academy of Science. Biological Markers of Reproductive Toxicology. Washington DC: National Academy Press, 1989:15–35.
2. Biomarker Definitions Working Group. Biomarkers and surrogate endpoints: preferred definitions and conceptual framework. Clin Pharmacol Ther 2001; 69:89–95.
3. Mayer FL, Versteeg DJ, McKee MJ, et al. Physiological and nonspecific biomarkers. In: Huggett RJ, Kimerle RA, Mehrle PM, eds. Biomarkers: Biochemical, Physiological, and Histological Markers of Anthropogenic Stress. Chelsea, MI: Lewis Publishers, 1992:5–85.
4. Olajos EJ, Salem H. Risk assessment and risk management: pathways toward process enhancement. In: Salem H, Olajos EJ, eds. Toxicology in Risk Assessment. Philadelphia, PA: Taylor & Francis, 2000:269–310.
5. Zajtchuk R, Bellamy RF, eds. Textbook of Military Medicine. Washington, DC: US Department of Army, Office of the Surgeon General and Borden Institute, 1997.

6. Noort D, Benschop HP, Black RM. Biomonitoring of exposure to chemical warfare agents: a review. Toxicol Appl Pharmacol 2002; 184:116–126.

7. Ellman GL, Courtney KD, Andres J, Featherstone RM. A new and rapid colorimetic determination of acetylcholinesterase activity. Biochem Pharmacol 1961; 7:88–95.

8. Cowan, FC, Broomfield CA, Stojilijkovic MP, Smith WJ. A review of multi-threat medical countermeasures against chemical warfare and terrorism. Military Med 2004; 169:850–855.

9. Technical Bulletin. Assay Techniques for Detection of Exposure to Sulfur Mustard, Cholinesterase Inhibitors, Sarin, Soman, GF, and Cyanide. TB MED 296. Department of the Army, Washington DC, 1996 (Available online at http:// usamricd.apgea.army.mil).

10. Polhuijs M, Langenberg JP, Benschop HP. New method for retrospective detection of exposure to organophosphorus anticholinesterases: application to alleged sarin victims of Japanese terrorists. Toxicol Appl Pharmacol 1997; 146:156–161.

11. Jakubowski EM, Heykamp LS, Durst HD, Thomson SA. Preliminary studies in the formation of ethyl methylphosphonofluoridate from rat and human serum exposed to VX and treated with fluoride ion. Anal Lett 2001; 34:727–737.

12. Jakubowski EM, McGuire JM, Evans RA, et al. Quantitation of fluoride ion released sarin in red blood cell samples by gas chromatography-chemical ionization mass spectrometry using isotope dilution and large-volume injection. J Anal Toxicol 2004; 28:357–363.

13. Degenhardt CE, Pleijsier K, van der Schans MJ, et al. Improvements of the fluoride reactivation method for the verification of nerve agent exposure. J Anal Toxicol 2004; 28:364–371.

14. Barr JR, Driskell WJ, Aston LS, Martinez RA. Quantitation of metabolites of the nerve agents sarin, soman, cyclohexylsarin, VX, and Russian VX in human urine using isotope-dilution gas chromatography-tandem mass spectrometry. J Anal Toxicol 2004; 28:372–378.

15. Black RM, Hambrook JL, Howells DJ, Read RW. Biological fate of sulfur mustard, 1,1′-thiobis(2-chloroethane). Urinary excretion profiles of hydrolysis products and beta-lyase metabolites of sulfur mustard after cutaneous application in rats. J Anal Toxicol 1992; 16:79–84.

16. Black RM, Read RW. Improved methodology for the detection and quantitation of urinary metabolites of sulphur mustard using gas chromatography-tandem mass spectrometry. J Chromatogr B Biomed Appl 1995; 665:97–105.

17. Black RM, Read RW. Biological fate of sulphur mustard, 1,1′-thiobis(2-chloroethane): identification of beta-lyase metabolites and hydrolysis products in human urine. Xenobiotica 1995; 25:167–173.

18. Fidder A, Moes GW, Scheffer AG, van der Schans GP, Baan RA, de Jong LP, Benschop HP. Synthesis, characterization, and quantitation of the major adducts formed between sulfur mustard and DNA of calf thymus and human blood. Chem Res Toxicol 1994; 7:199–204.

19. Fidder A, Noort D, de Jong LP, Benschop HP, Hulst AG. N7-(2-hydroxyethylthioethyl)-guanine: a novel urinary metabolite following exposure to sulphur mustard. Arch Toxicol 1996; 70:854–855.

20. van der Schans GP, Scheffer AG, Mars-Groenendijk RH, Fidder A, Benschop HP, Baan RA. Immunochemical detection of adducts of sulfur mustard to DNA of calf thymus and human white blood cells. Chem Res Toxicol 1994; 7:408–413.

21. Benschop HP, van der Schans GP, Noort D, Fidder A, Mars-Groenendijk RH, de Jong LP. Verification of exposure to sulfur mustard in two casualties of the Iran–Iraq conflict. J Anal Toxicol 1997; 21:249–251.

22. Noort D, Verheij ER, Hulst AG, de Jong LP, Benschop HP. Characterization of sulfur mustard induced structural modifications in human hemoglobin by liquid chromatography—tandem mass spectrometry. Chem Res Toxicol 1996; 9:781–787.

23. Black RM, Harrison JM, Read RW. Biological fate of sulphur mustard: in vitro alkylation of human haemoglobin by sulphur mustard. Xenobiotica 1997; 27:11–32.

24. Price EO, Smith JR, Clark CR, Schlager JJ, Shih ML. MALDI-ToF/MS as a diagnostic tool for the confirmation of sulfur mustard exposure. J Appl Toxicol 2000; 20(Suppl 1):S193–S197.

25. Noort D, Hulst AG, de Jong LP, Benschop HP. Alkylation of human serum albumin by sulfur mustard in vitro and in vivo: mass spectrometric analysis of a cysteine adduct as a sensitive biomarker of exposure. Chem Res Toxicol 1999; 12:715–721.

26. van der Schans GP, Noort D, Mars-Groenendijk RH, et al. Immunochemical detection of sulfur mustard adducts with keratins in the stratum corneum of human skin. Chem Res Toxicol 2002; 15:21–25.

27. Capacio BR, Smith JR, DeLion MT, et al. Monitoring sulfur mustard exposure by gas chromatography-mass spectrometry analysis of thiodiglycol cleaved from blood proteins. J Anal Toxicol 2004; 28:306–310.

28. Noort D, Fidder A, Benschop HP, De Jong LP, Smith JR. Procedure for monitoring exposure to sulfur mustard based on modified edman degradation of globin. J Anal Toxicol 2004; 28:311–315.

29. van der Schans GP, Mars-Groenendijk R, de Jong LP, Benschop HP, Noort D. Standard operating procedure for immunoslotblot assay for analysis of DNA/ sulfur mustard adducts in human blood and skin. J Anal Toxicol 2004; 28:316–319.

30. Boyer AE, Ash D, Barr DB, et al. Quantitation of the sulfur mustard metabolites 1,1'-sulfonylbis[2-(methylthio)ethane] and thiodiglycol in urine using isotope-dilution gas chromatography-tandem mass spectrometry. J Anal Toxicol 2004; 28:327–332.

31. Noort D, Fidder A, Hulst AG, Woolfitt AR, Ash D, Barr JR. Retrospective detection of exposure to sulfur mustard: improvements on an assay for liquid chromatography-tandem mass spectrometry analysis of albumin-sulfur mustard adducts. J Anal Toxicol 2004; 28:333–338.

32. Young CL, Ash D, Driskell WJ, et al. A rapid, sensitive method for the quantitation of specific metabolites of sulfur mustard in human urine using isotope-dilution gas chromatography-tandem mass spectrometry. J Anal Toxicol 2004; 28:339–345.

33. Read RW, Black RM. Analysis of beta-lyase metabolites of sulfur mustard in urine by electrospray liquid chromatography-tandem mass spectrometry. J Anal Toxicol 2004; 28:346–351.

34. Read RW, Black RM. Analysis of the sulfur mustard metabolite 1,1'-sulfonyl-bis [2-S-(N-acetylcysteinyl)ethane] in urine by negative ion electrospray liquid chromatography-tandem mass spectrometry. J Anal Toxicol 2004; 28:352–356.
35. Fowler WK, Stewart DC, Weinberg DS, Sarver EW. Gas chromatographic determination of the lewisite hydrolysate, 2-chlorovinyl arsonous acid, after derivatizaion with 1,2-ethanedithiol. J Chromatogr 1991; 558:235–246.
36. Logan TP, Smith JR, Jakubowski EM, Nielson RE. Verification of lewisite exposure by the analysis of 2-chlorovinyl arsonous acid in urine. Toxicol Methods 1999; 9:275–284.
37. Wooten JV, Ashley DL, Calafat AM. Quantitation of 2-chlorovinyl arsonous acid in human urine by automated solid-phase microextraction-gas chromato-graphy-mass spectrometry. J Chromatogr B Anal Technol Biomed Life Sci 2002; 772:147–153.
38. Fidder A, Noort D, Hulst AG, de Jong LP, Benschop HP. Biomonitoring of expo-sure to lewisite based on adducts to haemoglobin. Arch Toxicol 2000; 74:207–214.
39. Sciuto AM, Clapp DL, Hess ZA, Moran TS. The temporal profile of cytokines in the bronchoalveolar lavage fluid in mice exposed to the industrial gas phos-gene. Inhal Toxicol 2003; 15:687–700.
40. Sciuto AM, Cascio MB, Moran TS, Forster JS. The fate of antioxidant enzymes in bronchoalveolar lavage fluid over 7 days in mice with acute lung injury. Inhal Toxicol 2003; 15:675–685.
41. Sciuto AM, Carpin LB, Moran TS, Forster JS. Chronological changes in elec-trolyte levels in arterial blood and bronchoalveolar lavage fluid in mice after exposure to an edemagenic gas. Inhal Toxicol 2003; 15:663–674.
42. Duniho SM, Martin J, Forster JS, et al. Acute changes in lung histopathology and bronchoalveolar lavage parameters in mice exposed to the choking agent gas phosgene. Toxicol Pathol 2002; 30:339–349.
43. Noort D, Hulst AG, Fidder A, van Gurp RA, de Jong LP, Benschop HP. In vitro adduct formation of phosgene with albumin and hemoglobin in human blood. Chem Res Toxicol 2000; 13:719–726.
44. Groff WA, Stemler FW, Kaminskis A, Froehlich HL, Johnson RP. Plasma free cyanide and blood total cyanide: a rapid completely automated microdistilla-tion assay. J Toxicol Clin Toxicol 1985; 23:133–163.
45. Troup CM, Ballantyne B. Analysis of cyanide in biological fluids and tissues. In: Ballentyne B, Marrs TC, eds. Clinical and Experimental Toxicology of Cyanides. Bristol, England: Wright, 1987:22–40.
46. Baskin SI, Petrikovics I, Kurche JS, et al. Insights on cyanide toxicity and methods of treatment. In: Flora SJS, Romano JA, Baskin SI, Sekhar K, eds. Pharmacological Perspectives of Toxic Chemicals and Their Antidotes. New Delhi, India: Narosa, 2004:105–146.
47. Lundquist P, Kagedal B, Nilsson L, Rosling H. Analysis of the cyanide meta-bolite 2-aminothiazoline-4-carboxylic acid in urine by high-performance liquid chromatography. Anal Biochem 1995; 228:27–34.
48. Logue BA, Kirschten NP, Moser MA, Petrikovics I, Baskin SI. Determination of the cyanide metabolite 2-aminothiazoline-4-carboxylic acid in urine and plasma by gas chromatography-mass spectrometry. J Chromatogr B Analyt Technol Biomed Life Sci 2005; 819:237–244.

13

Applications of Biomarkers in Toxic Tort and Forensic Litigation

Gary E. Marchant

Center for the Study of Law, Science and Technology, Arizona State University College of Law, Tempe, Arizona, U.S.A.

INTRODUCTION

Biomarkers have the potential to fill critical evidentiary gaps that currently plague many types of litigation. For example, toxic tort litigation, which involves injuries allegedly caused by exposure to toxic agents, is limited by the current inability to associate particular exposures with subsequent health consequences in a specific individual. The consequence of this ignorance is the need to rely on crude assumptions and presumptions that frequently result in unjust outcomes, whether it be manufacturers of harmless products that are unfairly saddled with punitive monetary damages, or seriously injured citizens who are denied fair compensation because they cannot prove sufficiently that a particular exposure caused their injury. By providing an evidentiary link between exposures and health effects, toxicological biomarkers have the potential to shine objective scientific illumination on whether a specific toxic exposure did or did not cause a particular individual's injuries.

This chapter explores the potential uses of toxicological biomarkers in toxic tort and forensic litigation, and the scientific, legal, policy, and ethical challenges presented by these biomarker applications. It first discusses potential applications of biomarkers, drawing where available on existing precedents involving the use of toxicological biomarkers, or cases which provide a relevant analogy for the use of such biomarkers. It then addresses a series of issues relevant to the use of biomarkers in the litigation context, including the admissibility of biomarker evidence under the new legal standards for scientific evidence, as well as other practical and normative issues that will be presented by the use of biomarkers in litigation.

POTENTIAL APPLICATIONS OF BIOMARKERS IN LITIGATION

Toxic Torts

Toxic tort litigation is the legal forum in which toxicological biomarkers will likely have their greatest demand and utility. Biomarkers will have applications in demonstrating exposure, causation, risk, and susceptibility, which are legally important determinations that are currently woefully deficient of scientific support in most toxic tort litigation.

Exposure

A threshold issue in toxic tort litigation is that the plaintiff (the person who brought the lawsuit alleging injury) must demonstrate sufficient exposure to the toxic agent that allegedly caused injury. Many courts require the plaintiff to not only prove that exposure occurred, but also require some degree of quantification of that exposure. As one federal court of appeals stated, "there must be evidence from which the fact finder can conclude that the plaintiff was exposed to levels of that agent that are known to cause the kind of harm that the plaintiff claims to have suffered" (1). In other types of personal injury litigation, such as cases involving allegedly harmful medical devices or pharmaceuticals, proving exposure is usually not a problem because the exposed individual knowingly and deliberately undertook a carefully measured exposure (by agreeing to the implanting of a medical device or the administering of a pharmaceutical). In toxic tort cases involving, for example, alleged injuries from groundwater contamination or from an accidental explosion at an industrial facility, it is much more difficult to demonstrate and quantify exposure.

Toxicological biomarkers of exposure have the potential to provide objective evidence of individual exposure (or lack thereof). Courts have already indicated their receptivity to this application of biomarker data. For example, citizens living near the Three Mile Island (TMI) nuclear facility attempted to use chromosomal biomarkers to demonstrate and quantify exposure to a plume of radiation allegedly released during the 1979 TMI accident. The plaintiffs lacked adequate direct or modeling evidence of exposure, which the court described as the "critical issue" in the case (2). The plaintiffs therefore sought to prove exposure based on evidence of an increased frequency of dicentric chromosomes in the lymphocytes of citizens living near the facility. The court held that this use of biomarkers was "an accepted method, not simply for determining if the subject of the analysis was irradiated, but also for estimating radiation dose to the individual." Notwithstanding its finding that "[r]adiation dose estimation based on dicentric enumeration is a valid and reliable scientific methodology," the court rejected the evidence in that particular case because the "validity and reliability decrease as the time gap between the alleged irradiation and the dicentric count increases" and the plaintiffs had waited 15 years to assay dicentric chromosomes in the allegedly exposed population.

This judicial holding, while not helpful to the plaintiffs in that specific case, nevertheless does establish the more general proposition that chromosomal rearrangements can be used in the proper litigation context as biomarkers to both establish and quantify exposure. Other types of biomarkers, such as changes in gene expression, are also likely to be offered as biomarkers of exposure in future cases (3,4). As the TMI case demonstrates, the temporal relationship between the exposure event and the subsequent assay for elevated biomarkers will be a critical issue for producing a valid exposure estimate and hence judicial acceptance. Other important issues will be the specificity and sensitivity of the biomarker assay, and interindividual variations in biomarker levels for a given exposure (3).

Causation

The second, and usually most onerous, impediment that a toxic tort plaintiff must overcome is to demonstrate causation. The causation inquiry has two steps. The first step, general causation, inquires whether the toxic agent that the plaintiff was exposed to *is capable of causing* the health problems afflicting the plaintiff. The second step, specific causation, asks whether that exposure *actually did cause* the health effects in the individual plaintiff. Biomarkers can be useful for both inquiries, but are likely to be most significant for the specific causation inquiry.

The primary application of biomarkers for general causation will be to provide a linkage between a toxic agent and toxicological endpoint that has not been directly substantiated in standard toxicological studies. Often plaintiffs lack any data showing a direct association between the specific agent they were exposed to and the particular health effect they are alleging was caused by that exposure. By necessity, they often attempt to rely instead on data showing that the agent causes other related health effects (e.g., a tumor in a different organ of the body) or that a similar agent (perhaps from the same family of chemical compounds) does cause the specific health effect at issue. Courts generally reject such indirect data, ruling that a plaintiff must produce evidence showing a direct linkage between the specific exposure and particular health endpoint at issue in that case.

Biomarkers have the potential to provide such a connection. For example, a plaintiff with a kidney tumor may be able to rely on evidence showing that the toxic agent in question causes liver tumors if there is evidence that the agent produces similar biomarkers (e.g., DNA adducts, gene expression changes, or proteomic markers) in both the liver and kidney, and the liver biomarkers are in some way related to the liver tumors. The common biomarker in the liver and kidney might then allow the plaintiff to extrapolate the tumor findings in the liver to the kidney. Similarly, if a plaintiff has been exposed to an agent (compound A) that causes an elevated biomarker in the lung but has not been associated with any toxicological endpoint in a published study, the plaintiff may be able to rely on evidence showing that a related compound B causes the same biomarker elevation in the lung and the toxic endpoint present in the plaintiff. While this biomarker "bootstrapping" to prove general causation has yet to be considered by courts, several judicial statements and holdings suggest that courts might be amenable to such arguments. If so, it would greatly expand the universe of potential combinations of toxic agents and toxicological endpoints for which plaintiffs will be capable of demonstrating general causation.

The greatest utility of biomarkers in toxic tort litigation is likely to be in demonstrating specific causation. Specific causation is the "Achilles' heel" of many plaintiffs' claims because of the scientific difficulty in proving that a specific exposure caused disease in a particular individual. The only cases in which specific causation is not a major challenge are those involving "signature" diseases that are caused primarily or exclusively by a particular agent, such as mesothelioma caused by asbestos or clear cell adenocarcinoma caused by the drug DES. In most other causes, many toxic agents as well as other environmental exposures (e.g., foods, medicines, lifestyle factors, disease vectors) and intrinsic factors (e.g., genetic susceptibility) are capable of causing or contributing to the cause of the disease manifested in the individual plaintiff. Standard "black box" toxicology that looks at increased rates of disease in a population in response to a particular exposure is simply incapable of determining the cause of disease in a particular individual. Courts thus resort to methods such as differential diagnosis or statistical presumptions to adjudicate specific causation, which are based on conjecture rather than direct evidence of causation.

Biomarkers have the potential to provide direct evidence to link a specific exposure with health endpoints in an individual plaintiff. Specifically, strong evidence of specific causation will be provided by a finding that chemical-specific biomarkers of effect are elevated in a plaintiff who has been exposed to that agent and has developed disease known to be caused by that agent. Conversely, defendants can use the absence of biomarkers expected from such an exposure to refute any linkage to the plaintiffs' disease.

An example of the use of biomarkers to support causation is a federal appellate court decision overturning a trial court's dismissal of a case brought by parents of a young child claiming she had been harmed by exposure to formaldehyde from a new dresser. The trial court dismissed the case based on its finding that the parents had not made a sufficient showing that the dresser's emissions of formaldehyde caused the child's health problems, but the appellate court reversed and allowed the case to go forward based in part on evidence that the child had antibodies in her blood indicating a recent exposure to formaldehyde (5).

Only biomarkers that are specific for a specific toxic agent or family of compounds will be useful for demonstrating specific causation. For example, some mutagenic chemicals produce a chemical-specific spectra of mutations that can be used as a biomarker of exposure to that chemical (6). Similarly, gene expression changes may provide a chemical-specific "fingerprint" of exposure to a particular toxicant (7,8). In contrast, biomarkers such as chromosomal rearrangements are not agent-specific, and thus are unlikely to be helpful in proving or disproving specific causation, although they may be useful for proving exposure or general causation (discussed earlier).

Because specific causation will generally require biomarkers of effect, another contentious issue in such inquiries will be the tissue in which the biomarker is measured. For many toxicological endpoints, the target organ (e.g., the liver or brain) cannot be easily assayed for biomarkers. Researchers often use surrogate tissues (e.g., white blood cells) to assay for biomarkers (9). Parties are likely to dispute whether a biomarker measured in a more easily accessible tissue is an adequate surrogate for the target organ under the legal standards for causation.

Yet another area of likely dispute in using biomarkers to prove specific causation is the issue of whether the biomarker response detected in the individual plaintiff is indeed diagnostic for causation. Biomarkers are generally identified and validated in populations rather than individuals, and the baseline levels and changes in any single individual could be affected by a variety of intrinsic (e.g., genetics) and extrinsic (e.g., diet or medications) factors (10). Thus, even when a biomarker of effect that may suggest specific causation is detected in an individual plaintiff, the opposing party will likely seek to cast that finding into doubt by suggesting other exposures or factors that might explain the reported finding.

Risk

A relatively new trend in toxic tort litigation is for plaintiffs who have been exposed to a toxic agent to file lawsuits seeking compensation for their latent risks that have not yet manifested into health problems. These latent risk claims are of three general types: (i)"increased risk" claims in which exposed plaintiffs seek to recover for their asymptomatic increased risk of disease; (ii)"fear of disease" claims in which exposed plaintiffs seek compensation for their fear of developing a disease such as cancer, which they claim is an injury in and of itself; and (iii)"medical monitoring" claims in which plaintiffs seek to recover the future costs of periodic medical examinations to check for any developing disease. The motivation for bringing a claim under the first two theories (increased risk and fear of disease) is that the defendant company and relevant evidence may not be available if the plaintiff waits 15 or 20 years for the manifestation of latent disease. Medical monitoring claims are based on the premise that frequent medical examinations may result in early detection and hence more effective treatment of emerging clinical disease.

Because virtually every citizen has been exposed to some type of toxic agent, courts have searched for limiting principles to prevent being flooded by latent risk claims, while permitting the most compelling claims to proceed. Thus, most courts have required a plaintiff bringing an increased risk or fear of disease claim to demonstrate a "present injury" as a prerequisite to pursuing such a claim (11,12). Many courts have also required a demonstration, and in some cases a quantification, of a sufficient magnitude of increased risk (13). Most plaintiffs exposed to toxic agents are unable to meet these threshold requirements using traditional toxicological data.

Biomarkers of effect that indicate the progression of a disease process characteristic of exposure to the relevant agent may help to support latent risk claims in several ways. First, biomarkers may provide the requisite evidence of "present injury" necessary to sustain a latent risk claim. There is both scientific and legal disagreement about whether the presence of a biomarker is sufficient to indicate a present injury. For example, many changes in gene expression may simply indicate the body's reversible and adaptive response to a toxic exposure, while other gene expression changes may be a true indicator of real toxic injury (14). A recent expert review of DNA adducts concluded that "[i]n the absence of any other toxicological data, the formation of chemical-specific DNA adducts should be considered an adverse effect, i.e., one which potentially compromises the organism" (15). Yet, the same review observed that there are a number of examples of DNA adducts that do not appear to be associated with any detectable toxicological consequence.

While the courts are somewhat split on the significance to be accorded to asymptomatic biomarkers, at least some courts have recognized asymptomatic molecular changes that are part of the disease process as a sufficient present injury to support a latent risk claim. Other jurisdictions require symptomatic disease to satisfy the present injury requirement, primarily due to the difficulty up until now of objectively proving alleged subcellular injuries. The availability of biomarkers that have been validated as a reliable marker of disease progression may cause some courts to relax their requirement of symptomatic disease to support a latent risk claim.

Second, biomarkers of effect may assist plaintiffs in demonstrating and perhaps quantifying their increased risk. The detection of biomarkers of effect in the exposed plaintiff could qualitatively confirm the increased risk from the plaintiff's exposure, and if supported by adequate human studies, could even be used to quantify risk (as the court in the TMI litigation indicated, discussed earlier). Such a finding would also validate the plaintiff's fear of disease, whereas a finding of no increase in biomarkers would diminish such fears and discredit any associated legal claims.

Biomarkers of effect (or perhaps even exposure) could also be used to support medical monitoring claims in two respects. First, the detection of such biomarkers in an individual would verify that the disease process has commenced and that further periodic testing of that individual might be warranted. Biomarkers could also serve as the target as well as the justification for medical monitoring, in that the monitoring would focus on detecting biomarkers of effect in exposed individuals, which might justify increased preventive or prophylactic measures in those individuals. A requirement for a valid medical monitoring claim in most jurisdictions is that monitoring and diagnostic methods exist that make early detection and treatment of the disease both possible and beneficial (16). Biomarkers may satisfy this requirement by making possible early detection that may make treatment more effective.

Susceptibility

While biomarkers of exposure and effect have many potential applications for proving exposure, causation, and risk in toxic tort litigation, biomarkers of susceptibility will also have many potential applications. For example, some jurisdictions require plaintiffs to show that their relative risk of developing a health effect from exposure to a toxic agent is greater than two, in order to meet the "more likely than not" legal standard of proof in civil (i.e., noncriminal) litigation. Relatively few toxic exposures double background risk, especially for relatively common health effects, even though the exposure may be important from a public health perspective. A plaintiff who can demonstrate a unique sensitivity to the exposure because of a genetic or other biomarker of susceptibility may be able to overcome this formidable burden of proof even when the relative risk in the general population is less than two. In other words, even though the relative risk for an entire exposed population in an epidemiologic study may be less than two, there could very well be subjects within that population who have an individual relative risk greater than two due to genetic or some other type of susceptibility. Plaintiffs who can demonstrate such susceptibility may be able to move forward with a case that would otherwise be dismissed because of an overall population relative risk less than two (17).

Plaintiffs may also argue that the presence of susceptible subgroups within a population may trigger a duty to warn of such susceptibilities on the part of product manufacturers. Although some regulatory programs impose warning requirements on some products, tort law also imposes a general duty to provide reasonable warnings against foreseeable harms. As biomarkers of susceptibility become available and feasible to test for, susceptible individuals harmed by the product are likely to bring "failure to warn" cases against product manufacturers who do not warn consumers about genetic and other susceptibilities to their products. Some lawsuits based on this theory have already been filed. For example, some users of the Lymerix vaccine against Lyme disease brought lawsuits against the vaccine manufacturer alleging a genetic susceptibility to the vaccine, claiming that the manufacturer had a duty to warn recipients to obtain a genetic test for the relevant genetic biomarker before using the vaccine. The manufacturer and the Food and Drug Administration denied that there was any such genetic susceptibility to the product, and the lawsuits were settled, but not before the vaccine was withdrawn from the market in significant part because of the adverse publicity generated by the litigation (12).

Defendants are also likely to try to exploit biomarkers of susceptibility. A defendant might argue that it was a plaintiff's genetic predisposition to disease that explains the plaintiff's illness, rather than exposure to the defendant's product, process, or waste. A product manufacturer might also argue in a suitable case that it had no legal duty to protect an individual who was abnormally sensitive to its product because of a genetic polymorphism. Indeed, under a doctrine sometimes described as the "idiosyncratic response defense," courts have held that a defendant is not negligent for harming a highly susceptible individual because it only has a duty to protect a "normal" or "average" person. A defendant might also assert an assumption of risk defense based on the plaintiff's genetic susceptibility, arguing that such a plaintiff had a duty to avoid hazardous exposures given their susceptible condition. Another possible argument available to defendants is to suggest that a plaintiff with a genetic predisposition to disease had a shortened life expectancy, and thus any compensation the plaintiff receives (which is often based on life expectancy) must be discounted proportionately. Finally, defendants have successfully used the existence of different genetic susceptibilities to a product within the population to defeat attempts to certify a class of plaintiffs in a class action lawsuit, in which the common issues of law and fact must predominate in order to allow a large group of plaintiffs (a "class") to proceed collectively against a manufacturer in a single lawsuit (12).

Forensic Applications

Beyond toxic torts, biomarkers have many other potential litigation applications, particularly for forensic purposes. Markers for blood type and DNA loci have been used extensively in criminal litigation to inculpate guilty criminals and exonerate innocent suspects by checking for matches between crime scene samples and samples from suspects. In recent years, toxicological biomarkers have also increasingly been used for forensic purposes in both civil and criminal litigation.

Blood alcohol concentration is a biomarker that has been used for many years as direct evidence of intoxication for driving under the influence (DUI) convictions. More recently, metabolites in the urine have been used as biomarkers to support criminal charges for illegal drug use. An issue that has emerged in such litigation is whether the presence of the illicit drug or its metabolites is sufficient to establish all elements of the crime, in particular the requirement that there must be "knowing use" of the illegal drug. Courts have issued conflicting decisions on whether the presence of the biomarker is sufficient to support an inference of knowing use of the illegal drug (18).

One of the most important and fastest growing forensic uses of biomarkers is in the field of microbial forensics, which seeks to use genetic and other variations to identify the origin, relationships, or route of transmission of a bacterial or viral strain that has caused harm (19). An example is the use of viral DNA sequencing to indicate that a Florida dentist was the source of HIV infection in several patients with no other risk factors who were infected with the identical strain of the HIV virus (19,20). Microbial forensic biomarkers will also play a critical role in the investigation and prosecution of "biocrimes," such as biological terrorist attacks, in which a microorganism is used as a weapon in criminal acts (21). A recent high-profile application of forensic biomarkers was the attempt to use DNA matching to identify the source of the anthrax used in the 2001 U.S. letter attacks that killed five people and sickened 17 others. Scientists sequenced the DNA of the anthrax used in the mailings, and compared it to other isolates of *Bacillus anthracis*. This effort putatively identified the source of the anthrax used in the attacks as a strain developed by the U.S. Army to test anthrax vaccines at Fort Detrick, Maryland (22).

Forensic biomarkers can also be used to trace the source of other types of toxicants or hazardous agents. At least one U.S. law firm is now using DNA fingerprinting to trace the source of contaminated meats that cause food poisoning. The law firm compares the genetic fingerprints of samples from individuals who were sickened by food poisoning with the genetic fingerprints of strains associated with recalls of contaminated ground beef (which it posts on its Internet Web site) (23). A fingerprint match would help support a lawsuit against the food company that supplied the contaminated meat.

Forensic biomarkers can also be used to investigate other illicit activities. The source of oil spills can be investigated using biomarker compounds that are found only in certain oils, which can help resolve legal liability for the spill and support litigation against the culpable entity (24). Meats, fish, and other food products that are falsely marketed as a more desirable species or strain can be detected using genetic markers. For example, the United Kingdom is using DNA tests on rice sold in grocery stores to determine if products are being falsely labeled as basmati rice, which can result in a substantial fine (25). The identity and potential source of illegally traded endangered species can also be revealed using forensic biomarkers, which can be used in criminal proceedings for illegal poaching or smuggling.

Animal DNA evidence can also be used to link a criminal to a crime scene, and DNA from traces of animal hairs, blood, or feces have helped to convict at least 15 defendants in U.S. criminal cases ranging from animal abuse to murder as of March 2003 (26).

POTENTIAL OBSTACLES AND COMPLICATIONS

This section reviews several key challenges for the use of toxicological biomarkers in litigation.

Premature Use of Biomarkers

Litigation has several attributes that will create strong incentives for the premature use of unvalidated biomarkers. First, litigation decision-makers do not have the luxury enjoyed by regulatory agencies of being able to wait to make a decision until adequate data are available (or to change their position if necessary in light of subsequent information), as lawsuits generally proceed according to an ordered schedule that marches inevitably to a final decision. Second, because litigants usually only have one "bite at the apple," they have every reason to deploy any piece of evidence that could possibly support their case. Third, litigation frequently involves high stakes and strongly-held positions, which again makes parties and their attorneys eager to use any evidence that may be helpful to their case. Fourth, lawsuits are decided by lay decision-makers, whether they be judges or juries, who usually lack scientific training and expertise, and thus who may be vulnerable to being misled into accepting dubious biomarker evidence by a wily expert. Finally, the lack of other direct evidence of specific causation in most toxic tort cases often leaves parties little choice but to use whatever biomarker evidence might be available, regardless of how well (or little) it is validated.

For all these reasons, it is inevitable that some litigants will seek to rely on biomarker evidence prematurely. There have been other examples of dubious scientific concepts being successfully employed, at least initially, such as the claims put forward by "clinical ecologists" of "chemically induced AIDS," which was subsequently discredited in position statements adopted by leading scientific societies (17,27). Such examples suggest that both the legal system and the scientific community need to be vigilant against improper or premature introduction of biomarker evidence into toxic tort or forensic litigation.

Admissibility

A biomarker should be adequately validated before it is used in litigation. Validation involves demonstrating the specificity, sensitivity, and reproducibility of the biomarker response (28). The validation should also verify that the biomarker is consistently linked with a clinical endpoint (i.e., toxicological injury). In litigation, the threshold inquiry into whether a biomarker has been adequately validated to be used in a lawsuit will generally be determined by the trial judge in deciding whether the biomarker evidence can be admitted into evidence.

In 1993, the U.S. Supreme Court issued a decision known as *Daubert*, which fundamentally transformed the standard for admitting scientific and other technical evidence in federal courts (29). Many state courts have subsequently adopted similar standards (30). *Daubert* requires judges to act as "gatekeepers" for scientific evidence introduced into a lawsuit, by prescreening such evidence to ensure that it is reliable and relevant before it can be presented to a jury. The Supreme Court provided a nonexclusive list of four factors a trial judge should consider in determining whether proffered scientific evidence is reliable, including whether the evidence: (i) can and has been empirically tested; (ii) has a known rate of error; (iii) has been peer-reviewed and published; and (iv) is generally accepted within the relevant scientific field. In response to this new admissibility standard for scientific evidence, trial courts have been much more stringent in admitting scientific testimony and data, which often has the consequence of dismissing a case if the party bringing the lawsuit (who thus has the burden of proof) lacks scientific evidence that is admissible.

The *Daubert* criteria for scientific reliability comport well with the validation requirements of biomarkers in that they require evidence to be testable and tested with a known rate of error, peer reviewed and published, and generally accepted. Nevertheless, a trial judge faced with dueling experts disagreeing about whether a particular biomarker is adequately validated and meets the *Daubert* criteria may have a difficult time deciding whether to admit the evidence. The authors of many scientific studies reporting positive biomarker associations tend to emphasize (perhaps in some cases overemphasize) the importance of their findings, and these statements published in credible scientific journals will certainly be presented to the judge even if most scientists do not believe that the particular biomarker is adequately validated for the purpose for which it is being introduced in litigation.

An illustrative example of the premature acceptance of a biomarker by the courts was the claim that silicone breast implants resulted in the production of antinuclear antibodies and/or silicone antibodies, and that the elevated levels of those biomarkers in women with silicone breast implants supported an association between the implants and rheumatologic disease. Some of the initial court cases permitted such evidence to be presented, and this biomarker evidence was apparently quite influential in large jury awards to plaintiffs with implants (31,32). Over time, however, scientific bodies such as the Institute of Medicine of the U.S. National Academy of Sciences challenged the reliability and relevance of such biomarkers.

Subsequent judicial opinions began rejecting the admissibility of such evidence of elevated biomarkers under the *Daubert* criteria (33,34).

At the same time, the strict standards for the admission of new scientific evidence under the *Daubert* regime may impede the use of novel biomarkers that may be scientifically valid but have not yet been widely accepted or appreciated in the scientific community. As one court recently noted, "[t]horny problems of admissibility arise when an expert seeks to base his opinion on novel or unorthodox techniques that have yet to stand the tests of time to prove their validity" (35). Judges applying the strict scrutiny of scientific evidence that has become the norm following *Daubert* may be skeptical, perhaps unduly so, of emerging new biomarkers such as gene expression assays. This roadblock is likely to be only temporary, however, until one or more courts find that particular biomarkers are adequately validated and meet the *Daubert* criteria, at which point such biomarkers are likely to quickly become widely used in litigation.

In trying to decide whether particular biomarkers are adequately validated and therefore admissible under *Daubert*, trial judges will look for authoritative scientific criteria or standards for the validation of biomarkers by governmental agencies or scientific bodies. Yet, despite the frequent use of the term "validation" in the scientific literature, there is no consensus on the definition of validation or the "rules of evidence" for determining whether a biomarker has been validated (36). The lack of any such definitive criteria at the present time will complicate the judicial task, and will guarantee some inconsistent and questionable court decisions.

Privacy of Litigants

Judicially compelled assays for some biomarkers may present privacy issues to the extent that they involve sensitive personal medical information that could, if improperly disclosed, result in stigma, embarrassment, or discrimination for litigants. In some cases, the harm may not be caused by the perceptions or actions of others, but simply because litigants evaluated for biomarkers may have preferred not to know information about their own susceptibility or increased risk that is revealed by biomarker assays. Bioethicists have recognized a right "not to know" details of one's own health status or predispositions (37). Yet, the traditional rule in toxic tort and similar litigation is that when a plaintiff files a lawsuit seeking health-based damages, the plaintiff has placed personal health status in controversy, and the party who has been sued has the right to compel reasonable and relevant medical testing of the plaintiff. In federal courts, for example, the trial judge has discretion to compel medical tests requested by an opposing party unless the judge finds such tests to be unnecessary or unreasonable (17,38).

Privacy concerns about compelled testing for biomarkers in litigation are likely to be greatest for biomarkers of susceptibility, such as genetic predispositions to cancer or other serious diseases. Information on such susceptibilities could potentially be used outside of litigation to discriminate against the plaintiff in employment or insurance decisions. Public disclosure of such genetic susceptibility could also complicate or interfere with a plaintiff's marital and child-bearing prospects. In addition, many people would rather not know which genetic susceptibilities they carry, especially those with no effective treatment or prophylactic measures, but the option of deciding not to know of one's own susceptibilities would be eliminated if an opposing party in litigation were able to persuade the judge to compel such testing.

A party ordered to undergo biomarker evaluation who is concerned about privacy of medical information could seek a protective order from the court, which is a court-imposed confidentiality directive that requires sensitive information uncovered in litigation to be kept under seal and not disclosed outside of the trial proceedings. This protection is not absolute, however. For example, a plaintiff who was ordered by the court to undergo genetic testing for susceptibility polymorphisms would have no choice but to answer affirmatively if an insurer subsequently asked whether the individual had ever undergone genetic testing.

Privacy concerns could also be raised by tests for biomarkers of effect that indicate that the individual suffers from preclinical manifestations of a disease process. It is not difficult to imagine that an insurer or employer might view such information negatively and, based on that perception, consciously or unconsciously discriminate against the plaintiff. For example, an insurance company may treat the evidence of early disease progression as a preexisting condition not entitled to insurance coverage, even though the condition was asymptomatic at the time of testing and would never have been revealed but for the litigation-related testing. Biomarkers of exposure present the least privacy concerns, but even with these biomarkers, evidence of significant exposure to a very hazardous agent would indicate an increased risk of disease, which could again lead to discrimination against a plaintiff in insurance, employment, and other contexts.

Notwithstanding these privacy concerns, it will often be necessary to compel the testing of a plaintiff for biomarkers (or absence thereof) because, as discussed earlier, biomarkers have the potential, for example, to provide very useful and relevant information for determining exposure, causation, risk, and susceptibility in litigation. Indeed, plaintiffs are likely to increasingly obtain and rely on such biomarker information themselves when it is helpful to their case. Opposing parties should not be precluded from seeking similar information when it is helpful to their case.

There will nevertheless be a need for courts to be vigilant regarding the importance of protecting plaintiffs' privacy rights against unnecessary, irrelevant, or overly broad requests for compelled biomarker testing. For example, some have suggested that businesses sued in any toxic tort lawsuit should seek genetic testing of the plaintiffs for genetic susceptibilities to cancer and other serious diseases, since such predispositions adversely affect life expectancy on which damages are based (38). Courts should reject such "fishing expeditions" that are not directly related to the health effects for which the plaintiff has brought the lawsuit. Plaintiffs' attorneys also have an ethical obligation to notify their prospective clients that filing a personal injury lawsuit may subject them to intrusive and unwanted medical testing.

Doctrinal Implications

Most new applications of toxicological biomarkers will promote fairer and more scientifically defensible litigation outcomes, but will not otherwise have a major impact on legal doctrine. In some cases, however, new biomarker data have the potential to dramatically alter the legal system and legal doctrine. An example is claims for latent risk. Most of these claims, which involve lawsuits by individuals who are at increased risk from a toxic exposure but have yet to manifest any clinical symptoms, are precluded today by demanding evidentiary requirements imposed by the courts. Biomarker evidence has the potential to overcome many of these evidentiary barriers, such as by demonstrating a "present injury" or making it easier to quantify increased risk. Since a large percentage of the general public has had a significant exposure to one or more toxic agents (even if a relatively small proportion will actually develop disease as a result), the courts may be flooded with tidal waves of latent risk lawsuits if biomarker evidence succeeds in overcoming the existing evidentiary barriers. Legal and legislative decision-makers will then be confronted with difficult policy choices on whether and when to allow latent risk claims which have the potential to fundamentally transform the dynamics of the legal system.

Another area where new biomarker evidence could have a dramatic effect on legal doctrine is with respect to susceptibility biomarkers, such as genetic polymorphisms conferring increased sensitivity to certain toxic exposures. To date, the legal system has for the most part assumed that we are alike in our susceptibility to various toxic exposures, even though it has been known since at least the time of Pythagoras that there are major interindividual differences in susceptibility to many different substances in our environment. To date, in the relatively rare cases in which an individual plaintiff was able to demonstrate a unique susceptibility, the courts have considered such susceptibility on a case-by-case basis, in some cases using the plaintiff's susceptibility to favor the plaintiff, but in other cases against the plaintiff.

With the advent of genetic susceptibility testing, it may soon be possible to determine the particular genetic predisposition of every plaintiff. Existing legal doctrine remains ambiguous about how such genetic susceptibilities will be addressed. Will an expanded duty be placed on product manufacturers to protect these newly identified susceptible individuals, at the cost of imposing a substantial burden and cost on many products? Or will courts only require manufacturers to protect "average" consumers, leaving unprotected those individuals who through no fault of their own are saddled with higher susceptibility to a particular product or substance? While the legal system has been able to avoid addressing this dilemma in a systematic and generic manner up until now, that may no longer be possible in the genomic era.

CONCLUSION

Toxicological biomarkers will significantly transform toxic tort and forensic litigation over the next decade. By providing for the first time a direct, objective link between a toxicological exposure and resultant health effects, biomarkers have the potential to make such litigation more informed, reliable, and fair. At the same time, the widespread use of biomarkers has the potential to create difficult new challenges for the courts relating to admissibility, privacy of litigants, and legal doctrine.

ACKNOWLEDGMENT

The author acknowledges the useful research assistance of Jon Kappes in the preparation of this chapter.

REFERENCES

1. Wright v. Williamette Industries, Inc., 91 F.3d 1105, 1107 (8th Cir.), 1996.
2. In re TMI Litigation, 193 F.3d 613, 622 (3d Cir.), 1999, *cert. denied*, 120 S.Ct. 2238, 2000.
3. Marchant GE, Toxicogenomics, toxic torts. Trends in Biotech 2002; 20:329–332.
4. Marchant GE. Genomics and toxic substances: part I — toxicogenomics. Environ Law Rep 2003; 33:10071–10093.
5. Bednar V. Bassett Furniture Manufacturing Co., 147 F.3d 737 (8th Cir.), 1998.
6. Patlak M. Fingering carcinogens with genetic evidence. Environ Sci Tech 1997; 31:190A–192A.
7. Aardema MJ, MacGregor JT. Toxicology and genetic toxicology in the new era of "toxicogenomics": impacts of "-omics" technologies. Mutat Res 2002; 499:13–25.
8. Hamadeh HK, Busherl PR, Jayadev S, et al. Prediction of compound signature using high density gene expression profiling. Toxicol Sci 2002; 67:232–240.
9. Groopman JD, Kensler, TW. The light at the end of the tunnel for chemical-specific biomarkers: daylight or headlight? Carcinogenesis 1999; 20:1–11.
10. Ward JB, Henderson, RE. Identification of needs in biomarker research. Environ Health Perspect 1996; 104(suppl 5):895–900.
11. Ayers V. Township of Jackson, 525 A.2d 287, 287 (N.J.), 1987.

12. Marchant GE. Genetics and toxic torts. Seton Hall L Rev 2001; 31:949–982.
13. Bryson V. The Pillsbury Co., 573 N.W.2d 718 (Minn. Ct. App.), 1998.
14. Henry CJ, Phillips R, Carpanini F, et al. Use of genomics in toxicology and epidemiology: findings and recommendations of a workshop. Environ Health Perspect 2002; 110:1047–1050.
15. Pottenger LH, Penman M, Moore NP, Priston RAJ, Thomas M. Biological significance of DNA adducts: summary of discussion of expert panel. Regul Toxicol Pharmacol 2004; 39:403–408.
16. Hansen V. Mountain Fuel Supply Co., 858 P.2d 970, 979 (Utah), 1993.
17. Marchant GE. Genetic susceptibility and biomarkers in toxic injury litigation. Jurimetrics 2000; 41:67–109.
18. Fradella HF, O'Neill L, Fogarty A. The impact of Daubert on forensic science. Pepperdine Law Rev 2004; 31:323–361.
19. Cummings CA, Relman DA. Microbial forensics—"cross-examining pathogens." Science 2002; 296:1976–1979.
20. Centers for Disease Control and Prevention. Transmission of HIV infection during an invasive dental procedure—Florida. MMWR 1991; 40(2):21–27, 33.
21. American Academy of Microbiology. Microbial Forensics: A Scientific Assessment. Washington, D.C., 2003. Available at http://www.asm.org/Academy/index.asp?bid=17994.
22. Read TD, Salzberg SL, Pop M, et al. Comparative genome sequencing for discovery of novel polymorphisms in *Bacillus anthracis*. Science 2002; 296: 2028–2033.
23. Beers A. Marler Clark posting *E. coli* genetic fingerprints from recalls. Food Chem News 2002; 44(16):1.
24. Wang Z, Fingas MF. Development of oil hydrocarbon fingerprinting and identification techniques. Marine Pollut Bull 2003; 47:423–452.
25. Meikle J. Basmati rice cheats face crackdown. Guardian (U.K.), 2003; Feb. 26, 7.
26. Hansen M. Beastly evidence. Am Bar Assn J 2003; 80(March):20–21.
27. Marshall E. Immune system theories on trial. Science 1986; 234:1490.
28. Decaprio AP. Biomarkers: coming of age for environmental health and risk assessment. Environ Sci Tech 1997; 31:1837–1848.
29. Daubert V. Merrell Dow Pharmaceuticals, Inc., 509 U.S. 579 (1993).
30. Bernstein DE, Jackson JD. The *Daubert* trilogy in the states. Jurimetrics 2004; 44:351–366.
31. Hopkins V. Dow Corning Corp., 33 F.3d 1116 (9th Cir.), 1994.
32. Taubes G. Silicone in the System. Discover 1995: 65–71.
33. Allison V. McGhan Medical Corp., 184 F.3d 1300 (11th Cir.), 1999.
34. Clegg V. Medical Engineering Corp., 2004 WL 471694 (Fla. Cir. Ct), Feb. 25, 2004.
35. McCullock V. H.B. Fuller Co., 61 F.3d 1038 (2d Cir.), 1995.
36. Ransohoff DF. Rules of evidence for cancer molecular-marker discovery and validation. Nat Rev Cancer 2004; 4:309–314.
37. MacKay CM. Discussion points to consider in research related to the human genome. Human Gene Therapy 1993; 4:477–495.
38. Rothstein MA. Preventing the discovery of plaintiff genetic profiles by defendants seeking to limit damages in personal injury litigation. Indiana L J 1996; 71:877–909.

Index